Essentials of Physical Training and Sports Science

Essentials of Physical Training and Sports Science

Edited by Jacob Meyer

SYRAWOOD
PUBLISHING HOUSE
New York

Published by Syrawood Publishing House,
750 Third Avenue, 9th Floor,
New York, NY 10017, USA
www.syrawoodpublishinghouse.com

Essentials of Physical Training and Sports Science
Edited by Jacob Meyer

International Standard Book Number: 978-1-68286-564-4 (Hardback)

Cataloging-in-Publication Data

Essentials of physical training and sports science / edited by Jacob Meyer.
p. cm.
Includes bibliographical references and index.
ISBN 978-1-68286-564-4
1. Physical education and training. 2. Sports sciences. I. Meyer, Jacob.
GV341 .E87 2018
613.7--dc23

Printed in China.

TABLE OF CONTENTS

PREFACE

Over the recent decade, advancements and applications have progressed exponentially. This has led to the increased interest in this field and projects are being conducted to enhance knowledge. The main objective of this book is to present some of the critical challenges and provide insights into possible solutions. This book will answer the varied questions that arise in the field and also provide an increased scope for furthering studies.

The branch of medicine which is concerned with the well-being and fitness of sportspersons is known as sports medicine. Some of the common sports injuries that sports physicians have to deal with are muscle cramps, ACL tears, shin splints, concussion, etc. The main aim of athletic training and sports medicine is to promote wellness and prevent injury. This book explores all the important aspects of physical training and sports science in the present day scenario. It is a compilation of chapters that discuss the most vital concepts and emerging trends in this field. Researchers and students in this field will be assisted by this book.

I hope that this book, with its visionary approach, will be a valuable addition and will promote interest among readers. Each of the authors has provided their extraordinary competence in their specific fields by providing different perspectives as they come from diverse nations and regions. I thank them for their contributions.

Editor

Fitness knowledge, cardiorespiratory endurance and body composition of high school students

Skip M. Williams[1], Dan Phelps[2], Kelly R. Laurson[1], David Q. Thomas[1], Dale D. Brown[1]

[1] Illinois State University, [2] Hononegah High School, Illinois, USA

Summary

Study aim: The purpose of this study was to determine if high school physical education seniors' health-related fitness knowledge is related to their aerobic capacity and body composition.
Material and methods: The FitSmart test assessed students (n = 171) health-related fitness knowledge. Aerobic capacity was calculated based on the students PACER score. Body Composition was measured using the Tanita TBF 300A body composition analyzer.
Results: Aerobic fitness was a statistically significant predictor of exam score ($\beta = 0.563$, $p < 0.001$), but percent body fat was not ($\beta = 0.185$, $p = 0.074$). Comparing the health-related fitness exam scores by the FITNESSGRAM classification system, students who were classified as Very Lean and High Risk for body composition had lower exam scores than those classified in the healthy fitness zone.
Conclusions: The results confirmed previous findings that students have inadequate health-related fitness knowledge. Furthermore, the study extends these findings by identifying some associations of percent body fat and estimated VO_{2max} to health-related fitness knowledge.

Key words: Adolescent – Cardiovascular Health – Physical Fitness – Physical Activity – Physical Education

Introduction

Due to the increase in sedentary behavior [7] and obesity [20] among adolescents, public health initiatives (i.e. Comprehensive School Physical Activity Programs [3] and Healthy People 2020 [25]) have identified the school system, specifically the discipline of physical education, as a key contributor in helping educate youth in the adoption of a physically active lifestyle. The national standards for physical education have always supported this by identifying that students should demonstrate the knowledge and skills to achieve and maintain a health-enhancing level of physical activity (PA) and fitness [17].

Students can meet these goals by learning health-related fitness concepts, how to assess fitness, identify fitness goals, and design fitness programs. However, it has been identified that physical education programs need to be strengthened in regard to teaching health-related fitness [11, 14]. Although the national standards for physical education identify the importance of promoting PA in physical education, physical education has been an underused source [8] and more efforts are needed in this field [21] to help reduce sedentary behaviors and obesity among adolescents.

To adopt a physically active lifestyle it is critical to understand (i.e. apply) the principles and concepts of health-related fitness [1]. The attainment of health-related fitness knowledge is positively related to PA participation [12, 25]. Due to this relationship the mastery of health-related fitness concepts has emerged as an important area that needs to improve among adolescents [15, 19, 22]. The lack of health related fitness knowledge has been linked as a factor to obesity among middle school youth [28]. Additionally it has been proposed that health-related fitness knowledge could be a contributing component to establishing and maintaining a physically active lifestyle [29]. There is limited research that has linked knowledge with achieving a health-enhancing level of physical fitness [17]. The purpose of this study was to determine if high school physical education seniors' health-related fitness knowledge is related to their aerobic capacity and body composition. A secondary purpose was to examine gender differences between health-related fitness, aerobic capacity, and body composition.

Author's address Dr Skip M. Williams, School of Kinesiology and Recreation, Illinois State University, Campus Box 5120 Normal, IL 61790-5120, Illinois, USA

Material and Methods

Participants and Setting

Participants were 171 senior physical education students from one public high school in the Midwestern U.S. Male (n = 88) and female (n = 83) participants (ages from 17 to 18 years) were assessed in 3 areas: health-related fitness knowledge, body composition, and cardiovascular endurance. Permission was obtained from the University Institutional Review Board, the school administration, teachers, and students prior to data collection.

Instrumentation

Health-related fitness knowledge was measured through a modified version of the FitSmart [29] health-related fitness knowledge exam. The FitSmart is the only validated standardized multiple choice exam designed to assess secondary students health-related fitness knowledge in the following areas: concepts of fitness, scientific principles of exercise, components of physical fitness, effects of exercise on chronic disease risk factors, exercise prescription and nutrition, injury prevention, and consumer issues [29]. Due to time constraints in the physical education setting the primary researchers modified the 50 question exam to 40 questions.

The FITNESSGRAM [9] 20-meter PACER (Progressive Aerobic Cardiovascular Endurance Run) test was used to assess aerobic capacity. The PACER is a multistage fitness test that progressively gets faster while the participant runs continuously back forth across a 20-meter space. Students' PACER scores were converted to VO_{2max} using the following formula: $VO_{2max} = 32.57 + 0.27\text{ (laps)} + 3.25\text{ (gender)} + 0.03\text{ (age)}$ [5]. The PACER has demonstrated strong reliability and validity against measured VO_{2max} [9].

In a physical education setting there are three recommended methods to measure body composition (BMI, skinfolds and bioelectrical impedance (BIA)) [26]. These methods are recommended due to the feasibility (time and expense) of the assessment. In this study body composition was assessed using the Tanita TBF 300A BIA. There is some variability in results when comparing BIA to hydrostatic weighing, Bod Pod and Dexa. However, Terbizan, Rhee and Stasny [23] found that Tanita TBF 300A BIA provided accurate body fat percentage predictions.

Procedures

Four certified high school teachers were trained by one of the researchers on how to administer the health-related fitness exam, body composition assessment (BIA), and the aerobic endurance assessment (PACER). Teachers were then given a 6-week timespan to complete the body composition and aerobic capacity assessments. Participant estimated VO_{2max} and percent body fat were categorized into the healthy fitness zones set by the FitnessGram/ ActivityGram Test Administration Manual [9]. The health-related fitness knowledge exam was completed during the 6th week. Participants completed the 40 question health-related fitness exam on a computer through an online survey system during their physical education class. Exams were then scored using the percentage of questions answered correctly.

Statistical Analysis

Descriptive statistics were calculated and stratified by sex. Independent samples t-tests (for continuous variables) and chi-square tests of independence (for categorical variables) were used to identify differences in fitness (body composition and aerobic capacity) and exam performance between males and females. Partial correlations were conducted to estimate associations between exam score, body composition and aerobic fitness while controlling for age and sex. Following, a multiple linear regression model was used to predict exam score from %BF and estimated VO_{2max}, also controlling for age and sex. Because both body composition and aerobic fitness are associated with FITNESSGRAM Healthy Fitness Zone (HFZ) standards, comparisons between the fitness groups (HFZ vs. high risk, etc.) were completed using univariate ANOVA models controlling for age and sex. Finally, to create groups of equal size, students were split into quartiles based on exam scores (Q1: $\geq$ 55%, Q2: 45% to <55%, Q3: 38% to <45%, Q4: <38%). Continuous percent body fat and estimated VO_{2max} values were compared between quartiles using univariate ANOVA models controlling for age and sex. All analyses were conducted in IBM SPSS Version 20 (Somers, NY).

Results

Descriptive statistics are in Table 1 The partial correlations indicated a weak-moderate, negative relationship between %BF and estimated VO_{2max} ($r = -0.44$, $p < 0.001$). There was no association between %BF and exam score ($r = 0.01$, $p = 0.916$). However, there was a weak association between estimated VO_{2max} and the exam ($r = 0.256$, $p = 0.001$), where students with higher exam scores tended to also have higher aerobic fitness when controlling for age and sex. When %BF and estimated VO_{2max} were entered simultaneously into a multiple linear regression model similar results were found. Aerobic fitness (ml/kg/min) was a statistically significant predictor of exam score ($\beta = 0.563$, $p < 0.001$), but %BF was not ($\beta = 0.185$, $p = 0.074$). The entire model, controlling for age and sex, accounted for 8.6% of the variance in exam score.

The results of the univariate ANOVA models comparing exam score by the FITNESSGRAM classification system are located in Table 2 For body composition, in general, exam scores were lower for students with %BF values in the Very Lean and High Risk groups and highest in the HFZ and Some Risk stratifications. Considering only the significantly different groups, adjusted mean exam score differences ranged from approximately 5% to 7.5%. When comparing the groups on aerobic fitness FITNESSGRAM classifications, the students in the HFZ had the highest adjusted exam score and the High Risk group had the lowest, but these differences were 1.5-2.0% and were not statistically significant.

The results of the univariate ANOVA models comparing continuous %BF and VO_{2max} are located in Table 3. Because of ties within the exam score distribution, the four quartiles were similar in size, but not identical (varying between 20% and 29% of the total sample per group). There were no differences between the 4 groups by %BF (all $p > 0.05$). However, the top quartile (highest exam scores) were those students with the highest adjusted mean estimated VO_{2max}, by approximately 4-5 ml/kg/min.

Table 1. Aerobic fitness, body composition, and health-exam performance by sex

Variable	Males (n = 88)	Females (n = 83)	Combined (n = 171)
Age (years)	17.3 ± 0.5	17.2 ± 0.4	17.3 ± 0.4
Percent Body fat (%)	14.0 ± 8.4	24.7 ± 9.2*	19.2 ± 10.3
Percentage in Body Composition HFZ	69.3%	62.7%	66.1%
Estimated VO_{2max} (ml/kg/min)	52.8 ± 7.2	43.2 ± 5.1*	48.2 ± 7.9
Percentage in Aerobic Fitness HFZ	88.6%	78.3%	83.6%
Exam Score	45.0 ± 11.0	44.0 ± 10.9	44.6 ± 11.0

Values are mean ± SD, excluding percentages HFZ = FITNESSGRAM Healthy Fitness Zone

*Significant difference between sexes ($p < 0.05$)

Table 2. Health-related Fitness exam score by FITNESSGRAM body composition and aerobic fitness standard classification

Body Composition Classification	n (% of sample)	Adjusted Mean Exam Score (SE)
A) Very Lean	25 (14.6%)	39.8 ± 2.2B,C
B) Healthy Fitness Zone	113 (66.1%)	45.7 ± 1.0A
C) Needs Improvement: Some Risk	20 (11.7%)	47.2 ± 2.4 A,D
D) Needs Improvement: High Risk	13 (7.6%)	39.5 ± 3.0C

Aerobic Fitness Classification	n (% of sample)	Adjusted Mean Exam Score (SE)
A) Healthy Fitness Zone	143 (83.6%)	44.8 ± 0.9
B) Needs Improvement: Some Risk	19 (11.1%)	43.5 ± 2.6
C) Needs Improvement: High Risk	9 (5.2%)	42.8 ± 3.7

Means are adjusted for age and sex. Significantly different groups ($p < 0.05$) are differentiated by superscript letters. For example, the A) Very Lean group adjusted exam score is significantly different from the Healthy Fitness Zone and Some Risk groups.

Table 3. Mean percent body fat and estimated maximal oxygen consumption by health-exam score quartiles

	Quartile 1 (n = 48)	Quartile 2 (n = 49)	Quartile 3 (n = 34)	Quartile 4 (n = 40)
Mean Exam Score	57.4 ± 4.1	47.6 ± 2.3	40.1 ± 2.0	29.3 ± 4.7
Adjusted Percent Body Fat (%)	18.9 ± 9.2	19.9 ± 10.8	18.4 ± 10.4	19.4 ± 11.2
Adjusted VO_{2max} (ml/kg/min)	51.1 ± 0.9*	47.1 ± 0.9	47.2 ± 1.0	46.6 ± 1.0

*Significantly different from all other quartiles ($p < 0.05$)

Means (SE) are adjusted for age and sex, excluding exam score mean ± SD

In general males had a lower percent body fat and a higher estimated VO_{2max} than females. However, when using the age- and sex-specific FITNESSGRAM standards, a similar proportion of males and females tested into the HFZ. Further, the majority of students in the sample had body composition and aerobic fitness scores within the HFZ. Males and females also scored similarly on the exam, with a mean score near 45%.

Discussion

Given the significant health consequences due to inactivity among adolescents, there is a need to examine factors that could potentially promote PA in obtaining adequate fitness levels. Knowledge acquisition of health-related fitness concepts has been identified as a factor that could potentially increase PA and fitness among adolescents. Over the past decade there has been a greater emphasis placed on physical education to teach health-related fitness concepts. The purpose of this study was to determine if high school physical education seniors' health-related fitness knowledge was related to their aerobic capacity and body composition. Although this is not the first study to examine health-related fitness knowledge it is the first to compare knowledge to two specific fitness outcomes. The average health-related fitness exam score among males and females (44.6%) were a failing grade; however, the scores were comparable to other health-related fitness knowledge acquisition studies [10, 12, 15, 22, 24] despite the methodological differences (different health-related fitness exams) between the studies. These failing scores can be attributed to the lack of health-related fitness content covered in class, teacher variables (i.e. knowledge, teaching style), and lack of student accountability (i.e. the grade on the exam does not count towards the students' overall grade). Only one aforementioned study [24] examined students' knowledge that were actually enrolled in a health-related fitness concept-based physical education class.

An examination of %BF and estimated VO_{2max} among males and females showed that males had lower %BF and higher estimated VO_{2max} scores (14.0 ± 9.4 & 52.8.6 ± 7.2) than females (24.7 ± 9.2 & 43.2 ± 5.1). When %BF and estimated VO_{2max} scores were placed in the FITNESSGRAM healthy fitness zones a slightly greater percentage of males (69.3%) compared to females (62.7%) were in the HFZ for %BF and a greater percentage of males (88.6%) compared to females (78.3%) were in the HFZ for aerobic fitness. In a study measuring FITNESSGRAM achievement among Texas high school-aged youth 34.2% of males and 31.4% of females were classified in the HFZ for aerobic capacity and 70.6% of males and 70.0% of females were classified in the HFZ for body composition [27]. Although the body composition results were similar to the current study it should be noted that the aforementioned study assessed body composition through BMI measurement not %BF. The amount of individuals classified in the HFZ for aerobic capacity was significantly different than the current study. A possible explanation for this result could be that the participants in the current study had required daily physical education. The difference between the amount of males and females in this study that were classified in the HFZ for aerobic fitness was not a surprise. PA participation among females declines [4] dramatically between the ages of 12-18 years old. Due to this knowledge and previous research showing a moderate relationship between PA participation and aerobic fitness it was expected that more males than females would have been classified in the HFZ [13]. However, one must remember that there are many other factors besides PA participation that influences aerobic fitness such as age, genetics, developmental factors, body composition and motivation [18] that were not accounted for in the current study.

Despite the majority of the students failing the exam positive relationships did exist between exam scores, body composition and estimated VO_{2max} whether examining the data continuously or by grouping the data in the FITNESSGRAM health fitness zones. These relationships suggest that a by product of health-related fitness knowledge is healthy body composition and aerobic fitness. As this was the first study to compare HRF knowledge to aerobic fitness and body composition further research is needed among this population and elementary/junior high school students before these results can be generalized to other groups.

The implications of this study apply directly to physical education programs, teachers and physical education teacher preparation programs in the U.S. Physical education has been identified as a key setting to educate youth on health-related fitness concepts in hopes to reduce the obesity epidemic in the U.S. Although the results of this study show that the majority of students had good aerobic fitness and body composition the students demonstrated inadequate health-related fitness knowledge therefore cannot be deemed "physically educated". Responsibility to teach fitness knowledge falls on the PE teacher. It has been noted that Physical Education Teacher preparation programs at universities do not adequately train pre-service teachers in the area of health-related fitness [16]. Additionally, Castelli and Williams [6] identified that the main problem persists at the professional level because few physical education teachers participate in professional activities, such as attending conferences, reading professional journals, or participating in workshops that would provide current information regarding fitness knowledge [14]. Therefore if health-related fitness knowledge is important in sustaining and or adopting a healthy active lifestyle we need to hold the professionals in physical education accountable.

The limitations of this study are important to note. First, the students in this study may or may not have been enrolled in a PE class that taught health-related fitness concepts or had a teacher who addressed these concepts. A conceptually based PE course has been found to increase student knowledge [2]. Second, the exam was not part of their overall grade, some students might not have taken the exam seriously. Lastly, no other factors such as PA levels motivation or parental influence were accounted for. Exploring these additional variables might have given more insight to why the sample had adequate %BF and estimated VO_{2max} and inadequate HRF knowledge.

This was the first study to compare %BF and estimated VO_{2max} to health-related fitness knowledge. The results confirmed previous findings that students have inadequate HRF knowledge. Furthermore the study extends these findings by identifying some associations of %BF and estimated VO_{2ma}x to HRF knowledge. The results underscore that more efforts are needed to teach adolescents health-related fitness concepts and potentially mandating a concepts-based physical education course in schools.

References

1. Adams T.M., P. Bryntcson (1992) A comparison of attitudes and exercise habits of alumni from colleges with varying degrees of physical activity programs. *Res. Q. Exerc. Sport.*, 63(2):148-152.

2. Adams T.M., M.M. Graves, H.J. Adams (2006) The effectiveness of a university level conceptually based health-related fitness course on health-related fitness knowledge. *The Phys. Educator.*, 63(2):104-112.

3. American Alliance for Health, Physical Education, Recreation and Dance. (2013). *Comprehensive school physical activity programs: Helping students achieve 60 minutes of physical activity each day* [Position statement]. Reston, VA: Author.

4. Bengoechea E., C. Sabiston, C. Ahmed, M. Farnoush (2010) Exploring links to unorganized and organized physical activity during adolescence: The role of gender, socioeconomic status, weight status, and enjoyment of physical education. *Res. Q. Exerc. Sport.*, 81(1):7–16.

5. Boiarskaia E.A., M.S. Boscolo, W. Zhu, M.T. Mahar (2011) Cross-Validation of an Equating Method Linking Aerobic FITNESSGRAM Field Tests. *Am. J. Preventive Med.*, 41:124-130.

6. Castelli D., L. Williams (2007) Health-related fitness and physical education teachers' content knowledge. *JTPE.*, 26:3-19.

7. Centers for Disease Control and Prevention (2010) Youth Risk Behavior Survey. www.cdc.gov/yrbs. Accessed August 8, 2012.

8.Cone S.L. (2004) Pay me now or pay me later: 10 years later and have we seen any change? *JTPE.*, 23:271-280.

9.Cooper Institute (2010) FITNESSGRAM /ACTIVITYGRAM Test Administration Manual. Champaign, IL: Human Kinetics

10. Desmond S.M., J.H.Price, R.S. Lock, D. Smith, P.W. Stewart (1990) Urban black and white adolescents' physical fitness status and perceptions of exercise. *J. Sch. Health.*, 60(5):220-226.

11. Ferguson R., X. Keating, D. Bridges, J. Guan, C. Li (2007) California Secondary School Physical Education Teachers' Attitudes Toward the Mandated Use of the Fitnessgram. *JTPE.*, 26(2):161-176.

12. Keating X.D., L. Chen, J. Guan, L. Harrison, B. Dauenhauer (2009) Urban minority ninth-grade students health-related fitness knowledge. *Res. Q. Exerc. Sport.*, 80(4):747-755.

13. Kolle K., L.B. Steene-Johannessen, S.B. Andersen (2010) Objectively assessed physical activity and aerobic fitness in a population-based sample of Norwegian 9- and 15-year-olds. *Scandinavian J. Med. & Sci. in Sport.*, 20(1):1-7.

14. Kulinna P.H. (2004) Physical activity and HRF knowledge: How much 1-6 grade students know. *International J. of P.E.*, 41(3):111-121.

15. Merkle D.G., D.F. Treagust (1993) Student knowledge of health and fitness concepts and its relation to locus control. *Sch. Sci Math.*, 93:355-259.

16. Miller M.G., L. Housner (1998) A survey of helath-related physical fitness knowledge among preservice and inservice physical educators. *The Phys. Educator.*, 55(4):176-186.

17. National Association for Sport and Physical Education (2013) National Standards and Grade-Level Outcomes for K-12 Physical Education. Reston, VA. Available at http://www.aahperd.org/naspe/standards/ nationalStandards/PEstandards.cfm. Accessed August 8, 2013.

18. National Association for Sport and Physical Education (2001) The Physical Best Teacher's Guide: Physical Education for Lifelong Fitness. Champaign, IL: Human Kinetics.

19. National Center for Chronic Disease Prevention and Health Promotion (2000) *Promoting better health for young people through physical activity and sports: A report to the president from the secretary of health and human services and the secretary of education.* Silver Spring, MD: CDC at Healthy Youth.

20. Ogden C.L., M.D. Carrol, B K Kit, K.M. Flegal (2012) Prevalence of obesity and trends in body mass index among US children and adolescents, 1999-2010. *JAMA.*, 307(5):483-490.

21. Pate R.R., M.G. Davis, T.N. Robinson, E.J. Stone, T.L. McKenzie, J.C. Young (2006) Promoting physical activity in children and youth: A leadership role for school. *Circulation.*, 114(11):1214-1224.

22. Stewart S., M. Mitchel (2003) Chapter 4: Instructional variables and student knowledge and conceptions of fitness. *JTPE.*, 22:533-551.

23. Terbizan D., Y. Rhee, S. Stasny (2009) A comparison of different body composition assessment techniques. *Missouri J. of HPERD.*, 19:104-11.

24. Thompson A., J.C. Hannon (2012) Health-related fitness knowledge and physical activity of high school students. *The Phys. Educator.*, 69:71-88.

25. U.S. Department of Health and Human Services. Office of Disease Prevention and Health Promotion. Healthy People 2020. Washington, DC. Available at http://www.healthypeople.gov/2020/default.aspx. Accessed August 8, 20013.

26. Vehrs P., R. Hager (2006) Assessment in interpretation of body composition in physical education. *JOPERD.*, 77(7):46-51.

27. Welk G.J., M.D. Meredith, M. Ihmels, C. Seeger (2010) Distribution of health-related physical fitness in texas youth. A demographic and geographic analysis. *Res. Q. Exerc. Sport.*, 81(3):S6-S15.

28. Zapata L.B., C.A. Bryant, R.J. McDermott, J.A Hefelfinger (2008) Dietary and physical activity behaviors of middle school youth: The youth physical activity and nutrition survey. *J. Sch. Health.*, 78(1):9-18.

29. Zhu W., M. Safrit, A. Cohen (1999) Fitsmart Test User Manual: High School Edition. Champaign, IL: Human Kinetics.

2

Quality of life and functional fitness of the elderly

Anna Leś, Marta Gaworska

University of Physical Education, Warsaw, and European Association for Promoting Motor Activity 50+, Warsaw, Poland

Summary

Study aim: To assess the perceived life quality and functional fitness of elderly subjects.
Material and methods: Two groups of subjects, aged 70 – 92 years, were studied: residents of a nursing home (Group R; n = 53) and those attending daytime nursing homes (Group D; n = 76). The EuroQol 5D questionnaire, and Romberg's and The Fullerton Functional Fitness tests were applied.
Results: Subjects from Group D perceived their daily functioning and general feeling much higher than those from Group R. Group R seemed more homogenous in that respect than Group D since only in the former all three indices of the quality of life (daily functioning, general feeling and perceived health) were significantly intercorrelated ($p<0.05 - 0.001$).
Conclusions: Social aid for the elderly ought to be focused on stimulating them to be active instead of giving them a direct assistance only.

Key words: Elderly people – Nursing homes – Social care – Functional fitness – Quality of life

Introduction

Among the objectives of residential nursing homes (RH) and of daytime nursing homes (DH) for the elderly is their activisation and improvement of their life quality. However, the quality of life of those attending both kinds of homes is expected to be perceived differently. At present, 28 residential nursing homes and 13 daytime nursing homes (including 3 for the mentally disabled) are being run in Warsaw by local authorities or as private enterprises, total capacities of both kinds of homes amounting to about 2200 and 520, respectively. Subjects attending the DH units are being qualified by the local Centres of Social Aid which usually deal with the impoverished ones.

Professional assistance to the elderly is the prime objective of nursing homes. This is supposed to include motor activities but their implementation and practices are exceedingly difficult due to diverse barriers – financial, psycho-emotional (reluctance to actively spend time), cognitive (lack of appropriate knowledge, its deficient promotion and public reception) and cultural; all these barriers restrict participation, activity and creativity, especially pertaining to motor activities. Moreover, mutual encouragement plays an important, prompting role in the engagement in motor activities; that engagement in nursing homes amounts to about 50% of their charges [14].

Among the factors contributing to the perceived life quality of the elderly are motor fitness, health status, psycho-emotional well-being and self-dependence in daily activities [16]. The daily functioning of elderly subjects (walking, washing, dressing, eating, writing, reaching and picking objects) is determined by their motor fitness which enables them also practicing leisure activities [16,18].

The lack of such activities is one of the independent risk factors [2], classified also as the so-called Population-Attributable Risk (PAR) [4,12]. Restriction of motor activities is known to induce many civilisation-related diseases, e.g. obesity, diabetes, atherosclerosis, hypertension, locomotor and spine disorders, etc. Rationally applied motor activities enable maintaining functional and social self-dependence until old age and improve the perceived quality of life [10,15].

The aim of the study was to assess some elements of the perceived life quality (health, physical fitness and functional self-dependence) and functional fitness of elderly subjects, residents of nursing homes or attending the daytime nursing homes.

Author's address Dr Anna Leś, Department of Recreational Motor Activity, University of Physical Education, Marymoncka 34, 00-968 Warsaw, Poland

Material and Methods

Subjects: A group of 129 subjects aged over 70 years consented to participate in the study. This included 53 nursing homes residents (Group R), who volunteered to join the all-year activities aimed at functional improvement, and 76 subjects attending daytime homes (Group D).*Methodology*: EuroQol questionnaire (Polish version, certified and admitted to use by The EuroQol Group [16]) was applied to study participants. The questionnaire consisted of 5 items pertaining to the life quality of the elderly and included a 0 – 100 points scale of perceived health at the time of being interviewed. The questions included the following topics: self-dependence in moving and in daily functioning, ease in daily functioning (leisure activities, housework), perception of pain and discomfort, of anxiety and of depression. Three optional answers were available and were assigned point ratings: a – I have no problems, no discomfort or depression (1 pt.); b – I can feel some problems sometimes (0 pts.); c – Such problems are permanent (-1 pt.). For further analysis, the values of daily functioning (Questions 1 – 3) and of general feeling (Questions 4 – 5) were averaged. In addition, the perceived health was determined by a 0 – 100 points scale ("thermometer").

Student's *t*-test for independent groups was used in data analysis. The level of $p \le 0.05$ was considered significant.

Results

Mean values (±SD) of age, body mass and BMI of nursing home residents (Group R) and of subjects attending daytime homes (Group D) are presented in Table 1 and the data pertaining to the declared functional fitness of the elderly in Fig. 1.

Table 1. Mean values (±SD) of age, body mass and BMI of nursing home residents (R) and of subjects attending daytime homes (D)

Variable Group	n	Age	Body mass	BMI
R-Men	12	81.3 ± 4.3	73.7 ± 7.9	25.2 ± 2.7
R-Women	39	80.0 ± 5.0	75.1 ± 14.0	30.0 ± 6.2
D-Men	17	78.6 ± 3.8	73.8 ± 13.0	26.7 ± 4.0
D-Women	57	78.9 ± 5.9	71.4 ± 11.5	27.6 ± 4.3

Women from Group R significantly ($p<0.05$) differed from Group D with respect to BMI which reflected the difference in percentages of obese subjects in those groups (46 and 25%, respectively). No such difference was noted for men.

Women from Group R functioned significantly ($p<0.05$) worse than men with respect to daily tasks other than moving or self-care (Question 3) and to feeling anxiety or depression. No gender-related differences were noted in Group D. Men and women from Group D significantly ($p<0.05 – 0.001$) more frequently declared better functional fitness and general feeling than the residents of nursing homes (Group R). However, women from Group R significantly ($p<0.001$) more frequently reported serious discomfort and anxiety (Questions 4 and 5) than those from Group D (Fig. 1).

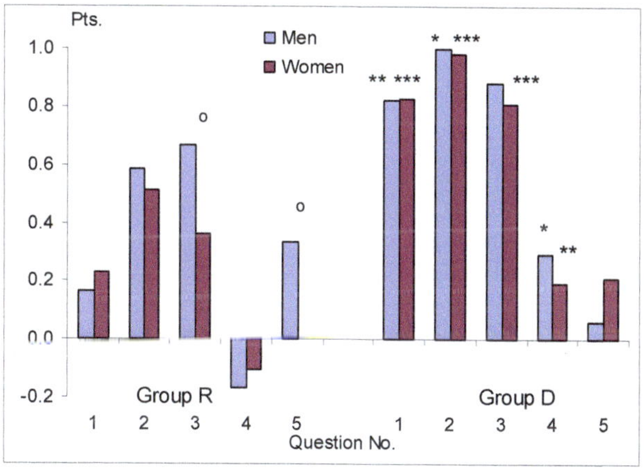

Fig. 1. Perceived quality of life of nursing home residents (n = 12 and 39, men and women respectively) and of subjects attending daytime homes (n = 17 and 57, men and women respectively)

Legend: 1 – Daily moving; 2 – Daily self-care; 3 – Other daily tasks (work, learning, household, leisure activities); 4 – Feeling discomfort; 5 – Anxiety, depression; ° Significant ($p<0.05$) difference between men and women; Significantly different from the respective value in Group R: * $p<0.05$; ** $p<0.01$; *** $p<0.001$

Table 2. Mean values (±SD) of the perceived quality of life of nursing home residents (R) and of subjects attending daytime homes (D)

Variable Group	n	Daily functioning	General feeling	Perceived health
R-Men	12	0.47 ± 0.63	0.08 ± 0.47	56.3 ± 22.0
R-Women	39	0.37 ± 0.44	-0.05 ± 0.51	47.7 ± 21.9
D-Men	17	0.90 ± 0.20*	0.18 ± 0.39	42.6 ± 15.3
D-Women	57	0.87±0.20***	0.19±0.36***	41.9 ± 11.4

Significantly different from Group R: * $p<0.05$; *** $p<0.001$

Women attending daytime homes declared a markedly better ($p<0.001$) daily functioning and general feeling than their mates from residential homes, while in case of men this was true only for daily functioning ($p<0.05$). No between-group or between-gender differences were found for the perceived health (Table 2) although R-men tended to rate their health higher than their D-mates ($p = 0.06$).

All three indices of the perceived quality of life were significantly intercorrelated ($p<0.05 - 0.001$) only in nursing home residents; this means that subjects who declared a better functional fitness and general feeling considered themselves healthier than those less fit. In those attending daytime homes only the daily functioning and general feeling were weakly correlated ($p<0.05$; Table 2). No significant partial correlations were noted.

Table 2. Coefficients of correlation between declared daily functioning, general feeling and perceived health

Correlated variables / Group	R n = 51	D n = 74
Daily funct. – General feeling	0.529***	0.250*
Daily funct. – Perceived health	0.490***	-0.058
General feeling – Perceived health	0.277*	-0.062

* $p<0.05$; *** $p<0.001$

Discussion

The presented differences between nursing home residents (Group R) and those attending daytime homes (Group D) might have been due not only to the type of the nursing home and the provided services but to the fact that residential homes lodge mainly those who are incapable of attending daytime centres and that incapability is one of the criterions of recruiting residents. Apart from that, the accessibility of residential homes is limited and many elderly subjects attend daytime homes while awaiting admission to the residential one. It may thus seem that nursing home residents represent a more homogenous population than those attending daytime homes; that issue calls for further studies. At any rate, those attending daytime homes (Group D) may be expected to be better fit functionally than their residential mates (Group R) ant that was indeed demonstrated in this study.

Subjects from Group D perceived their daily functioning and general feeling (expressed by the declared lack of discomfort) higher than R-subjects. In contrast to that, the health status tended to be perceived even higher by male R-subjects than by the D-ones. As follows from the report of Płaszewska-Żywko *et al.* [13], elderly subjects leading an independent life, i.e. not having to make use of nursing homes, rated their quality of life significantly higher than those studied by us; for example, their perceived health was as high as 72.1 points.

It ought to be emphasised that the abovementioned higher homogeneity of the R-group compared with D-subjects was reflected in correlation coefficients – all three elements studied – daily functioning, general feeling and perceived health were significantly correlated with each other in Group R while in Group D only one, weak correlation between daily functioning and general feeling was noted.

Summing up, those respondents making use of nursing homes, who are relatively self-sufficient, not relying on an extensive assistance of others, rated their quality of life higher than the aid-dependent ones. Thus, apart from giving the necessary assistance in daily functioning, preventive steps should be taken aimed at increasing the self-sufficiency of the elderly. The most efficient are efforts based on practicing motor activities adjusted to subject's capacity [1,3-9,11,17] and this ought to be one of principal roles of nursing homes and of other institutions providing social care. All actions directed at the elderly ought to be based on the auxiliarity principle, the starting point being the family. Social aid for the elderly ought thus to be focused on stimulating them to be active instead of giving them a direct assistance only.

References

1. Alexandre T., R.Cordeiro, L.Ramos (2009) Factors associated to quality of life in active elderly. *Revista de Saúde Pública* 43:613-621.

2. American Heart Association, Committee on Exercise Circulation (1992).

3. Baumann A. (1998) Use of population-attributable risk (PAR) in understanding the health benefits of physical activity. *Br.J.Sports Med.* 32:279-280.

4. Bauman A, J.Sallis, D.Dzewaltowski, N.Owen (2002) Toward a better understanding of the influences on physical activity: the role of determinants, correlates, causal variables, mediators, moderators and confounders. *Am.J.Prev.Med.* 23:5-14.

5. Brender E. (2006) Fitness for older adults. *JAMA Patient Page* 296(2):242 DOI: 10.1001/jama.296.2.242.

6. Canada's Physical Activity Guide to Healthy Active Living for Older Adults (2005) http://hepac.ca

7. Christensen U., N.Stovring, K.Schultz-Larsen, M.Schroll, K.Avlund (2006) Functional ability at 75: is there an impact of physical inactivity from middle age to early old age? *Scand.J.Med.Sci.Sports* 16:245-251.

8. Crespo C, M.Palmieri, R.Perdomo, D.McGee, E.Smit, C.Sempos, I.Lee, P.Sorlie (2002) The relationship of physical activity and body weight with all-cause mortality: Results from the Puerto Rico heart health program. *Ann.Epidemiol.* 12:543-552.

9. Improving the quality of life of elderly and disabled people in human settlements - A Resource Book of Policy and Programmes from around the World (1993) United Nations Centre for Human Settlements (Habitat).

10. Jancey J, A.Clarke, P.Howat, A.Lee, T.Shilton, J.Fisher (2008) A physical activity program to mobilize older people: A practical and sustainable approach. *The Gerontologist*, 48:251-257.

11. Last J.M. (2000). Dictionary of Epidemiology (4th ed.) Oxford University Press, New York.

12. Matuso M., J.Nagasawa, A.Yoshino, K.Hiramatsu, K.Kurashiki (2003) Effects of activity participation of the elderly on quality of life. *Yonago Acta Medica* 46:17-24.

13. Płaszewska-Żywko L., P.Brzuzan, I.Malinowska-Lipień, T.Gabryś (2008), Functional capability in persons of advanced age in homes for the elderly. Probl.Hig.Epidemiol. 89:62-66.

14. Spirduso W.W., K.L.Francis, P.G.Macrae (2005) Physical Dimensions of Aging. Human Kinetics, Champaign IL.

15. The Euroquol Group (2009) www.euroqol.org/

16. Thomas J.B. (2007) Institutionalization of elderly – 10 real expectations for quality of life in a well managed long term care facility. www.workingcaregiver.com/articles/senior-living-options/longtermcarequality

17. Webb D., E.Ward (2007) Getting more physical activity as a senior. http://health.howstuffworks.com/wellness/aging/senior-health/lose-weight-senior3.htm

18. Wiener J.M., R.Clark (1990) Measuring the activities of daily living: comparisons across national surveys. U.S. Department of Health and Human Services.

The influence of juggling on mental rotation performance in children

Petra Jansen [1], Léonie F. Lange [2], Martin Heil [3]

[1] Institute of Sport Science, University of Regensburg; [2] Department of Anaesthesiology, Charité University of Medicine, Berlin; [3] Institute of Experimental Psychology, University of Düsseldorf, Germany

Summary

Study aim: To assess the influence of juggling training on mental rotation performance in children.
Material and methods: Two groups of girls aged 6 – 14 years were studied: experimental (EG; n = 26) and control (CG; n = 24). All girls solved a mental rotation task with 3-D block figures on computer screen (pre-test). After the initial test, EG girls participated in juggling training for 3 months; the CG girls participated in light strength training with theraband stretch bands. After 3 months, all girls solved the mental rotation task again (post-test). The post-pre differences in the mental rotation performance were recorded.
Results: Children who learned juggling performed the mental rotation task significantly ($p<0.05 - 0.01$) faster, in terms of reaction time, at non-zero angular disparity than their mates who were strength-trained.
Conclusions: Since mental rotation skills enhance spatial imagination, problem solving and mathematical skills, it may be assumed that juggling training enhances also other cognitive domains and is worth implementing in the education process.

Key words: Motor behaviour – Spatial performance – Juggling – Mental rotation – Children

Introduction

Research in the developmental, as well as in cognitive science, is focused on the relations between motor abilities and cognitive performance. Since Piaget's work [19], it has been assumed that the sensorimotor system is important for mental representation. Evidence supporting this assumption came recently from modality theories which emphasise the importance not only of a central control executive function, but also of modal functions [7]. It was shown that a dysfunction in motor development is often associated with a dysfunction in cognitive development and *vice versa* [8]. This relates to the specific assumption [3] that motor development and movement experience are relevant factors for cognitive performance, especially for spatial abilities [1]. Spatial abilities are cognitive processes that involve visualisation, orientation, and mental rotation [17]. Thereby, mental rotation is the ability to imagine how an object would look if rotated away from the orientation in which it is actually presented [21].

The influence of motor processes on solving a mental rotation task in adults was already demonstrated [22]. Mental rotation tests result in faster times and fewer errors when manual and mental rotations were compatible. In another study with adults [24], it could be shown that mental rotation could be trained with the help of a manual rotation programme, where mental rotation was trained *via* motor rotation consisting of moving a joystick.

The effects of motor processes on solving a mental rotation task were also investigated in children. A sample of 5, 8, and 11-year old children and of adults performed a mental rotation task while simultaneously rotating their hand, guided with a handle, in the direction compatible/ incompatible with the mental rotation task. The 5 and 8-year old children solved the mental rotation task, compatible with the motor task, easier than the 11-year old or adults, showing association between motor and mental rotations in younger children [6]. In contrast to that, a motor effect during mental transformations of body parts was only found in one of two experiments (performed with children aged 5 - 6 years, 7 years, and adults) and this effect was less pronounced in younger children [16].

An experimental study of body-oriented motor training, without using a handle or a joystick, on visual spatial tasks in children is missing until now. In a study on adults it was shown that juggling training over a period

Author's address Prof. Petra Jansen, Institute of Sport Science, Universitätsstr. 31, 93053 Regensburg, Germany

of 3 months improved mental rotation performance compared with a control, untrained group [12]. That result is valid from a neurological point of view because increase in brain plasticity was shown after juggling training [4] in exactly that brain area (intraparietal sulcus) which is involved in mental rotation [15].

It is not yet known if motor and imagery processes in children and adults are alike [6,16]. The main goal of this study was to find out if coordinative motor training (here: juggling training) would lead to an enhancement of mental rotation performance in children as shown earlier for adults [12]. Beyond that, the present study expands on that former study. Because a purely motor benefit could also explain the reported differences in the reaction velocity in juggling subjects compared to the control ones [12], the control group in this study was subjected to another conditional form of motor training, namely strength training with theraband stretch-bands. The study included only girls for the well-known gender differences in mental rotation performance, even in children [18], were not our objective.

Material and Methods

Participants: A group of 57 girls aged 6 – 14 years participated in this study; 29 of them were randomly assigned to the juggling group and 28 to the strength training group. Seven girls did not participate in the post-test, thus the experimental group (EG) counted 26, and the control group (CG) 24 subjects. The girls were trained in gymnastics, in Wesel, Germany, during their regular gym classes. The girls from each group were trained by two instructors at different corners of the gym. The parents of children gave their informed consent for children's participation and data utilisation after having been made familiar with the objective and protocol of the study which was approved by the local Committee of Ethics. In addition, the club committee and the gymnastics instructors agreed to carry out the experiments during the lessons. The children received juggling balls or the theraband stretch bands as gifts and the entire gymnastics group received €300 for their participation. The girls had normal or appropriately corrected visual acuity. None of the children were able to juggle before participating in this study.

Procedure: All participants were subjected to timed pre- and post-study mental rotation tasks which took place in a quiet locker room or in a first-aid room, in two different gyms in Wesel, in groups of three children. Each girl worked with her own laptop (15-inch monitor at about 50-cm distance) not seeing her mates and had her personal test leader. The experimental stimuli consisted of 18 perspective line drawings of three-dimensional forms (each one composed of 10 cubes) [13,21] and were 3D-rotated around the horizontal or vertical axis. Each form had a maximum size of 7 × 7 cm on the screen spaced by 14 cm. In each trial, two drawings of the same form were presented together. The stimulus presented on the right side of the monitor was either identical to the left side or mirror-reversed. The angular disparity between the two stimuli was 0, 90 or 180° (see Fig. 1 as an example). The subjects responded "same" by pressing the left touchpad button with index finger and "different" by pressing the right touchpad button with the middle finger.

Individual sessions lasted about 50 min each; every trial started with a grey-background screen and after 500 ms the pair of stimuli appeared and the subject had to decide whether the two stimuli were "same" or "different" (mirror-reversed). The stimuli remained on the screen until the subject responded by pressing a touchpad-button. The participants were instructed to react as quickly and as accurately as possible. The "+" or "–" sign was displayed for 500 ms in the centre of the screen to indicate the correctness of given response. The trials were spaced by 1500-ms grey-background screen intervals. After a block of 27 trials, the participants could choose to take a short break. They were asked to start the new block by pressing the space key. Each combination of objects (18 different drawings), normal or mirror-reversed, and angular disparity (0, 90 or 180°) was presented 4 times during the test, which resulted in a total number of 432 trials. In order to make the participants familiar with the test sequence, 54 unrecorded test trials were performed at the beginning of the experiment. The stimulus items were the same in the pre- and post-study mental rotation tests separated by a 3-month interval. In that time period, the children of the experimental group (EG, juggling) were subjected to juggling training twice weekly, 15 min at the beginning and 15 min at the end of regular gymnastics classes. The training was based on the Rehoruli's method and designed by a German juggler, Stephan Ehlers [5]. The children practiced various throw-and-catch tasks, their difficulty increasing every week. The children were instructed to train at home for about 10 min daily. At every session, the exercise time and the numbers of successful throws were recorded – how often a ball was successfully thrown from one hand to the other during the juggle performance.

Control children subjected to strength training (CG) were underwent a light strength training with theraband stretch bands. The following exercises were applied: "Biceps curls"– the girl stood with one foot on the theraband, its ends being grasped with one hand each and wrapped up until tight, then both arms were bent alternately, and

"Knee bend" – the girl stood on both feet on the theraband, shoulder length apart, then bent down and wrapped the ends of the theraband round her hands; after that, she sat up and stretched up her arms simultaneously. Control girls were also asked to train at home for 10 min a day and the numbers of repetitions of the "Knee bend" exercise they were able to perform were recorded during the training sessions.

The motor training effect in the juggling group (EG) was expressed as the difference between the first and the last training sessions in the numbers of successful throws. That effect in the strength-training group (CG) was expressed as the difference in the numbers of "knee band" exercise.

Data analysis: Only trials with correct response were used for reaction time (RT) analysis which was further restricted to "same" responses only, for angular disparity could not be unequivocally defined for "different" responses [14]. Moreover, all RT values outside the mean ± 2SD interval were eliminated prior to the analysis. Nevertheless, the analysis of all data combined revealed identical results.

The percent differences in the error rate scores (difference score error) and the post-pre RT differences (difference score RT) were dependent variables [24]. The data were subjected to one-way ANOVA for each group separately, the significance levels being corrected according to Huynh and Feldt [11] in order to compensate for non-sphericity of the data. Pearson's coefficients of correlation were computed for age, mental rotation performance and motor behaviour (difference score between the first and last training session for juggling or strength performance). The level of $p \le 0.05$ was considered significant.

Results

No significant between-group difference in the reaction time (mental rotation task) was found at baseline. In the experimental group, juggling performance significantly ($p<0.01$) increased following the 3-month training compared with the pre-training status (baseline). The same was true for the control group performing "knee bend" exercises (Table 1). An example of the items of the mental rotation task is presented in Fig. 1.

The results of the training-induced differences in the reaction time are presented in Fig. 2. Significantly ($p<0.01$) better results were attained by girls from the experimental group (EG) than from the control one (CG) at angular disparities equal to 90 or 180°. Moreover, mean RT improvement in EG was significantly ($p<0.01$) highest at 90°. No significant angle-related differences were noted in CG. Regarding the error rate scores, no significant differences either between groups or between angular disparities were found.

Table 1. Mean values (±SD) of age, reaction time pre-training and of training effects

Variable / Group	Juggling n = 26	Strength n = 24
Age (years)	10.4 ± 2.2	10.5 ± 2.4
Reaction time (ms) pre	3704 ± 1055	3297 ± 1061
Motor training effect	16.8 ± 30.8**	2.33 ± 1.76**
Range	0 – 117	0 – 6

** p<0.01

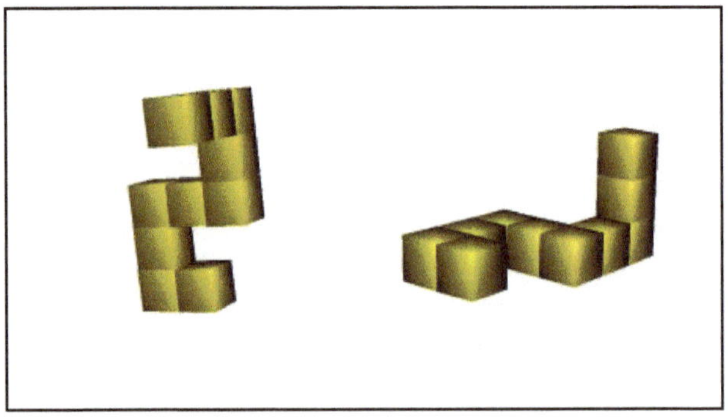

Fig. 1. An example of the items of the mental rotation task

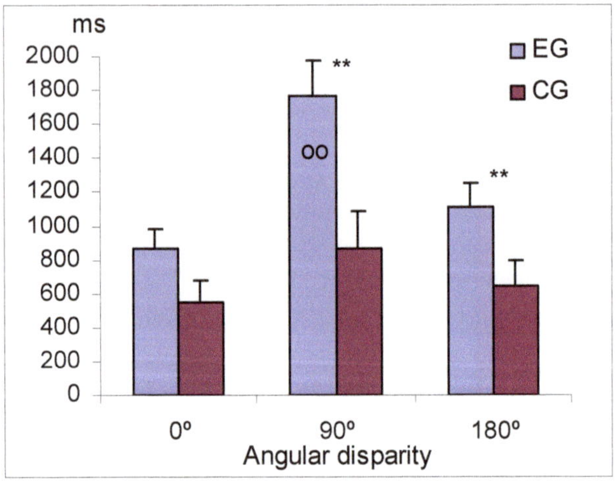

Fig. 2. Post-pre differences in reaction time in the mental rotation task (Means ±SE)

** Significant (p<0.01) difference between groups; °° Significantly (p<0.01) different from mans at 0 and 180°

Training effects were significantly ($p<0.05$) correlated with age in both groups but no significant correlations were noted with either difference scores in RT or with error rates (Table 2). Multiple regression calculus applied to data in the experimental group showed that a significant contribution to the mental rotation task had only age ($p<0.05$), that of motor performance remaining non-significant.

Table 2. Coefficients of correlation of training effects with age or difference scores in the mental rotation task

Group / Correlated variable	Juggling n = 26	Strength n = 24
Age	0.466*	0.443*
Difference score (RT)	-0.012	0.160
Difference score (Error)	-0.142	0.216

* $p<0.05$

Discussion

This study was a continuation of our earlier report on juggling [12] and showed the relations between juggling and the mental rotation performance in schoolchildren. The results indicated that the training effect was specific for juggling and not for a general motor effect. The juggling training affected the reaction time (RT) in trials, in which the angular disparity was 90 or 180°, that at 0° remaining unchanged. Of course, no mental rotation is required to compare the two stimuli at 0° disparity, that condition serving thus as a kind of reference for the other two. In contrast to RT, there was no effect of juggling training on error rates. This finding is in accordance with many other studies showing that reaction time is the substantially more sensitive measurement for mental rotation effects than error rates [10].

This study confirmed the results of an earlier study [23] that manual rotation training can improve the mental rotation performance of school-aged children but the results depended on age [6]. It was demonstrated that only those aged 5 or 8 years but not the 11 years old had shorter RT in mental rotation tasks when the spinning of a hand crank matched the assumed path of mental rotation, rather than the other way round. When mental rotation of pictures showing body parts were studied, motor effects in mental rotation were not stable [16] and it was concluded that imagery and motor planning shared common resources. This is in accordance with the view that mental representations such as mental rotation are controlled by different modal functions connected to sensory and action systems [16,19]. When interpreting the results of mental rotation processes in terms of embodiment [25] and modal functions, the experimental design has to be very precise. It might be speculated why juggling and not a strength task is effective in mental rotation. Both motor tasks imply a performance feedback; girls from both groups received feedback from their training improvement, although the feedback in the juggling group was coordinative and that in the strength group was a strength one; it could be assumed that juggling and mental rotation shared common features, since both juggling and mental rotation required a cyclic activity and had temporal and spatial constraints [12]. In juggling, the hands move along more or less elliptical trajectories while throwing and catching balls move in a regular fashion [20]. In mental rotation, one object is brought along a cyclic trajectory around the three axes to bring it in the position of the standard object. While juggling may be thought of as a "spatial clock" [20], mental rotation seems to be a covert manual rotation [26]. The latter authors showed that rotational hand movements interfered with mental rotation and *vice versa*. Furthermore, juggling requires mirrored movements of hands while mental rotation requires the decision of whether two rotated objects are superimposable or mirrored. Further studies are needed to compare the effects of mental rotation and of other motor tasks involving cyclic arms or body activity, e.g. swimming or discus throwing.

The here presented data suggest that the age, not motor development, is the key factor in the improvement. This assumption has to be investigated in further studies with cognitive development monitoring in order to more precisely assess the effects of the cognitive and motor processes on mental rotation performance. That latter is not influenced automatically by the motor system but since it shares common features with higher motor processes, such as juggling, it might be influenced by a specific motor task. Another issue to be investigated into are the known gender-related differences (cf. [13]); a stronger activation of motor cortex was noted in women than in men when observing hand vs. dot movement, in men the situation being reversed [2].

Furthermore, the role of hormones ought to be discussed in more detail. The girls in this study were 6 – 14 years old and differed in their hormonal status. Because at least the effect of testosterone level on mental rotation performance has been shown [9], the varying hormonal status before and during puberty has to be regarded in further studies.

Summing up, a relation between juggling and mental rotation performance and, in a broader sense, between motor and cognitive performance was demonstrated. Further studies are needed to evaluate, in detail, the effects of age, gender and training duration on how cognitive the motor tasks need to be to have a positive influence on other higher-level cognitive tasks such as problem-solving, as well the stability of such effects.

References

1. Campos J.J., D.I.Anderson, M.A.Barbu Roth, E.M.Hubbard, M.J.Hertenstein, S.Witherington (2000) Travel broadens the mind. *Infancy* 1:149-219.

2. Cheng Y.W, O.J.L.Tzeng, J.Decety, T.Imada, J.C.Hsieh (2006) Gender differences in the human mirror system: a magnetencephalography study. *Neuroreport* 17:1115-1119.

3. Diamond A. (2007) Interrelated and interdependent. *Dev.Sci.* 10:152-158.

4. Draganski B., C.Gaser, V.Busch, G.Schuierer, U.Bogdahn, A.May (2004). Nuroplasticity: changes in grey matter induced by training. *Nature* 427:311-312.

5. Ehlers S. (2005) REHORULI – Jonglieren lernen mit Erfolgsgarantie. Books on Demand.

6. Frick A., M.M.Daum, S.Walser, F.W.Mast (2009) Motor processes in children`s mental rotation. *J.Cogn.Dev.* 10:18-40.

7. Gallese V., M.Lakoff (2005) The brain`s concept. The role of the sensory-motor system in conceptual knowledge. *Cogn.Neuropsychol* 22:455-479.

8. Gillberg C. (2003) Deficits in attention, motor control, and perception: a brief review. *Arch.Dis.Child.* 88:904-910.

9. Hausmann M, O.Güntürkün (2000) Steroid fluctuations modify functional cerebral asymmetries: the hypotheses of progesterone-mediated interhemispheric decoupling. *Neuropsych.* 38:1362-1374.

10. Heil M., F.Rösler, M.Link, J.Bajric (1998) What is improved, if a mental rotation task is repeated - efficiency of memory access, or the speed of a transformation routine? *Psychol.Res.* 61:99-108.

11. Huynh H., L.S.Feldt (1976) Estimation of the Box correction for degrees of freedom from sample data in randomized block and split-plot designs. *J.Educ.Stat.* 1:69-82.

12. Jansen P., C.Titze, M.Heil (2009) The influence of juggling on mental rotation performance. *IJSP* 4:351-359.

13. Jansen-Osmann P., M.Heil (2007) Suitable stimuli to obtain (no) gender differences in the speed of cognitive processes involved in mental rotation. *Brain Cognit.* 6:217-227.

14. Jolicoeur P., S.Regehr, L.B.Smith, G.N.Smith (1985) Mental rotation of representations of two-dimensional and three-dimensional objects. *Can.J.Psychol.* 39:100-129.

15. Jordan K., H.J.Heinze, K.Lutz, K.M.Kanowski, L.Jäncke (2001) Cortical activations during the mental rotation of different visual objects. *NeuroImage* 13:143-152.

16. Krüger M., H.Krist (2009) Imagery and motor processes - when are they connected? The mental rotation of body parts in development. *J.Cogn.Dev,* 10:239-261.

17. Linn M.C., A.C.Petersen (1985) Emergence and characterization of sex differences in spatial ability: A meta-analysis. *Child Dev.* 56:1479-1498.

18. Neuburger, S.P.Jansen, M.Heil, C.Quaiser-Pohl (in press) Gender differences in pre-adolescents'mental rotation performance: do they depend on grade and stimuli? *Personality and Individual Differences.*

19. Piaget J. (1954) Construction of Reality in the Child. Basic Books, New York.

20. Post A.A., A.Daffertshofer, P.J.Beek (2000) Principal components in three-ball cascade juggling. *Biol.Cyber.* 82:143-152.

21. Shepard R.N., J.Metzler (1971) Mental rotation of three-dimensional objects. *Science* 171:701-703.

22. Wexler M., S.M.Kosslyn, A.Berthoz (1998) Motor processes in mental rotation. *Cognition* 68:77-94.

23. Wiedenbauer G., P.Jansen-Osmann (2008) Manual training of mental rotation in children. *Learn.Instr.* 18:30-41.

24. Wiedenbauer G., J.Schmid, P.Jansen Osmann (2007) Manual training of mental rotation. *Eur.J.Cogn.Psychol.* 19:17-36.

25. Wilson M. (2002) Six views of embodied rotation and the planning of hand movements. *Psychon.Bull.Rev.* 9:625-636.

26. Wohlschläger A., A.Wohlschläger (1998) Mental and manual rotation. *J.Exp.Psychol.Hum.* 24:397-412.

4

Flexibility: components, proprioceptive mechanisms and methods

Estélio H.M. Dantas [1], Rejane Daoud [1], Alexis Trott [2], Rudy J. Nodari Jr. [3], Mario C.S.C. Conceição [1]

[1] Human Motricity Biosciences Laboratory (LABIMH), Federal University of the State of Rio de Janeiro (UNIRIO), RJ; [2] Laboratory of Molecular Aspects Associated to Genetic Diseases, University of Western Santa Catarina (UNOESC), SC; [3] Laboratory of Prognostic Aspects of Intervention and Care in Health and Human Performance, UNOESC, SC, Brazil

Summary

A literature review on physical flexibility was presented and discussed. This included definitions and components that influence the performance of movements requiring large joint motion ranges and muscle elasticity. Flexibility was discussed with reference to specific age groups, e.g. children and the elderly. Proprioceptive mechanisms and components directly related to flexibility were overviewed, as well as suitable approaches towards flexibilisation, i.e. maintaining and/or enhancing flexibility.

Key words: Flexibility – Stretching – Flexibilising

Introduction

Flexibility is an important component of physical aptitude. According to the American College of Sports Medicine [16], it is one of the essential qualities for acquiring and developing human physical conditioning. An improved flexibility brings certain benefits, e.g. reduced risk of injuries and enhanced athletic performance [15]. For these and other reasons, flexibility becomes increasingly incorporated into physical activity prescription programmes. This prompted us to review the available literature on flexibility and to dispel common misconceptions frequently associated with this physical quality.

Definition and Limits of Flexibility

Flexibility was defined by Dantas [8] as '*physical feature responsible for the voluntary execution of maximum joint range* of motion, by a single or multiple *joints, within morphological limits, without a risk of injury*'. Thus, good flexibility may result in significant benefits for both athletes and non-athletes. However, unlike other physical features, it is better not to strive for maximum flexibility, but rather to attain the "optimal limit", i.e. only that needed for good performance of given movement. An excessive flexibility may fail to protect the joints, thus causing injuries like permanent sprains, ligament laxity, etc. [9]. In extreme cases, joints may be damaged to the point where tendons become torn, with serious consequences for the organism [19]. Thus, it is just as much of a problem having an excessive flexibility which increases the risk of diminished joint stability and leading to sprains, as it is to have insufficient flexibility which may lead to muscle strains [9]. Flexibility cannot be considered a general characteristic, since it may be joint-specific. For example, individuals might exhibit good flexibility in the shoulder complex, but not be as flexible in the hip joint. For this reason, improving overall flexibility could result in important benefits for the organism [19].

Stretching promotes muscle relaxation, defined as suspension of muscle tension. Muscle tension may also increase blood pressure and hinder muscle irrigation, leading to diminished oxygenation and nutrient supply. This compromises the removal of elements resulting from muscle work, which increases the amount of toxic residues accumulated in cells and predisposes muscles to fatigue and pain [18].

A contracted muscle also spends energy needlessly. If constantly contracted, it becomes shortened, less flexible and more vulnerable to injuries caused by sudden movements requiring greater range of motion [2]. Muscle contraction can be voluntary or involuntary and painful, as in cramps. These are generally of neural, not muscular

Author's address Prof. Estélio H.M. Dantas, Human Motricity Biosciences Laboratory (LABIMH), Federal University of the State of Rio de Janeiro (UNIRIO) – RJ, Brazil

origin, initiating when a muscle is in a shortened position and contracts even more. Cramps disappear when the affected muscle is passively stretched or when its antagonist is contracted. This technique is used in proprioceptive neuromuscular facilitation methods, due to stimulation of the Golgi tendon organ [11].

Flexibility is applicable at every age, provided the physiological transformations at given age are observed, especially in children and in the elderly [7]. Since children are in the longitudinal growth phase, their bones and soft tissues do not grow at the same rate. Bones may grow more rapidly than muscles and their conjunctive tissues, thereby increasing muscle tension. At certain stages of development, conjunctive tissue may exceed bone growth, causing hypermobility and leaving the joint vulnerable to sprains.

According to Weineck [27], mobility training at early school age must be undertaken very carefully; he stated that 'Contradictory tendencies can be identified during mobility development in this age group. On one hand, flexion capacity of the hip and shoulder joint, as well as the spine shows highest mobility at 8 – 9 years of age. On the other, a decrease is observed in capacity to extend the legs apart at the hip joint and dorsally directed mobility in the shoulder joint.' ([27] p.277). He further reported that muscles and ligaments do not accompany accelerated bone growth at the onset of adolescence because of rapid height growth and reduced mechanical strength in the passive locomotor apparatus. His conclusion was: 'Care must be taken to ensure a balanced relationship between load and the capacity to support them, avoiding exercises performed with partners, unilateral and twisting movements, as well as torso hyperflexion and hyperextension.'

A study conducted by Farinatti et al. [10] on 487 boys and 414 girls aged 5 – 15 years by using the flexitest, revealed that younger children exhibited more flexibility than the older ones due to greater articular mobility since their ligaments and joints were not completely developed. Advancing age causes an increase in ultimate tensile strength in these structures and a gradual decrease in flexibility potential. The authors report that intrinsic and extrinsic factors act together.

With respect to ageing, the joint motion ranges decrease due to enriched connective tissue (tendons and ligaments) and reduced muscle fibre elasticity. Reduced mobility may contribute to lower range of motion and pathologies related to the osteomuscular system, more common in the elderly. Functional decline occurs with the participation of various systems, leading to e.g. sensory and motor control losses. Weineck ([27], p.328) stated that during the ageing process 'Alterations in *active and passive locomotor apparatuses, cardiocirculatory and cardiopulmonary systems are mainly responsible for decreased physical performance capacity.*' Many of these disorders are irreversible, although physical activity may partially restore functional skills and psychological capacity of the elderly.

Dantas ([8], p. 204) studied the ageing-related reduction of flexibility and found that muscle elasticity and joint mobility losses contributed to 54 and 46%, respectively, of that reduction. Ueno et al. [24] applied a physical capacity development programme, including stretching sessions, to 13 men and 25 women aged 60 years or more, with the aim of improving performance of daily activities. At the end of the programme, the participants experienced less pain, as well as enhanced quality and improved performance of daily movements.

Pereira [7] compared two age groups (31 – 45 and 61 – 75 years) with respect to 10 joint movements measured by goniometry and found that cervical spine rotation and hip flexion showed greatest losses of motion ranges. Applying stretching adequate for the elderly might contribute to preventing or minimising ageing effects, provided the exercises correctly and safely adjusted individually.

Factors Influencing Flexibility

The major problem with the study of flexibility is its extreme complexity, largely due to the diversity of intervening components. Four factors are primarily responsible for the degree of joint flexibility: mobility, elasticity, plasticity and pliability [8].

Joint mobility is the degree of joint movement, accounting for 47% of flexibility resistance. Elasticity refers to the stretching of muscle components, contributing to 41% of flexibility resistance. Plasticity refers to the level of plastic component deformation during flexibility exercises, its residual post-exercise deformation being called hysteresis. Pliability refers to skin changes in the segment required for the movement. Resistance flexibility accounts for only 2%.

Proprioception Mechanisms

The locomotor apparatus is not the only factor influencing flexibility. Controlling the range of motion and muscle tension, and limiting the arc of joint motion, aimed at preventing injuries, is mostly due to the action of the nervous system. Proprioception in this system may be associated with joints or muscles [12].

Joint proprioceptors are formed by Pacinian and Ruffini corpuscles. Their function is to provide joint position sense, velocity of movement and information on resistance that opposes the movement. Several different types of sensitive receptors are found in the joint capsules and ligaments [11]. Muscle proprioceptors are formed by the muscle spindle and the Golgi tendon organ (GTO). The muscle spindle is located in muscle fibre. When a muscle is stretched, the central portion of the muscle spindle called the nuclear bag accompanies the movement and is pulled back, activating the sensitive terminals called annulospiral endings. These send impulses to the medulla, where synapses are made with α-motoneurons. After stimulation, they send commands to contract extrafusal fibres (myotatic reflex) [13].

The Golgi tendon organ is located near the insertion point of muscle fibre in the tendon. On average, 10 to 15 muscle fibres are connected in a direct line to each GTO, which responds to the tension produced by the bundle of muscle fibres. Nerve impulses discharged by the GTO are transmitted by fast conducting afferent axons to the spinal medulla and cerebellum. Upon reaching the medulla, those impulses excite inhibitory interneurons that secrete an inhibitory neuromediator, γ-aminobutyric acid (GABA). This acts on α-motoneurons, provoking muscle relaxation.

Components of Flexibility

Flexibility performance depends directly on different structures. Joints are formed by one or more bones, and movable joints are the most important for flexibility. Ligaments are another important structure that influences flexibility. These are strong fibrous cords of connective tissue, flexible but inelastic, which connect two bones. Their primary function is to sustain a joint. Ligaments are composed of bundles of collagen fibres placed parallel or intertwined around each other; they are pliable and flexible, offering freedom of movement, but strong and inextensible enough not to yield to the applied forces. The joint capsule and ligaments account for 47% of the total resistance to movement [2].

Tendons are formed by fibrous tissue responsible for connecting a muscle to bone. They are practically inextensible, offering approximately 10% of total resistance to movement. Their main function is to transmit muscle tension to the bones, thereby producing movement. This structure is composed mainly of firmly compressed parallel collagen fascicles of varying length and width [2].

Muscles are an essential component of flexibility owing to their elastic properties. They are active organs composed of fibre bundles that bring about voluntary and involuntary movement because of their contracting capacity, thus being the principal structure in flexibility performance [3]. Muscle fibres are covered by membrane (sarcolemma), overlaid by conjunctive tissue (endomysium). The sarcolemma contains contractile proteins, enzymes, food substrates, nuclei, organelles and the sarcoplasmic reticulum, where the muscle contraction process initiates [20]. Muscle fibre clusters form bundles (fascicles) surrounded by perimysium. A set of fascicles is covered by a sheath (epimysium), forming a muscle [20]. Fibres at muscle endings become increasingly scarce and the conjunctive tissue layers that surround the muscles begin to compact, forming tendons, which insert themselves into the bones. The functional unit of a muscle is the sarcomere, composed of myofilaments of actin (thin) and myosin (thick), bordered by the Z-line. Each sarcomere contains approximately 450 thick filaments at the centre and 900 thin filaments at the ends. Several sarcomeres form the myofibril, filaments that slide over each other causing muscle contraction [1].

The two previously described filaments are inextensible and only participate in muscle contraction, without changing their length during sarcomere extension. However, recent studies [14,20,21,23] revealed a third filament, thinner than actin, called titin, which takes part in the extension of a smaller functional muscle unit. The thick filament (myosin) is connected to both ends of the Z-line via titin, responsible for increased sarcomere length. The length of this filament is what determines the amount of sarcomere stretching. According to Trinick and Tskhovrebora [23], titin molecule resembles a chain and consists mainly of immunoglobulin and fibronectin. It forms a connection between the Z-line and A-band and is the third type of sarcomeric filament. Titin is responsible for muscle constitution and elasticity, thus being an important component in muscle stretching due to unfolding inside sarcomeres, the smaller functional units of a muscle [20].

From a mechanical point of view, the locomotor apparatus can be divided into elastic, plastic and inextensible components. During stretching, elastic and plastic muscle components are deformed, since the inextensible ones do not undergo significant deformation. Elastic com ponents formed by conjunctive tissue and myofilaments are those that return to their original form after muscle relaxation. Conjunctive tissue, because of its disposition both in series and parallel, provokes participation of parallel elastic components (PEC) surrounding both the sarcolemma/endomysium and fascicles (perimysium), and series elastic components (SEC) [25]. Plastic components, composed of mitochondria, reticulum, the tubular system, ligaments and intervertebral discs, do not return to their original form after stretching. Inextensible components are made up of the bones (totally inextensible) and tendons (partially inextensible). Tendons are not affected by training; ligaments, however adapt to stretching, since they do not return to their original form as elastic components do. Therefore, a ligament that is constantly injured may become loose and not perform its functional role.

Types of flexibility: There are four types of flexibility: static, dynamic, ballistic and controlled. Static flexibility occurs when the individual maintains a position, moving the segment slowly and gradually until the maximum articular arc has been reached. This type of flexibility is most frequently used to evaluate flexibility. It is characterised by the maximum range of motion attained during movement execution and is used extensively in physical education practices. Ballistic flexibility forces the limb into an extended range of motion when the muscle is not relaxed enough to enter it. It involves fast bouncing movements and is widely used by ballerinas and gymnasts.

Stretching vs. flexibilising: Specific methods are used to improve joint mobility and increasingly extend muscle fibres within physiologically feasible levels. However, if the objective is to maintain flexibility, the most widely indicated methodology uses muscle stretching with normal joint range of motion. This is a sub-maximal exercise aimed at maintaining flexibility obtained and performing normal range of motion with the least amount of physical restriction possible [5]. On the other hand, if the goal is an enhanced flexibility (greater joint range of motion arc), muscle elasticity and joint range of motion must extend to their maximum limits. This is achieved by flexibilising exercises [6].

Since stretching involves low intensity demands on flexibility components, it does not activate proprioception mechanisms. However, flexibilising constantly excites these mechanisms depending on the velocity of the movement. In compensation, stretching almost totally deforms plastic components. Quick movements stimulate muscle spindle, triggering the myotatic reflex and calling for muscle contraction. Slow and gradual muscle flexibilising activates the Golgi tendon organ, leading to muscle relaxation. Dynamic stretching, therefore, acts primarily on muscles, whereas static stretching has a greater effect on joint mobility.

Because of proprioceptor mechanisms, stretching and flexibilising must be applied according to the desired objective. If a response is required immediately after flexibility exercises, as in athletic competitions, stretching should be used only to prepare joint and muscle plastic components for the activity to be performed immediately. When the aim is to enhance flexibility, i.e. to acquire chronic deformation in plastic and muscle components, flexibilising should be used in specific sessions.

Flexibility Training Methods

As mentioned earlier, flexibility can be shaped using two processes: stretching and flexibilising by applying a variety of techniques. Stretching can be applied as elongation, suspension or release. Elongation aims at deforming the plastic components using movements within the normal joint arc. The suspension technique uses the action of gravity to stretch ligaments and muscles. Their objective is to eliminate various catabolites following muscle contraction. Release consists of balancing limbs or muscles, resulting in muscle relaxation and muscle spindle deactivation.

Flexibilising can be applied by different approaches, like active, passive or proprioceptive neuromuscular facilitation (PNF) [4]. The active method uses dynamic (ballistic) speed exercises, reaching maximum range of motion, that activates the muscle spindle and provokes a myotactic reflex. This method emphasises muscle elasticity and increases long-term flexibility levels. The passive method or static flexibilising aims at slowly, steadily reaching the largest range of joint motion and maintaining the position for 10 – 15 s, repeating the routine 3 to 6 times with a decontracting interval [6,22,26]. This technique emphasises joint mobility and activates the Golgi tendon organ, resulting in muscle relaxation, that does not require excessive muscle contractions immediately after its application and risk compromising joint components.

The Proprioceptive neuromuscular facilitation relies on the muscle spindle and Golgi tendon organ and its antagonist to obtain greater range of motion. Among the most commonly used techniques are Scientific Stretching for Sports-3S processes – hold-relax, contract-relax-antagonist and the slow-reversal one.

Concluding Remarks

This review aimed at emphasising the complexity and multifaceted nature of flexibility. Further studies are needed on this physical feature, so important for all those engaged in motor activities, i.e. both athletes and non-athletes. The steadily increasing sedentariness contributes to the inactivity-related diseases apart from decreasing the joint ranges of motion.

It is reassuring for professionals involved in flexibility training to know that young athletes will not be adversely affected, at least in the spine, as demonstrated by Raty *et al.* [17]. Flexibility has to be included in all training programmes, irrespectively of their objectives, since its importance for children, adolescents, adults and the elderly is undoubted.

References

1. Allen D., B.Zhang, N.Whitehead (2010) Stretch-induced membrane damage in muscle: comparison of wild-type and mdx mice. *Muscle Biophys.* 682:297-313.

2. Alter M. Alter M. (2004) Science of Flexibility (3rd ed.) Human Kinetics, Champaign IL.

3. Barbanti V. (2003) Dicionário de educação física e do esporte. Manole, São Paulo.

4. Bradley P., P.Olsen, M.Portas (2007) The effect of static, ballistic, and proprioceptive neuromuscular facilitation stretching on vertical jump performance. *J.Strengt Condit.Res.* 21: 223-226.

5. Conceição M., J.Novaes, E.Dantas, S.Melegário (2003) Flexibilidade, método passivo e tempo de insistência: uma revisão de literatura. Federation Internationale d'Education Physique.

6. Conceição M., R.Vale, M.Bottaro, E.Dantas, J.Novaes (2008) Effects of four different permanence times of the static overstretching on the flexibility's young adults. *Fitn.Perform-.J.* 7:88-92.

7. Dantas E.H.M., S.A.M.Pereira, J.C.Aragão, A.H.Ota (2002) The preponderance of decreased joint mobility or muscular elasticity in the loss of flexibility in the aging process. *Fitn.Perform.J.* 1(3):12-19.

8. Dantas E.H.M. (2005) Alongamento e Flexionamento. Shape, Rio de Janeiro.

9. Farinatti P. (2000) Flexibilidade e esporte: uma revisão de literatura. *Revista Paulista de Educação Física* 14:85-96.

10. Farinatti P., A.Nóbrega, C.Araújo (1998) Perfil da flexibilidade em crianças de 5 a 15 anos de idade. *Revista de Educação Física e Desporto* 14:23-31.

11. Guissard N., J.Duchateau (2006) Neural aspects of muscle stretching. *Exerc.Sport Sci.Rev.* 34:154-158.

12. Hong J., M.Velez, A.Moland, J.Sullivan (2010) Acute effects of whole body vibration on shoulder muscular strength and joint position sense. *J.Hum.Kinet.* 25:17-25.

13. Hsieh F., Y.Wang, T.Lu, A.Wang, C.Huang, C.Hsieh (2009) The Effects of Passive Warm-up with Ultrasound in Exercise Performance and Muscle Damage. Springer, pp. 1149-1152.

14. Linke W. (2000) Invited Reviews-Stretching molecular springs: Elasticity of titin filaments in vertebrate striated muscle. *Histol.Histopathol.* 15:799-812.

15. Nelson R., W.Bandy (2005) An update on flexibility. *Strength Condit.J.* 27:10-16.

16. Pollock M., G.Gaesser, J.Butcher, J.Despres, R.Dishman, B.Franklin, C.Garber (1998) ACSM Position Stand: The recommended quantity and quality of exercise for developing and maintaining cardiorespiratory and muscular fitness, and flexibility in healthy adults. *Med.Sci.Sports Exerc.* 30:975-991.

17. Räty H., M.Battié, T.Videman, S.Sarna (1997) Lumbar mobility in former elite male weight-lifters, soccer players, long-distance runners and shooters. *Clin.Biomech.* 12:325-330.

18. Rubini E., A.Costa, P.Gomes (2007) The effects of stretching on strength performance. *Sports Med.* 37:213-224.

19. Shrier I. (2004) Does stretching improve performance? A systematic and critical review of the literature. *Clin.J.Sport Med.* 14:267-273.

20. Silva E., W.Z.Freitas, M.L.D.Ferrão, J.Fernandes Filho, E.H.M.Dantas (2003) Flexibility levels in terms of the muscular fiber type. *Fitn.Perform.J.* 2(3):157-164.

21. Sorimachi H., A.Freiburg, B.Kolmerer, S.Ishiura, G.Stier, C.Gregorio, D.Labeit, W.Linke, K.Suzuki, S.Labeit (1997) Tissue-specific expression and α-actinin binding properties of the Z-disc titin: implications for the nature of vertebrate Z-discs 1. *J.Molec.Biol.* 270:688-695.

22. Torres J., M.Conceição, A.Sampaio, E.Dantas (2009) Acute effects of static stretching on muscle strength. *Biomed.Hum.Kinet.* 1:52-55.

23. Trinick J., L.Tskhovrebova (1999) Titin: a molecular control freak. *Trends Cell Biol.* 9:377-380.

24. Ueno L., S.Okuma, M.Miranda, W.Jacob Filho, L.Lee Ho (2000) Análise dos efeitos quantitativos e qualitativos de um programa de educação física sobre a flexibilidade do quadril em indivíduos com mais de 60 anos. *Motriz* 6:9-16.

25. Fung Y.C. (1993) Biomechanics: Mechanical Properties of Living Tissues (2nd ed.) Springer-Verlag, New York.

26. Voigt L, R.G.S.Vale, D.W.Abdala, W.Z.Freitas, J.S.Novaes, E.H.M.Dantas (2007) Effects of a ten seconds repetition of incentive of the static method for the development of the young adult men's flexibility. *Fitn.Perform.J.* 6(6):352-356.

27. Weineck J. (2004) Sportbiologie. Spitta (Auslieferung WMI).

Effects of a regular motor activity on somatic and fitness variables in boys aged 17 – 18 years

Joanna Piotrowska

Warsaw Academy of Tourism, Food and Hospitality, Warsaw, Poland

Summary

Study aim: To assess the somatic and fitness changes in semisedentary boys persuaded to undertake Nordic Walking activities throughout a school year.

Material and methods: Two groups of schoolboys aged 17 – 18 years were studied: regularly attending physical education (PE) classes (Group A; n = 46) and those who avoided PE classes by submitting sick note ors excuses signed by parents (Group N; n = 29). The latter ones undertook Nordic Walking training (3 sessions a week throughout the school year). Group A undertook no motor activities except regular PE classes. At the beginning (Pre) and at the end of the study (Post) all boys were subjected to 7 fitness tests: 50-m run (50 m), shuttle run 4×10 m (SR4), 1000-m run (LDR), sit-ups (SUP), standing broad jump (SBJ), pull-ups (PUP) and stand-and-reach (STR).

Results: Mean Post-Pre changes in Group N evidenced significant improvements, compared with Group A, in most studied variables – body mass, body fat content, 50-m dash velocity, PUP, SUP, STR, SR4 velocity, no significant, unfavourable changes being noted.

Conclusions: Nordic Walking, being an attractive form of activity, may be an easy way to encourage people to undertake motor activities thus improving the health status.

Key words: Nordic Walking – Motor fitness – Physical activity

Introduction

Motor activity, directed at health-related fitness, needs not be intense but ought to shape sport habits from the earliest age as these carry over the effects to the adult age [9,10] and such activities are known to represent preventive measures against many a disorder [4]. Abstaining from motor activities restricts a normal functioning of young individuals and optimal functioning of adults [6,10]. Yet, children and youths lead nowadays increasingly more sedentary life and the sedentary activities reduce the motor activities beyond the required level [10]. According to the National Health Project (2007 – 2015) [3], only about 30% of children and youths meet the motor activity requirements; that problem was, however, reported also for other countries [6]. This is the result of upbringing children without prompting them to undertake motor activities which, in turn, leads to a high percentage of schoolchildren avoiding motor activities despite their being obligatory.

Among the recently fashionable motor activities is Nordic Walking that becomes increasingly popular as it may be practiced at practically every age [2,5], even by those with disabilities. That activity, when properly performed, engages up to 90% of muscles; an appropriate engagement of shoulders and arms protects from falling and reduces the load exerted on the spine and on the ankle, knee and hip joints [4,8].

Students of upper secondary schools select the lifelong sports or resign from motor activities for various reasons, including laziness. Since the activity schedule in Nordic Walking is so designed as to bring about improvements in body composition, motor coordination, strength and agility, and is attractive for both individual and group practicing, it seems extremely well suited to attract those who habitually abstain from physical activities. The aim of this study was thus to assess the somatic and fitness changes in sedentary or semisedentary young men, aged 17 – 18 years, persuaded to undertake Nordic Walking throughout a school year.

Author's address Dr Joanna Piotrowska, Chodakowska 50, 03-816 Warsaw, Poland

Material and Methods

Two groups of schoolboys aged 17 – 18 years volunteered to participate in the study: Group A (n = 46), consisting of boys regularly attending physical education (PE) classes, and Group N (n = 29), who avoided PE classes by submitting sick note ors excuses signed by parents. Boys from that latter group were suggested to receive a credit for PE classes by attending a Nordic Walking project financed by local municipality in 2009, aimed at popularising that form of motor activity among youths. The project lasted one school year and consisted of three 45-min sessions a week. The sessions included walking at a distance averaging 5.2 km at an average velocity of 5.6 km/h, as well as strength and coordination exercises. Sports Tracker software was used to measure the distance and velocity via mobile phone equipped with GPS module and GPS Garmin Forerunner 310 XT (Taiwan) device. The project included also competitive walking at 2-km distance.

Boys from Group A attended only the curricular PE classes consisting predominantly of training team sports (volleyball, basketball, football, unihockey). Total time spent on motor activities was in both groups alike, the only reason of absence being illness. None of the boys from both groups undertook any other motor activities.

The boys were examined twice: in September, after having returned from vacation (Pre), and in June, at the end of the school year (Post). All boys were subjected to 7 tests from the International Fitness Test battery: 50-m run (50 m), shuttle run 4×10 m (SR4), 1000-m run (LDR), sit-ups (SUP), standing broad jump (SBJ), pull-ups (PUP) and stand-and-reach (STR). The results of running tests were converted to velocities (m/s). Body composition was assessed by BIA technique using the Tanita TBF-300A (Japan) device.

Student's *t*-test for dependent data was used to assess the Post-Pre differences. The data were also standardised against Polish population data by employing age functions of the respective means and standard deviations [7]. The level of $p \leq 0.05$ was considered significant.

Results

The results of the study are presented in Table 1 and in Figs. 1 and 2. Figure 1 shows multivariate profiles of both groups, i.e. standardised against Polish population data, at the beginning of the study (Pre). As compared with the Polish population of male youths, those from this study were markedly inferior in SBJ, LDR, PUP and STR but superior in 50-m dash, SR4 and SUP. With respect to BMI, over 60% of boys from both groups were within normal limits and only two boys were obese.

Table 1. Mean values (±SD) of somatic and fitness variables and of the Post-Pre changes (Δ) in boys aged 17 – 18 years

Group	N (n = 29)		A (n = 46)	
Variable	Pre	Δ	Pre	Δ
Body mass (kg)	74.1 ± 13.3	-0.1 ± 2.5	68.5 ± 12.5	4.0 ± 2.6 ^{ooo}
BMI	22.4 ± 3.5	0.0 ± 1.1	21.6 ± 3.2	1.3 ± 4.0 ^{o}
Body fat content (%)	11.8 ± 5.6	-0.8 ± 1.0 ^{ooo}	9.3 ± 3.2*	1.4 ± 2.3 ^{ooo}
Body water (%)	62.6 ± 6.2	1.9 ± 2.2 ^{ooo}	64.8 ± 10.0	-0.2 ± 3.2
50-m run (m/s)	6.83 ± 0.43	0.08 ± 0.15 ^{oo}	6.92 ± 0.41	-0.14 ± 0.24 ^{ooo}
SBJ (cm)	197 ± 26	-1.0 ± 7.6	202 ± 22	-2.5 ± 4.7 ^{oo}
LDR (m/s)	3.77 ± 0.50	0.03 ± 0.17	3.82 ± 0.45	-0.07 ± 0.27
PUP (s)	6.72 ± 5.05	0.62 ± 1.93	8.52 ± 5.76	-1.41 ± 1.41 ^{ooo}
SR4 (m/s)	3.85 ± 0.25	0.02 ± 0.06	3.90 ± 0.23	-0.05 ± 0.06 ^{ooo}
SUP (n)	28.9 ± 5.4	0.0 ± 1.9	29.9 ± 4.4	-1.8 ± 1.4 ^{ooo}
STR (cm)	-2.0 ± 8.7	1.1 ± 1.7 ^{oo}	3.6 ± 6.9**	-1.0 ± 1.2 ^{ooo}

Legend: SBJ – Standing broad jump; LDR – Long-distance run (1000 m); PUP – Pull-ups; SR4 – Shuttle run (4×10 m); SUP – Sit-ups; STR – Stand-and-reach; Significantly ($p<0.01$) different from Group N: * $p<0.05$; ** $p<0.01$; Significant Post-Pre changes: ^{o} $p<0.05$; ^{oo} $p<0.01$; ^{ooo} $p<0.001$

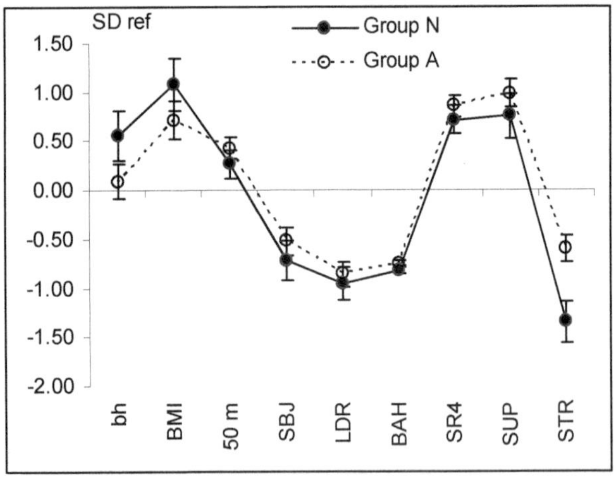

Fig. 1. Mean values (±SE) of somatic and fitness variables standardised against Polish population of male youths (X-axis)

Legend: bh – Body height; 50 m – 50-m run (velocity); SBJ – Standing broad jump; LDR – Long-distance run (1000 m; velocity); PUP – Pull-ups; SR4 – Shuttle run (4×10 m; velocity); SUP – Sit-ups; STR – Stand-and-reach

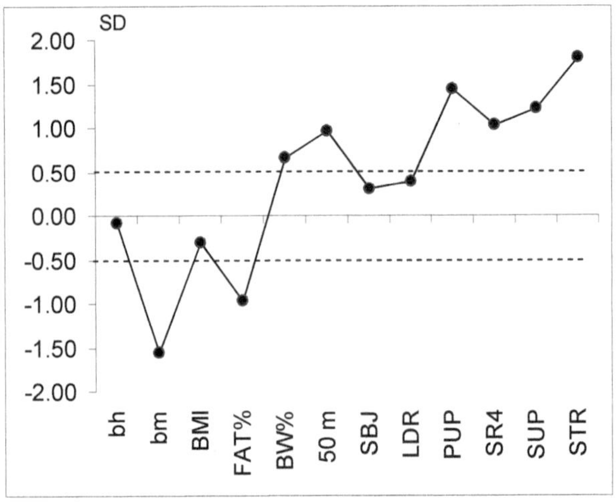

Fig. 2. Multivariate profile of Group N standardised against Group A ("control")

Legend: bh – Body height; bm – Body mass; BW – Body water content; 50 m – 50-m run; SBJ – Standing broad jump; LDR – Long-distance run (1000 m); PUP – Pull-ups; SR4 – Shuttle run (4×10 m); SUP – Sit-ups; STR – Stand-and-reach; Dotted lines correspond to $p<0.05$

It is worth noticing that boys from Group A ("control") had lower body fat content at the beginning of the study than their sedentary mates. Yet, at the end of the school year, the control boys significantly gained in body mass, BMI and body fat content while boys from Group N significantly lost body fat. In effect, no significant between-group differences were noted post-study in any variable, except flexibility (STR), boys from Group N remaining significantly ($p<0.05$) inferior to Group A boys (by 3.5 cm on the average).

On the other hand, when considering the effects of regularly practicing Nordic Walking throughout a school year, significant improvements (body fat content, by nearly 7%; 50-m dash velocity, by 1%) or a lack of significant changes (body mass, BMI, SBJ,PUP, SR4, SUP) were noted in contrast to the A-group, in which no significant improvement was observed in any variable studied. Moreover, in that latter group significant, unfavourable changes were noted in all fitness variables except LDR and in the somatic ones (body mass, BMI, body fat content) as shown in Table 1.

In Fig. 1 are shown changes recorded in Group N standardised against those in Group A. Thus, the changes are expressed in SD units of the respective individual Post-Pre changes in Group A. Mean changes in both groups did not differ significantly only in case of body height, BMI, SBJ and LDR. All other changes evidenced a significant improvement in Group N.

Discussion

The nearly adult students who led a semisedentary life and avoided regular PE classes but consented, upon persuasion, to undertake Nordic Walking activities throughout a whole school year, exhibited marked improvement not only in their fitness but in their body composition as well. That improvement could be attributed to the specificity of Nordic Walking, i.e. engagement of almost all muscles that enabled a more intense workout at a lower perceived fatigue [1,5]. It should be emphasised that although a significant improvement in that group (N) was noted only for the 50-m dash (speed) and for the stand-and-reach test (flexibility), the training-induced changes in Group N showed significant improvements in all variables except BMI and SBJ when compared with Group A that could be regarded as a reference, control group.

The deviations in several fitness variables in relation to the respective population means could be due to local specificity, like daily habits at school and at home, since representative cohorts studied every decade showed no such deviations [6]. The observed deviations may also point to the need of modifying the curricular PE classes and of promoting non-sedentary life styles. The results presented for Group N and the experience in running Nordic Walking sessions with those youths, seem highly promising. It would be interesting to assess the motivation of those boys who seemed truly committed to those activities. It is also necessary to conduct repeated studies in order to assess the long-term engagement and persistence. Nordic Walking, with its motor novelty is very well suited to attract people of any age.

Summing up, Nordic Walking, being an attractive form of activity, may be an easy way to encourage people to undertake motor activities thus improving their motor fitness and a general health status.

References

1. Church T.S., C.P.Earnest, G.M.Morss (2002) Field testing of physiological responses associated with Nordic Walking. *Res.Q.Exerc.Sport* 73:296-300.

2. INWA Instructor Manual (2009) 5th ed.

3. Jopkiewicz A. (2007) The importance of physical fitness in the promotion of health Man Zeszyty Naukowe ALMAMER 3 (47).

4. Morss G.M., T.S.Church, C.P.Earnest, A.N.Jordan (2001) Field test comparing the metabolic cost of normal walking versus Nordic Walking. *Med.Sci.Sports Exerc.* 33:S23.

5. Piech K., B.Raczyńska (2010) Nordic Walking – a versatile physical activity. *Polish Journal of Sport and Tourism* 17:69-78.

6. Przewęda R., J.Dobosz (2007) Growth and Physical Fitness of Polish Youths. AWF Warsaw.

7. Stupnicki R., J.Dobosz, P.Tomaszewski, K.Milde (2005) Standardisation of somatic and fitness variables. *Phys.Educ.Sport* 49:72-79.

8. Willson J., M.Torry, M.Decker, T.Kernozek, J.Steadman (2001) Effects of walking poles on lower extremity gait mechanics. *Med.Sci.Sports Exerc.* 33:142-147.

9. World Health Organization (1990) Prevention in childhood and youth of adult cardiovascular diseases: time for action (WHO Technical Report Series, No. 792).

10. Young M.L. (1985) World Health Organization Switzerland. Estimation of fitness and physical ability physical performance, and self-concept among adolescent *J.Sport Med.* 25: 50-144.

6

The prevalence of injuries in professional Turkish soccer players

Faruk Yamaner [1], Hayrettin Gümüşdağ [1], Alparslan Kartal [1], M. Gümüş [2], A. Güllü [3], O. Imamoğlu [4]

[1] Hitit University, School of Physical Education and Sports, Çorum; [2] Zonguldak Karaelmas University, School of Physical Education and Sports, Zonguldak; [3] İnönü University, School of Physical Education and Sports, Malatya; [4] 19 Mayıs University, School of Physical Education and Sport, Samsun, Turkey

Summary

Study aim: To assess the prevalence and anatomical sites of injuries in professional soccer players in one game season.
Material and methods: A cohort of 510 professional male soccer players consisting of 48 goalkeepers, 194 defence players, 189 mid-field players and 79 forward players of the 1st and 2nd Turkish Professional Soccer Leagues in 2005 -2006 season were requested to submit questionnaire reports on all injuries they experienced.
Results: About 60% of all injuries pertained to lower extremities, another 25% to upper extremities, the most frequent being skin abrasions (about 24%). The percentage of players who sustained injuries was lowest among mid-field players (about 47%) compared with other categories (nearly 70%) but the average number of injuries per player was highest among them (8.1 vs. about 4.5). The risk of sustaining injury when playing a match amounted to 9.8% for mid-field players; that was significantly ($p<0.01$) lower (11.7 – 13.0%) than for other categories of players.
Conclusions: Football injuries are the major factor affecting players' performance. Thus, appropriate strategies, aimed at reducing injuries, ought to be implemented.

Key words: Football – Injuries – Injury risk – Anatomical sites

Introduction

Football is one of the most popular sports in the world [1,4,8,12], as many as about 200 million individuals playing that game, including about 200.000 professional players [10]. The popularity of professional football creates a big financial effect [14]. At the same time, football players are at a high risk of injuries [2,7,9], that risk in professional football being about thousand times higher than in industry workers [1]. Every elite male football player is supposed to be exposed to injury at least once in a year, which affects his performance [2,8]. Sustained injuries are associated with health expenses; they decrease football club incomes because of the absence of top players and, thus, club success [14].

It is evident that knowing the type of injury, its anatomical localisation and playing position of the player is important not only to prevent injuries but also for selecting appropriate treatment. Thus, the aim of the study was to determine the prevalence of various types of injuries in relation to body parts and playing positions.

Material and Methods

A cohort of 510 professional male football players aged 22 – 29 years was studied in the season 2005 – 2006. The cohort consisted of 48 goalkeepers, 194 defence players, 189 mid-field players and 79 forward players of the 1st and 2nd Turkish Professional Football Leagues. After having been informed about the scope and protocol of the study, the players were requested to fill questionnaires containing demographic questions and those pertaining to details of injuries they experienced; the players were interviewed by their club physicians. The clubs made the players' records available for the purpose of the study. All players gave their informed consents to participate. All matches were played on grass fields. The SPSS for Windows software was used in data analysis, the level of $p \le 0.05$ being considered significant.

Results

The results of the study are presented in Tables 1 – 4. As follows from Table 1, most players had over 10 years

Author's address Dr Faruk Yamaner, School of Physical Education and Sports, Hitit University, Çorum, Turkey

of training experience and during the season 2005 – 2006 all of them played nearly 30 matches, on average (Table 2). About 70% of goal keepers, defence and mid-field players sustained injuries; the respective percentage of forward players was significantly ($p<0.001$) lower but they sustained significantly ($p<0.001$) more injuries per injured player compared with other categories (8.1 vs. 4.1 – 4.6). The risk of sustaining injury when playing a match amounted to 9.8% for mid-field players; that was significantly ($p<0.01$) lower (11.7 – 13.0%) than for other categories (Table 2).

Table 1. Demographic data (%) of professional football players aged 22 – 29 years (n = 510)

Variable	Category	%
Education	Primary	10.2
	Secondary	42.7
	University	47.1
Marital status	Married	40.6
	Single	59.4
Training experience	5 – 10	26.5
	11 – 15	41.2
	Over 15	32.3

Table 2. Numbers of players, played matches and sustained injuries

Category of players Variable	Keepers n = 48	Defence n = 194	Mid-field n = 189	Forward n = 79	Total n = 510
Players (n)	48	194	189	79	510
Players injured (%)	75.0	69.6	68.8	46.8***	66.3
Injuries, total (n)	167	639	533	299	1638
Players×matches (n)	1284	5396	5436	2553	14669
Mean No. of matches played (n)	26.8	27.8	28.8	32.3	28.8
Mean No. of injuries/injured player (n)	4.6	4.7	4.1	8.1***	4.8
Injury risk, per played match (%)	13.0	11.8	9.8**	11.7	11.2

Legend: Players×matches – Total number of matches every subject played; Significantly different from all other categories of players: ** $p<0.01$; *** $p<0.001$

Table 3. Percent distribution of injuries by body parts and player categories

Category Body part	Keepers n = 48	Defence n = 194	Mid-field n = 189	Forward n = 79
Head/neck	4.8	5.2	9.0	11.0
Upper extremity	29.3	27.5	22.5	21.7
Trunk	4.8	7.5	8.1	5.4
Lower extremity	61.1	59.8	60.4	61.9

The distribution of injuries by body parts was in all categories of players alike except the forwards, in whom the proportion of head/neck to trunk injuries was significantly ($p<0.05$) higher. On average, the frequencies of injuries of lower and upper extremities amounted to about 60 and 25%, respectively (cf. Table 3).

A detailed analysis of the latter injuries (Table 4) revealed that, generally, hand and foot injuries dominated but interesting between-category differences were noted. Hand injuries were most pronounced in mid-field players and were exceeded about threefold injury frequencies of other segments of upper extremities. As to lower extremities, foot injuries dominated in all categories. Hip injuries were least frequent in mid-field players and most frequent in the forwards ($p<0.001$), and knee injuries were more frequent ($p<0.05$) in mid-field and forward players compared with other ones.

Table 4. Detailed percent distribution of injuries of upper and lower extremities

Category Body part	Keepers n = 48	Defence n = 194	Mid-field n = 189	Forward n = 79
Upper extremity				
Shoulder	18.4^{b}	27.3	18.3^{b}	24.6
Arm	24.5	21.6	13.3^{b}	16.9^{b}
Forearm	20.4	22.7	18.3^{b}	18.5^{b}
Hand	36.7	28.4	50.0	40.0
Lower extremity				
Hip	1.0	3.7	0.6	7.0
Thigh	13.7°	16.8°	13.4°	14.1°
Knee	19.6°	19.9°	$26.7^{\circ\wedge}$	$23.8^{\circ\wedge}$
Lower leg	$26.5^{\circ\wedge}$	$25.9^{\circ\wedge}$	$27.3^{\circ\wedge}$	$22.7^{\circ\wedge}$
Foot	$39.2^{\circ\wedge}$	$33.8^{\circ\wedge}$	$32.0^{\circ\wedge}$	$32.4^{\circ\wedge}$

Significantly ($p<0.05$ – 0.001) different from: ^{b} Hand; $^{\circ}$ Hip; ^ Knee

Table 5. Percent distribution of injuries by body components and player categories

Category Body part	Keepers n = 48	Defence n = 194	Mid-field n = 189	Forward n = 79
Bones	1.2	0.8	1.5	2.0
Joints	9.0	12.7	11.1	17.4*
Tendons	15.0	15.6	16.1	13.7
Muscles	18.6	15.8	18.9	15.4
Skin	56.3	55.1	52.3	51.5

* Significantly (p<0.05) higher than in other categories combined

Table 6. Detailed percent distribution of injuries of body components

Category Body part	Keepers n = 48	Defence n = 194	Mid-field n = 189	Forward n = 79
Joints				
Sprain	73.3	80.2	62.7**	75.0
Dislocation	26.7	19.8	37.3**	25.0
Tendons				
Strain	84.0	84.0	77.9	78.0
Tear	16.0	16.0	22.1	22.0
Skin				
Abrasion	43.6	46.0	43.7	39.6
Laceration	23.4	25.9	16.8	27.3
Haematoma	19.1	16.5	23.7***	16.9
Ecchymosis	13.8	11.6	15.8	16.2

Significantly different from other categories combined: ** p<0.01; *** p<0.001

When classifying injuries by body components, skin was the most frequently affected and accounted for over 50% of all injuries (Table 5), other components being rather evenly represented (13 – 17%, on average) except bones (1.3%). No significant between-category differences were noted except mid-field players, in whom the frequency of joint injuries was significantly (p<0.01) more frequent than in other players.

A detailed analysis of those injuries (Table 6) revealed rather uniform distribution of injuries among player categories, mid-field players being again an exception; the frequencies of joint dislocations and of haematomas were in them significantly higher than in other categories combined (p<0.01 and p<0.001, respectively).

Discussion

The presented results reflect the incidence and pattern of injuries sustained by professional Turkish football players over one game season. Cromwell *et al.* [3], in a study on 107 professional Welsh players, reported that 77% of injuries affected lower extremities, mainly soft tissues at the ankle being affected. Similar or higher frequencies were reported also by other authors [1,5,14], thus, the 60.5% reported here was not an exceeding figure. Yoon *et al.* [13], in a study on 401 Asian players, reported 18.5% of knee injuries, 17.3% of lower leg and 14.2% of ankle injuries, with contusions dominating. Similar values were found in this study; knee injuries amounted to 19.8% in goal keepers and defence players but were significantly higher in mid-field and forward players (26%). Moreover, the most frequent injuries found by us were skin abrasions and muscle strains. Our results differed from those of Yon which might have been due to differences in terminology used in the questionnaires.

Hawkins *et al.* [5] reported 6030 injuries in 91 professional football clubs throughout two seasons, 37% of those injuries being muscle strains, 19% ligamentous sprains, 7% muscle sprains, 4% bone fractures and only 3 skin abrasions. In our study, among skin injuries which exceeded 50% of all injuries, abrasions ranged from 40 to 46%, and the frequencies of muscle and tendon injuries were lower than in Hawkins' report.

In the study of Woods *et al.* [14], in which the preseason injuries (n = 6030) in the English professional football league were evaluated, 23% were related to thighs, 17% to knees, 17% to ankles, 12% to lower legs, 6% to feet and toes, 2% to hips and 3% to upper extremities; in our study, the thigh injuries were markedly less frequent (about 15%) and those of the knee, lower leg and foot were much higher with inverted trend along the lower extremity. Regarding the types of injuries, Wood reported muscle strains (37%), muscle contusions (7%), tendon injuries (5%) and bone fractures (5%). In our study, the percentage of tendon injuries was higher and those of bone fractures or muscle injuries markedly lower. The differences between the two studies might have, however, originated from different questionnaires and, perhaps, from different game styles.

Inklaar *et al.* [7] reported that thigh (23%), knee (22%) and ankle (23%) were the most frequently injured, the distribution of injuries being not age-related; the most frequent injury types were sprains (31%), contusions (28%) and strains (19%). In our study, the percentage of lower extremity injuries was similar (60.5%) and that of strains and sprains (tendons and muscles combined) higher. Again, the differences could have been due to different conditions of playing fields. Moreover, Inklaar stated that sprain and strain injuries tended to afflict the same body parts resulting in continuous sufferings.

The same observation was made by us and the likely reasons were most of the struggle taking place in the midfield, high fatigue and higher exposure to intervention.

Hoy *et al.* [6] studied 646 male and 69 female football players and reported that the most frequent were joint injuries (49%) and skin lesions (30%). Fractures were detected in 18% of the cohort, both upper and lower extremities being equally afflicted. In this study, joint injuries were decidedly lower and skin lesions were dominating in all player categories.

Schmidt-Olsen *et al.* [11] studied 496 male footballers aged 12 – 18 years; they found that most of the injuries affected lower extremities (70%), especially knee (26%) and ankle (23.1%); head and neck injuries amounted to 1.2%, upper extremity injuries 10.3% and back problems constituted 14% of all injuries. As much as 4% of injuries were bone fractures, mostly of upper extremities, the fractures being most likely due to the lack of experience of young players in falling down [11]. The incidence of fractures was significantly ($p<0.001$) higher than in our study while that of head/neck injuries significantly ($p<0.001$) lower.

Summing up, the study showed that injuries in football are a serious problem. As the coaches have a good practical knowledge of field incidents, a detailed overview of injuries may help them in taking appropriate preventive steps. It would appear that the approaches towards reducing the incidents, violence and repeated injuries ought to be supervised by physicians and physiotherapists, the coaches playing a key role.

References

1. Adamczyk G., L.Luboinski., (2002) Epidemiology of football – related injuries (Part I) *A.Clin.* 2:236-250.
2. Arnason A., S.B.Sigurdsson, A.Gudmundsson, I.Holme, L.Engebretsen, R.Bahr (2004) Physical fitness, injuries and team performance in football. *Med.Sci.Sports Exerc.* 36: 278-285.
3. Cromwell F., J.Walsh, J.Gormley (2000) A pilot study examining injuries in elite Gaelic footballers. *Br.J.Sports Med.* 34:104-108 DOI:10.1136/bjsm.34.2.104.
4. Drovak J., A.Junge (2000) Football injuries and physical symptoms, a review of the literature. *Am.J.Sports Med.* 2:3-9.
5. Hawkins R.D., M.A.Hulse, C.Wilkinson, A.Hodson, M.Gibson (2001) The association football medical research programme: an audit of injuries in professional football. *Br.J. Sports Med.* 35: 43-47 DOI:10.1136/bjsm.35.1.43.
6. Hoy K., B.E.Lindblad, C.J.Terkelsen, H.E.Helleland, C.J. Terkelsen (2003) European football injuries - a prospective epidemiologic and socioeconomic study. *Am.J.Sports Med.* 20: 318-322 DOI:10.1177/036354659202000314.
7. Inklaar H., E.Bol, S.L.Schmikli, W.L.Mosterd (1996) Injuries in male football players: team risk analysis. *Int.J.Sports Med.* 17: 229-234.
8. Junge A., J.Drovak (2004) Football injuries, a review on incidence and prevention. *Sports Med.* 34: 929-938.
9. Price R.J., R.D.Hawkins, M.A.Hulse, A.Hodson (2004) The football association medical research programme: an audit of injuries in academy youth football. *Br.J.Sports Med.* 38:466-471 DOI:10.1136/bjsm.2003.005165.
10. Rahmana N., T.Reilly, A.Lees (2002) Injury risk associated with playing actions during competitive football. *Br.J.Sports Med.* 36: 354-359.
11. Schmidt-Olsen S., U.Jorgensen, S.Kaalund, J.Sorensen (1991) Injuries among young football players. *Am.J.Sports Med.* 19:273-275.
12. Tumulty D. (1993) Physiological characteristics of elite football players. *Sports Med.* 16:80-96.
13. Yoon Y.S., M.Chai, D.W.Shin (2004) Football injuries at Asian tournaments. *Am.J.Sports Med.* 32:36-42.
14. Woods C., R.Hawkins, M.Hulse, A.Hodson (2002) The football association medical research programme: an audit of injuries in professional football-analysis of preseason injuries. *Br.J.Sports Med.* 36:436-441.

Overcoming psychosocial barriers to maternal exercise: intervention strategies to improve participation and adherence

Brad Schoenfeld, Gül Tiryaki-Sönmez

Lehman College, Department of Health Sciences, The City University of New York, Bronx, NY, USA

Summary

Poor adherence to physical activity programmes during pregnancy is a serious national issue, one that has detrimental effects on a large percentage of the population. Not only does a lack of activity result in a decrease in quality of life for women during term, but the effects can carry over well after pregnancy, potentially leading to increased morbidity and mortality. What's more, reduced prenatal activity can cause adverse effects on the foetus, with impairments seen in physical health as well as cognition. Accordingly, the purpose of this paper is twofold: first, to examine the socio-demographic data and psychosocial influences that modify exercise behaviours in pregnant women and, second, to make recommendations as to effective intervention strategies that can be adopted by health and fitness professionals to help improve maternal exercise participation and adherence.

Key words: Pregnancy exercise – Pregnancy fitness – Exercise psychology

Introduction

Leisure time physical activity (LTPA) is universally regarded as positive mediator on health and wellness, with beneficial effects seen on incidence of disease, functional capacity, and mental health. Yet, despite the overwhelming body of research supporting its efficacy, a large percentage of the population remains sedentary and less than half meet minimum participation guidelines set forth by the American College of Sports Medicine (ACSM) [20].

On average, women are less active than men, especially in terms of performing moderate-to-vigorous activity [34]. This is even more apparent with respect to the exercise habits of pregnant women – a subgroup that has much to gain from staying active. So much so that the Institute of Medicine has identified pregnancy as a period of critical risk for inactivity and overweight, and categorised women who fall into these categories at an increased risk for various chronic disease states and premature mortality [14]. Accordingly, the purpose of this paper is twofold: first, to examine the socio-demographic data and psychosocial influences that modify exercise behaviours in pregnant women and, second, to make recommendations as to effective intervention strategies that can be adopted by health and fitness professionals to help improve maternal exercise participation and adherence.

Socio-demographic Influences on Maternal Exercise

Participation in LTPA is highest in developed nations such as the United States and United Kingdom [6,10] and lowest in third-world countries [7]. Precise measurements of participation in the United States have been difficult to qualify, with figures varying between studies. For example, Evenson *et al.* [10] reported that approximately 2/3 of American women perform at least some LTPA during pregnancy while Zhang *et al.* [36] found that nearly 60% were sedentary. These differences are perhaps attributable to limitations in study designs. Most protocols use a questionnaire format and the phrasing of questions can influence the perception as to what actually constitutes LTPA. For instance, some women might not realise that gardening and various household chores are forms of physical activity if the questionnaire does not specifically state as such. What is clear from all studies is that LTPA during pregnancy is suboptimal to provide desired benefits for health and wellness [10], with only 15.1% of pregnant women estimated to meet ACSM guidelines for physical activity [20].

Leisure time physical activity declines once a woman becomes pregnant and progressively drops off as the term advances [6,7,10,24,36]. Clapp and Dickstein [5] found

Author's address Prof. Gül Tiryaki-Sönmez, Lehman College, The City University of New York, Department of Health Sciences, 250 Bedford Park Blv. West, Bronx, NY 10468, USA

that 60% of women who exercised vigorously pre-term, markedly reduced their activity levels early in pregnancy and ceased training by the 18th week. Sternfeld *et al.* [30] found that the participation of 41% of women who performed aerobic exercise before pregnancy steadily declined and only 14% were still active by the 3rd trimester, and Pereira *et al.* [25], showed a decrease of LTPA during pregnancy from 9.6 to 6.9 h/week from the first to second trimester, a majority of the reduction being seen in moderate and vigorous activities.

Types of activities: Walking is by far the most popular mode of LTPA. Evenson *et al.* [10] reported that 53% of pregnant women declared having walked at some time during pregnancy. Zhang *et al.* [36] reported 43% – well above the next two activities cited (swimming and aerobics), both being declared by 12% of the population. Only a small percentage of women reported participation in resistance training activities, which could be highly beneficial for maintenance of functional capacity as the pregnancy progresses [12,35]. In third world countries, the percentage of women who declared walking as a source of exercise jumped to 70% [7]. This could be attributed to a lack of adequate fitness facilities and/or transportation to these facilities in less developed nations, thus limiting options for other modes of exercise. Regardless of the activity chosen, most women opt to train at low intensities. This was born out in a study by Ning *et al.* [23] , who found that less than half of the 61% of women reporting to have participated in LTPA during pregnancy were regularly engaged in high intensity activities (defined as greater than 6 METs).

Education: There appears to be a direct link between the level of education and maternal LTPA participation [7,16,24]. Evenson *et al.* [10] found that the number of college-educated women who performed any LTPA during pregnancy was significantly greater compared with those who had less than a high-school education (79 vs. 42%, respectively). A similar relation was found for exercise volume and intensity, with 19% of college-educated women reporting to have met ACOG guidelines vs. only 4% for those with less than a high-school education. It is possible that educated women have a better awareness of the benefits of exercise or, alternatively, that they may display an increased propensity to seek out information on the subject and understand its complexities.

Income status: An inverse association exists between household income and exercise during pregnancy [7,23]. This relationship appears to hold true independently of the education level, and is correlated both with volume and intensity of training. Poverty might contribute to a reduced participation in LTPA during pregnancy due to an inability to afford membership to fitness facilities or to have a convenient source of transportation to travel to such a facility.

Ethnicity: Studies on the relationship between ethnicity and maternal LTPA are somewhat equivocal. On the whole, there seems to be a tendency for whites to have a slightly greater LTPA level during pregnancy than non-whites [7,10,28], with Asians performing the least maternal exercise [36]. This, perhaps, can be explained, at least in part, by differing customs and beliefs within each ethnic group. Exercise seems to be more ingrained in certain cultures than in other ones, possibly due to long-standing cultural values held over many generations. Such belief systems could have an impact on attitudes of pregnant women toward exercising during pregnancy as well as their perception of the benefits associated with maternal fitness. However, Marshall *et al.* [22] noted that most of the ethnic variability in exercise participation is moderated by social class, making it difficult to tease out the actual impact of ethnicity.

Age: Studies on the association between maternal age and exercise frequency are contradictory. Some authors reported them to be positively correlated [16,24] while others reported a negative correlation [10,26]. Ning *et al.* [23] found that women under 35 years of age were more likely than their seniors to participate in high-intensity activities. In those latter ones this could be possibly attributed to fear that intense exercise might harm the foetus and that it then may be difficult to get pregnant again at an advanced biological age.

Psychosocial Factors Affecting Maternal Exercise

The LTPA behaviour during pregnancy is driven by a variety of social, psychological and physical factors. Clarke *et al.* [6] reported that a combination of these factors may ultimately discourage otherwise healthy, pregnant women from exercise. Moreover, women's reasons for exercising or not exercising vary across pregnancy, indicating that there is a continual reassessment of exercise priorities as pregnancy progresses. According to the Theory of Planned Behaviour, psychosocial factors can be classified into three basic categories: attitude, subjective norm, and perceived behavioural control; these will be discussed with respect to their application to maternal LTPA.

Attitudinal factors: A woman's attitude toward exercise plays a dominant role in whether or not she will be physically active throughout pregnancy; it is regarded as the strongest determinant of exercise participation across all three trimesters [8,15]. Those with positive attitudes will tend to continue with existing programmes or begin new ones, while those with negative attitudes will tend to remain sedentary. Perplexingly, Domingues *et al.* [7] found that despite the overwhelming belief that maternal exercise made labour easier and led to a healthier baby (by 83 and 76%, respectively), only 13% of pregnant women participated in LTPA.

A primary factor that shapes a woman's attitude toward exercise is previous training experience. Research shows that participation in a regimented maternal fitness programme is highly correlated to whether or not a woman has exercised in the past. Ning *et al.* [23] found that women who were physically active as teenagers were 4 times as likely to be active during pregnancy and more than 12 times as likely to engage in intense LTPA. Owe *et al.* [24] reported that women who exercised pre-pregnancy were almost 10 times more likely to continue regular LTPA while pregnant. This demonstrates a clear need to get women exercising early in life to shape and strengthen enduring lifelong habits.

Concerns about safety are another significant attitudinal influence on exercise behaviour. Many women continue to cling to the misguided belief that maternal exercise may be harmful. Clarke *et al.* [6] found that approximately ⅓ of women who reduced exercise during pregnancy mentioned potential danger to the foetus as the primary reason. Moreover, Duncombe *et al.* [9] found that although only 8% of women queried cited safety issues as a barrier to performing light exercise, the vast majority believed weight bearing activity to be unsafe. The study went on to conclude that safety concerns predicted both the amount and intensity of a woman's exercise patterns during pregnancy.

In contrast to non-pregnant women, motivation to stay thin does not seem to be a significant motivator for a majority of expectant mothers. Symons-Downs *et al.* [31] found that the most common behavioural advantage during pregnancy was that exercise improved mood, weight management being of just marginal consequence. Only in the immediate postpartum period did weight loss become a significant attitudinal motivator that influenced a woman's intention to work out.

Subjective norm factors: Exercise factors related to subjective norms consist of social influences on the pregnant woman. Subjective norm was found to be correlated with the intention to exercise during pregnancy only moderately – less than the factors associated with attitude and the perceived behavioural control. However, this should not be taken to mean that social influences are trivial. Women with a supportive network of family and friends are more inclined to exercise than those with less supportive networks [8]. In a study of women in the United Kingdom, Clarke *et al.* [6] reported that 96% of participants received advice about LTPA at least once during the pregnancy and 49% on at least 3 occasions. The importance of social influences appears particularly strong in the Latino community. Thornton *et al.* [33] found husbands and female relatives the primary sources of emotional, instrumental, and informational support for Latino women, and an absence of these influences to provide advice and companionship with respect to exercise were prominent barriers that limited their desire to maintain an active lifestyle.

Research is unclear as to who provides the majority of social influence to exercise during pregnancy. Symons-Downs *et al.* [31] found that the most common normative influence for women came from husbands/fiancés, and that clinicians did not play a prominent role. Clarke *et al.* [6] noted similar findings, reporting that the primary source of advice came from friends and family, with only 18% receiving guidance directly from their health care professional. In contrast, Krans *et al.* [19] reported that nearly half of those surveyed mentioned their physicians as having the greatest influence over their exercise habits.

Regardless of the source of advice, the influences of subjective norms are all-too-often overly negative with respect to maternal exercise. The majority of friends and family provide discouragement based on an inadequate knowledge of the facts on the subject, with 85% of pregnant women reporting that they were dissuaded from participating in LTPA by Week 34 [6]. Physicians are only marginally better in conferring the importance of prenatal exercise. Although Krans *et al.* [19] found that women who were encouraged to exercise by their physicians were more likely to exercise than those who were not so encouraged, less than 10% of women said their doctors helped them develop an exercise programme but almost 70% of them placed exercise restrictions on expectant mothers based on outdated, invalid guidelines. As Clarke *et al.* [6] aptly summed up, our health education system is doing a poor job correcting misperceptions about the risks and benefits of maternal exercise.

Perceived behavioural control factors: The Perceived Behavioural Control (PBC) refers to the ease or difficulty of performing a task as perceived by given woman, and is independently associated with exercise intention during pregnancy [13]. Hausenblaus *et al.* [15] reported that PBC was a stronger predictor of exercise behaviour than motivation. However, because of the various physiological and sociological ramifications of pregnancy, pregnant women tend to sense of a lack of behavioural control over their exercise programmes.

Health-related factors are the most important behavioural control issues, with women who are in good health significantly more likely to exercise than those in poor health [10]. Duncombe *et al.* [9] noted that women performing little or no exercise during pregnancy reported feeling tired and/or unwell as the primary reasons. In the latter stages of pregnancy, discomfort and lack of energy seem to be the primary health-related PBC barriers to exercise [9], as increased weight gain, impaired sleep, and general fatigue take an increasingly greater toll on a woman's psyche. Owe et al. [24] found that women with pregnancy-related disorders such as pelvic girdle pain, nausea, musculoskeletal pain were less likely to exercise regularly than non-symptomatic women. Other disorders negatively associated with exercise participation include leg cramps, body soreness, and short breath.

Another significant PBC barrier is the time constraint brought on by pregnancy. In a study by Duncombe *et al.* [9], being too busy was reported by women as one of the main reasons for reducing LTPA while pregnant. Job-related issues are at the forefront of these beliefs. Pereira *et al.* [25] found that pregnant women who worked full-time were 3 – 5 times more likely to become inactive than those who were not employed.

Having children at home also contributes to the perceived lack of time to exercise. The number of pregnancies was inversely correlated with exercise volume, the primiaparae being more likely to exercise than women having at least one child [10,23,24]. The odds ratio of becoming inactive was found to be significantly greater in women with at least one child already in the home as compared to the childless ones [25]. This was presumably due to the fact that since the first-time mothers did not have children to occupy their leisure time, they were more apt to spend their free hours exercising [7].

Child care can also be a significant barrier of perceived behavioural control over exercise. While the evidence that primiparae are more active than women with children is most often attributed to time constraints, the lack of child care must also be considered a possible contributor. Pereira *et al.* [25] found that women who considered childcare an issue, were 1.7-fold more likely to become inactive compared to those that had no child care issues.

Intervention Studies

There is a paucity of research on the effects of exercise interventions for pregnant women. Only a handful of studies have specifically addressed their efficacy, with varying degrees of success. The first such intervention study was conducted by Gray-Donald et al. [11] and aimed at improving the dietary intake during pregnancy, at optimising the gestational weight gain, glycaemia levels and birth weight, and at avoiding unnecessary post-partum weight retention. A counselling protocol, based on the Social Learning Theory, was utilised by health care professionals. The employed strategies included modelling, skill training, contracting and self-monitoring. The effects on LTPA levels in the intervention and control groups were alike, the former having actually a much greater percentage of participants classified as sedentary compared with controls. The authors suggested this could be due to the fact that subjects from the interventional group were counselled on exercise thus being more in tune with activity levels; the study, however, was methodologically somewhat inconsistent with other reports. First, the study was more nutrition- than exercise-oriented, with counselling carried out by nutritionists who emphasised the dietary component for weight loss rather than for the importance of LTPA. The interviews revealed that in the Cree's culture being plump was desirable while exercising during pregnancy was not. Additionally, the protocol did not take a stage-matched approach, which has been shown to be more successful in modifying exercise behaviour [3]. Finally, pregnant women in general are not significantly motivated to lose weight [31], which was the primary objective of that study, all that making it difficult to draw conclusions as to the potential benefits of intervention on maternal exercise behaviour.

Polley, *et al.* [27] conducted a similar trial to evaluate a behavioural intervention designed to reduce excessive maternal weight gain. Women were given written and oral information on exercise and nutrition at set counselling sessions. After each clinical visit, the patients received a personalised graph of their weight gain. Those whose weight exceeded recommendations were given additional individualised counselling. A stepped care approach was utilised, where women who gained more than recommended were given increasingly structured behaviour goals with each visit and a between visits telephone follow-up was initiated. The results of the study were mixed regarding the interventional impact on weight gain. Among normal weight women, those in intervention group were markedly less likely to gain excessive weight compared with controls (58 vs. 33%, respectively). Among overweight women, however, the treatment had a negligible effect and actually showed a tendency toward increased weight gain. With respect to exercise, the intervention was of little benefit, showing similar participation rates in both groups. That study, however, had similar methodological issues as that discussed above [11]. Namely, it was more nutritionally than exercise-oriented and focused on promoting weight management rather than on exercise benefits specific to the needs of pregnant women.

Hausenblas *et al.* [14] was the first to employ an intervention that showed potential for altering the exercise behaviour patterns of pregnant women. In their trial, the researchers employed a multimedia CD-ROM designed to encourage exercising during pregnancy. The content of the CD-ROM incorporated social/cognitive theories of the Transtheoretical Model and the Theory of Planned Behaviour; it contained a blend of theory, practical content and detailed information personally tailored to users, based on their stage of exercise change profile. Interactive components such as true/false quizzes, audio and video clips of pregnant women exercising, and personal accounts from women detailing the physical and psychosocial benefits of exercise were integrated into the presentation. The results were promising, the intervention group reporting significantly higher self-efficacy and exercise knowledge at post-test compared to the control group. The drawback of the study was that it did not track subjects post-testing. Thus, there was no way to determine whether or not the intervention had an enduring effect on women's exercise habits throughout pregnancy.

Aittasalo *et al.* [2] conducted what is to-date the most comprehensive intervention specifically designed to increase participation in maternal exercise. The counselling protocol was based on the Transtheoretical Model and took into account a woman's stages of change. A total of 5 counselling sessions (one primary and 4 booster sessions) were integrated into routine health care visits. Booster sessions were used to assess the compliance as well as to discuss any adverse events related to LTPA, and barriers and incentives affecting compliance. Health care advisors were instructed to consider each woman's readiness to increase exercise participation within their stages of change. The counselling was supported with an option for supervised exercise in close proximity to clinics in order to facilitate behavioural changes. At the end of gestation, both frequency and duration of at least moderate intensity LTPA was significantly higher throughout the pregnancy in the intervention group compared with controls (by 43 and 154%, respectively). These figures prevailed despite the fact that subjects from the intervention group had higher BMI and were less educated – factors bearing an inverse relationship to maternal LTPA [10,24]. Moreover, participants from the intervention group more often reported that counselling provided an incentive to initiate or maintain LTPA than those from the control group (81 vs. 43%, respectively). The one confounding finding of the study was that only 28% of interventional subjects adhered to the group exercise programme. The authors posited that this might have been due to the fact that pregnant women felt less in need for peer support than the postpartum women. It is also conceivable that the limited scheduling of group activities might have been inconvenient for many of the participants, thereby reducing its appeal.

Practical Applications

A poor adherence to physical activity programmes during pregnancy is a serious national issue, one that has detrimental effects on a large percentage of the population. Not only does it result in a decrease in life quality of pregnant women, but the effects can carry over well after pregnancy, potentially leading to increased morbidity and mortality [1,17,18]. A reduced gestational activity can also bring about adverse effects in the foetus, with impairments in physical health as well as in cognition [6].

Properly employed intervention strategies can significantly increase maternal LTPA participation and adherence [2,14]. A face-to-face counselling can provide greater individualised attention than non-personal modes, and is particularly beneficial for lower-income and/or less educated women who might not own a computer and/or are potentially unskilled in modern technologies [7]. Stage-based interventions using the Transtheoretical Model of Behaviour proved to be more successful than traditional approaches in this regard [21], and can facilitate forward-stage progression and increased exercise participation in pregnant women [29]. Expectant mothers should be asked to complete a Stages of Change questionnaire that assesses readiness to exercise. Based on their score, interventions then should be individualised to a woman's current stage of change.

Intervention programmes must be flexible enough to accommodate individual needs. Behaviour beliefs about exercise have been shown to vary across populations, and the practitioners need to take these unique beliefs into account when designing specific LTPA interventions [31]. Moreover, a woman's physical and mental state tends to change across pregnancy, resulting in a continual reassessment of exercise priorities as the pregnancy progresses [6]. Accordingly, recommendations should consider the nutritional intake, BMI before pregnancy and exercise history, personalising a prescription to the participant.

To increase the adherence, individualised counselling can be supplemented with technology-based interventions. Computer interventions have been found to increase knowledge and self-efficacy in pregnant women with respect to exercise [14]. E-mail interventions can be a particularly time-efficient, cost-effective strategy to improve maternal LTPA participation. Computer-generated e-mails with motivational tips and pertinent information have been shown to be as effective as human e-mail counselling, at least in weight loss trials [32]. Personalised e-mails addressing specific issues can be included in the intervention if and when a follow-up appears necessary.

References

1. ACOG Committee Obstetric Practice (2002) ACOG Com-mittee Opinion, No. 267, January 2002: exercise during pregnancy and the postpartum period. *Obstet.Gynecol.* 99:171-173.

2. Aittasalo M., M.Pasanen, M.Fogelholm, T.I.Kinnune, K. Ojala, R.Luoto (2008) Physical activity counseling in mater-nity and child health care - a controlled trial. *BMC Womens Health* 14:8-14.

3. Blissmer B., E.McAuley (2002) Testing the requirements of stages of physical activity among adults: the comparative effectiveness of stage-matched, mismatched, standard care, and control interventions. *Ann.Behav.Med.* 24:181-189.

4. Clapp J.F. (2003) The effects of maternal exercise on fe-tal oxygenation and feto-placental growth. *Eur.J.Obstet.Gyne-col.Reprod.Biol.* 22:110(Suppl. 1):S80-S85.

5. Clapp J.F., S.Dickstein (1984) Endurance exercise and pregnancy outcome. *Med.Sci.Sports Exerc.* 16:556-562.

6. Clarke P.E., H.Gross (2004) Women's behaviour, beliefs and information sources about physical exercise in pregnancy. *Midwifery* 20:133-141.

7. Domingues M.R., A.J.Barros (2007) Leisure-time physi-cal activity during pregnancy in the 2004 Pelotas Birth Cohort Study. *Rev.Saude Publica* 41:173-180.

8. Downs D.S., H.A.Hausenblas (2003) Exercising for two: examining pregnant women's second trimester exercise intention and behaviour using the framework of the theory of plan-ned behaviour. *Womens Health Issues* 13:222-228.

9. Dumcombe D., E.H.Werheim, H.Skouteris (2007) Fac-tors related to exercise over the course of pregnancy including women's beliefs about the safety of exercise during preg-nancy. *Midwifery* 25:430-438.

10. Evenson KR, D.A.Savitz, S.L.Huston (2004) Leisure-time physical activity among pregnant women in the US. *Perinat.Epidemiol.* 18:400-407.

11. Gray-Donald K, E.Robinson, A.Collier, K.David, L.Re-naud, S.Rodrigues (2000) Intervening to reduce weight gain in pregnancy and gestational diabetes mellitus in Cree com-munities: an evaluation. *CMAJ* 10:1247-1251.

12. Haskell WL, I.M.Lee, R.R.Pate, K.E.Powell, S.N.Blair, B.A.Franklin, C.A.Macera, G.W.Heath, P.D.Thompson, A.Bau-man (2007) Physical activity and public health. Updated rec-ommendation for adults from the American College of Sports Medicine and the American Heart Association. *Circulation* 116:1081-1093.

13. Hausenblas H., D.S.Downs, P.Giacobbi, D.Tuccitto, B. Cook (2008) A multilevel examination of exercise intention and behavior during pregnancy. *Soc.Sci.Med.* 66:2555-2561.

14. Hausenblas H.A.,B.W.Brewer, J.L.Van Raalte, B.Cook, D.D.Downs, C.A.Weiss, C.Niggs, A.Cruz (2008) Development and evaluation of a multimedia CD-ROM for exercise during pregnancy and postpartum. *Patient Educ.Couns.* 70:215-219.

15. Hausenblas H.A., D.S.Downs (2004) Prospective ex-amination of the theory of planned behavior applied to exer-cise behavior during women's first trimester of pregnancy. *J.Reprod.Infant Psychol.* 22:199-210.

16. Hinton P.S., C.M.Olson (2001) Predictors of preg-nancy-associated change in physical activity in a rural white population. *Matern.Child Health J.* 5:14-17.

17. Horton E.S. (1995) NIDDM: the devastating disease. *Diabetes Res.Clin.Pract.* 28(Suppl):S3S11.

18. Kinnunen T.I., M.Pasanen, M.Aittasalo, M.Fogelholm, E.Weiderpass,R.Luoto (2007) Reducing postpartum weight re-tention – a pilot trial in primary health care. *Nutr.J.* 6:21.

19. Krans E.E., J.G.Gearhart, P.M.Dubbert, P.M.Klar, A.L. Miller, W.H.Reploqle (2005) Pregnant women's beliefs and influences regarding exercise during pregnancy. *J.Miss.State Med.Assoc.* 46:67-73.

20. Lewis B., M.Avery, E.Jennings, N.Sherwood, B.Martin-son, A.L.Crain (2008) The effect of exercise during pregnancy on maternal outcomes: Practical implications for practice. *Am.J. Lifestyle Med.* 2:441-455.

21. Marcus B.H., L.H.Forsyth (2003). Motivating People to be Physically Active. Human Kinetics, Champaign IL, p. 9.

22. Marshall S.J., D.A.Jones, B.E.Ainsworth, J.P.Resi, S.S. Levy, C.A.Macera (2007) Race/ ethnicity, social class, and leisure-time physical inactivity. *Med.Sci.Sports Exerc.* 39:44-51.

23 Ning Y., M.A.Williams, J.C.Dempsey, T.K.Sorensen, I.O. Frederick, D.A. Luthy (2003) Correlates of recreational physical activity in early pregnancy. *J.Matern.Fetal Neo-nat.Med.* 13: 385-393.

24. Owe K.M., W.Nystad, K.Bo (2009) Correlates of regu-lar exercise during pregnancy: the Norwegian Mother and Child Cohort Study. *Scand.J.Med.Sci. Sports* 19:637-645.

25. Pereira M.A., S.L.Rifas-Shiman, K.P.Kleinman, J.W.Rich-Edwards, K.E.Peterson, M.W.Gillman (2007) Pre-dictors of change in physical activity during and after preg-nancy: Project Viva. *Am.J.Prev.Med.* 32:312-319.

26. Petersen A.M., T.L.Leet, R.C.Brownson (2005) Corre-lates of physical activity among pregnant women in the United States. *Med Sci Sports Exerc.* 37:1748–1753.

27. Polley B.A., R.R.Wing, C.J.Sims (2002) Randomized controlled trial to prevent excessive weight gain in pregnant women. *Int.J.Obes.Relat.Metab.Disord.* 26:1494-1502.

28. Schmidt M.D., P.Pekow, P.S.Freedson, G.Markenson, L.Chason-Taber (2006) Physical activity patterns during pregnancy in a diverse population of women. *J.Womens Health* 15: 909-918.

29. Spencer L., T.B.Adams, S.Malone, L.Roy, E.Yost (2006) Applying the transtheoretical model to exercise: a systematic and comprehensive review of the literature. *Health Promot. Pract.* 7:428-443.

30. Sternfeld B., C.P.Quesenberry, B.Eskanazi, L.A.Newman (1995) Exercise during pregnancy and pregnancy outcome. *Med.Sci.Sports Exerc.* 27:634-640.

31. Symons-Downs D., H.A.Hausenblas (2004) Women's exercise beliefs and behaviors during their pregnancy and postpartum. *J.Midwifery Women's Health* 49:138-144.

32. Tate D.F., E.H.Jackvony, R.R.Wing (2006) A randomized trial comparing human e-mail counseling, computer-automated tailored counseling, and no counseling in an Internet weight loss program. *Arch.Intern.Med.* 15:1620-1625.

33. Thornton P.L., E.C.Kieffer, Y.Salabarria-Pena, A.Odoms-Young, S.K.Willis, H.Kim, M.A.Salinas (2006) Weight, diet, and physical activity-related beliefs and practices among preg-nant and postpartum Latino women: the role of social support. *Matern.Child Health J.* 10:95-104.

34. Trost S.G., N.Owen, A.E.Bauman, J.F.Sallis, W.Brown (2002) Correlates of adults' participation in physical activity: review and update. *Med.Sci.Sports Exerc.* 34:1996-2001.

35. Wolfe L.A., G.A.Davies (2003) Canadian guidelines for exercise in pregnancy. *Clin.Obstet.Gynecol.* 46:488-495.

36. Zhang J., D.A.Savitz (1996) Exercise during pregnancy among US women. *Ann.Epidemiol.* 6:53-59.

8

Health and physical education: a new global statement of consensus (from a Polish perspective)

Christopher R. Edgington [1], Ming-kai Chin [2], Michał Bronikowski [3]

[1] School of Health, Physical Education and Leisure Services, University of Northern Iowa, Cedar Falls IA, USA; [2] HOPSports, Inc., Valencia CA, USA; [3] Methodology of Teaching Physical Education Department, Physical Education University, Poznań, Poland

Summary

Physical education has found itself in a difficult position; increasingly more voices are questioning its legitimisation on school curricula. There is an obvious need for performance standards and ways to measure the impact of physical education. Linking the benefits and outcomes of physical education to 21st Century core learning areas such as critical thinking, problem solving, the ability to operate with agility and adaptability, the ability to analyse information, communicate effectively and the ability to act innovatively, will be essential. One of the ways of enhancing its social value (and recognition) might be including and relaying more on health education. This paper draws some lines of direction for the pedagogy of these both subjects in the 21st Century referring to the Global Forum on Physical Education Pedagogy 2010 (GoFPEP 2010) and presenting its *Statement of Consensus*.

Key words: Physical education – Health education – Health pedagogy

Introduction

Significant changes in physical education have taken place over the past 40 years with a transition from a traditional sports skill-orientation to a broader emphasis on health-related fitness and lifelong physical activity [2,9,11]. However, throughout the world, physical education programmes are being reduced, minimised and/or outright eliminated from elementary and secondary curricula [5,12]. It is increasingly apparent that the value of physical education programmes is being tested worldwide.

In an age of increased accountability, the lack of effective measures to demonstrate the importance of physical education in the development of learners is a serious challenge to the future of the profession [10]. Linking the benefits and outcomes of physical education to the 21st Century core learning areas such as critical thinking, problem solving, ability to operate with agility and adaptability, ability to analyse information, communicate effectively and the ability to act innovatively, will be essential if physical education is to continue to be valued as a part of the basic school curriculum [1]. If, in fact, physical education can be linked to such core learning areas, then the importance of physical education will be more fully embraced. Can we demonstrate that physical education is as important as other basic areas, such as reading, writing and mathematics, as a necessary lifelong vocational and non-vocational requirement?

It is evident that there is a need to develop a more effective assessment leading to greater accountability. Physical education programmes must generate data that can make the profession's efforts much more accountable for programme interventions. The lack of accountability in physical education prevents programmes from becoming a part of the health care system of any community. There is an obvious need for performance standards and ways to measure the impact of physical education. The need for physical education programmes to enable students demonstrating their basic proficiencies is paramount in an increasingly standardised educational world. Just as there is a need to improve basic skills such as reading, mathematics and science, there is a need to justify the existence of physical education programmes. The physical education teacher is increasingly being called upon to demonstrate student's proficiency in developing the skills to achieve a healthy, active lifestyle.

Author's address Prof. Christopher Edginton, 203, WRC, School of HPELS, University of Northern Iowa, Cedar Falls, IA 50614-0241, USA

We now live in a time when obesity and overweight, especially among children and youths, has become a major health concern on a worldwide basis [8,14]. It has been well documented that patterns developed in the childhood will, in fact, carry forward to one's adult life [4]. The emerging epidemic of obesity among children and youths thus becomes a concern for future adult populations. The challenge is a complex one that requires more holistic and multidisciplinary thinking to address the problem. Health, leisure and physical education professionals worldwide have a key role to play in formulating strategies to address this problem. There is a need to employ new forms of pedagogy, integrate health and physical education programmes in a more effective fashion, support the development of healthy, active lifestyles, explore ways to employ technology in the teaching of physical education, link school-based activities to informal community programmes and review the way in which physical education teachers are prepared [3].

These are, indeed, difficult and complex challenges, problems and issues that require multiple perspectives and, increasingly, views that are global, reflecting successful methods, strategies and procedures from throughout the world. The Global Forum on Physical Education Pedagogy 2010 (GoFPEP 2010) was established and structured to explore ways of rethinking, reforming and reframing health and physical education pedagogy as well as preparation of physical education teachers.

The Global Forum on Physical Education Pedagogy 2010 (GoFPEP 2010)

Organised to examine new forms of pedagogy, GoFPEP 2010 sought to review the use of technology, ways of linking practice to theory and the importance of contextually-based education embedded in community life as a way to reshape and redesign the future of health and physical education. GoFPEP 2010 explored several basic areas including the following:

1. Reframing health and physical education pedagogy internationally by promoting dialogue and discussion on critical themes and issues;
2. Exploring a new model of pedagogy for preparing health and physical education teachers which promotes accountability, builds community life, employs a greater use of reflection to improve practice and embeds learning in practice;
3. Examining the extension of health- and physical education-based school programmes into community life;
4. Reviewing the application of technology as related to the teaching of health and physical education;
5. Promoting the establishment of partnerships between the school, community, university, nongovernmental organisations and commercial enterprises;
6. Rethinking the relationship between health and physical education as a strategy for promoting lifelong active living; and
7. Stimulating forward thinking.

The GoFPEP 2010 invited international voices in a dynamic programme designed for educators, health professionals, administrators, policymakers and citizens the opportunity to discuss the future of physical education pedagogy. The forum provided unique opportunities for professional enhancement, drawing together leading educational and professional experts from throughout the world; GoFPEP 2010 saw 70 invited delegates from 25 countries representing 64 universities, institutions and schools participate in the event lasting two days that included keynote, invited presentations and workshops, and discussion groups.

The primary goal of GoFPEP 2010 was drafting a Consensus Statement focused on "Health and Physical Education Pedagogy in the 21St Century". The consensus statement was rooted in previous documents: International Charter for Physical Education and Sport adopted at its General Conference in Paris, 1978 [13], The Berlin Agenda for Action for Government Ministers, accepted at the 1st World Summit of Physical Education, 1999 [6] and the Magglingen Commitment for Physical Education approved in 2005 in Switzerland [7]. The uniqueness of GoFPEP 2010 was that it was deeply embedded in the actual context of a school setting and its community environment. This enabled a focused dialogue and discussion in real time as the school day unfolded, providing the opportunity for a more authentic analysis of challenges, problems, issues and solutions.

Each delegate to GoFPEP 2010 was asked to offer suggestions and recommendations formatted to poster presentations in advance of the event. Recommendations were sought in the following areas:

1. Innovative strategies employed in the teaching of health and physical education at the elementary, secondary and /or post-secondary levels,
2. Innovative approaches employed in the preparation of health and physical education teachers and
3. Three to five of their most important recommendations that could be used in formulating the GoFPEP 2010 Consensus Statement. Information from the discussion groups and poster presentations was analysed using the Qualrus qualitative analysis software package. In turn, this yielded subjects that were highlighted in the final drafting of the document.

The GoFPEP 2010 Consensus Statement provided multifaceted recommendations focused on improving physical education pedagogy and the preparation of physical education teachers. Recommendations advanced the importance of healthy, active lifestyles, integrating health and physical education, promoting good practices, advancing the knowledge and skills around physical literacy, assessment of students and teachers, and community partnerships. The core of the Consensus Statement (see below) calls for enhancing and maintaining the health and well-being of individuals. Actions of students, physical educators, health and leisure professionals, policymakers, citizens and business leaders were called for to provide programmes that would promote a committed effort, addressing the ever increasing worldwide concern of obesity and overweight among children and youths.

Physical education programmes in the 21st Century can inspire, motivate and prepare learners to live in an ever changing world, increasingly marked by the epidemic of obesity and overweight. Globalisation, explosion of knowledge and changing demographics have an increasingly significant impact on the knowledge, skills and dispositions required to live, work and play in the 21st Century. Children and youths will be required to gain critical thinking and problem solving skills, operate with agility and adaptability, effectively analyse information, communicate in various oral and written forms, reflect greater curiosity, imagination and innovation in their thinking, and develop healthy, active lifestyles.

Worldwide, physical education programmes, as well as physical education teacher preparation programmes, need to be rethought and reformed. Hosted by the University of Northern Iowa (USA) and the Grundy Center, Iowa (USA) Community Schools, the Global Forum for Physical Education Pedagogy 2010 (GoFPEP 2010) was organised to examine a new pedagogy for preparing physical education teachers, utilisation of technology to help teach physical education and the building of school, university, community and corporate partnerships. The GoFPEP 2010 drew 70 invited delegates from 25 countries representing 64 universities, schools, business and community organisations, as well as professional organisations and societies.

Conclusions

Despite global trends, the situation in various countries is influenced by regional (country-specific) conditions. This has been broadly researched and described in numerous reports which make it clear that countries and nations characterised as 'well-developed' and having a high socio-economic status, i.e. high standards of daily living, are on the front line of civilisation changes. On the other side, countries like Poland, which underwent drastic changes in the living mode due to recent geopolitical turnovers, are only learning the rules of social and economic 'free society' living. Some areas, e.g. business, politics, culture, are catching-up quicker than other ones, e.g. education or health care, which are slow and difficult to change due to high financial demands, as well as to deeply rooted habits of individuals, used to be told how to live their lives accordingly to certain politically influenced philosophy. And although in both these areas the changes are progressing, this takes time; but looking at the frontrunners of democratic societies may help avoiding some 'blind paths' which well-developed countries have already tried out. Bringing Poland as an example of how the changes are happening and in what direction they are heading, may serve as a signpost for other post-communist countries.

In Poland, the changes brought a reform of the school education system introduced in 2009. A new curriculum has been implemented with new ideas for physical education and its organisation. According to the curriculum, two classes (45 min each) of physical education are included in the weekly timetable. Additionally, schoolchildren may choose two more classes of extracurricular activities, e.g. sports, from a range of activities offered by given school. This applies to primary and lower secondary schools. In upper secondary schools there is only one class weekly of physical education, two more classes being available in extracurricular time. A novelty in new curricula is health education, included in regular curricula of physical education in lower (13 – 16 years of age) and upper (16 – 19 years of age) secondary schools with a 30-h mandatory module to be included once over the three year period. In that module, schoolchildren will learn about health and health-enhancing behaviours, as well as learn to plan health-related activities, to cope with stress and to reduce negative emotions. Introducing such contents into teaching of physical education will require adjustments in the teacher training system of physical education professionals, which now deals with physical education as a school subject only! It will have to be extended to give new competences, skills and knowledge, enabling also teaching health education at schools (and possibly elsewhere). This concerns also teaching methods and techniques and also teaching styles, going more into the interactive ones.

The first institutions of higher education which will introduce these changes into their curricula will probably drain the market from the potential students, but sooner or later most of the universities certifying qualifications in physical education will have to provide them also in health-related professions. The existing system of academic education (and the majority of staff) in East European countries, that want to maintain the present status (no changes in curricula, easy going atmosphere, relatively low academic criteria, in some cases the same teaching materials for years), will be disappearing from the map of higher education institutions authorised to issue certificates and diplomas. The changes have to be deep, but not just administratively; they would rather touch the didactic approaches, and new segments of professional needs of the labour market will have to be included. Open-mindedness and creative teaching of academic staff, though reflective in thinking, will be highly demanded. All that requires a clear sense of direction. Some changes concerning preparation of physical and health education teachers have already been implemented at the University School of Physical Education in Poznań. Linking knowledge (theory) with practice, involving a number of workshops where students exchange their ideas with in-service teachers, introducing new study options like nutrition, sport or active tourism and recreation, developing projects promoting local partners – sport clubs, city municipalities, educational boards and schools with teachers, children and their parents. New materials (guide books, manuals) are published, emphasising methodologies aimed at developing healthy and active behaviour patterns. Such changes are slowly taking place.

****

Statement of the Global Forum for Physical Education Pedagogy 2010: Health and Physical Education Pedagogy in the 21st Century

---

A STATEMENT OF CONSENSUS

Physical Education Pedagogy

Focusing on content and methodologies to develop healthy active lifestyles for children and youth. This requires the integration of skill development, physical fitness, health, nutrition and planning for leisure.

Redesigning the physical education curriculum to promote active student-centred learning and empowering individuals to develop life skills that lead to lifelong, self-directed engagement in physical activity.

Accentuating the importance of co-operation of stakeholders in the community (teachers, administrators, parents, community members, business leaders and others) to advocate, promote, educate and develop individuals to incorporate physical activities into their daily life through formal and informal education.

Establishing physical education and health programmes as models of social justice which foster a safe learning environment, promote the joyful participation of physical activity with appreciation of cultural, racial, ethnic and social and economic differences.

Linking knowledge, skills and dispositions required by 21st Century learners with programme outcomes such physical competency (skills and fitness), health literacy and leisure planning throughout all subject matter and disciplines in the school.

Using technology to support individualised learning processes and assessment.

Re-conceptualising the strategies of assessment with appropriate measurable and performance-based goals and objectives tied to standards which promote greater accountability.

Ensuring that qualified professionals teach physical education and health, physical activities, and sport and leisure.

Physical Education Teacher Preparation

Emphasising the acquisition of teaching techniques and strategies for assisting individuals in developing a healthy, active lifestyle; one which recognises the importance of the integration of health and physical education.

Advocating policies and a broad continuum of programmes including healthy nutrition, weight management, physical activity and leisure planning.

Creating a positive learner-centred environment reflecting good practices to encourage students to become active participants in the learning process.

Promoting the development of partnerships with parents, schools and community organisations to embed and provide contextually based programme elements which enhance physical education teacher preparation.

Developing sensitivity for one's role in addressing racial, ethnic and cultural differences, socio-economic levels, funding levels, access to equipment and facilities, as well as approaches to mitigate these issues.

Including assessment and educational strategies which would provide programme accountability, as well as focus on educational processes and individual developmental outcomes.

Linking practice to theory, promoting the use of reflection and the use of effective technology to accentuate learning opportunities.

Linking the evaluation of students in physical education teacher preparation programmes to relevant knowledge, skills and dispositions directly tied to good practices.

References

1. Bailey R. (2006) Physical education and sport in schools: A review of benefits and outcomes. *J.School Health* 76:397-401.

2. Bocarro J., M.A.Kanters, J.Casper, S.Forrester (2008) School physical education, extracurricular sports and lifelong active living. *J.Teach.Phys.Educ.* 27:155-166.

3. Edginton C.R., B.Kirkpatrick, R.Schupach, C.Philips, M.K.Chin, P.Chen (2011) A dynamic pedagogy of physical education teacher preparation: Linking practice with theory. *Asian J.Phys.Educ.Recreat.* 16(2):7-23.

4. Freedman D.S., Z.Mei, S.R.Srinivasan, G.S.Berenson, W.H.Dieta (2007) Cardiovascular risk factors and excess adiposity among overweight children and adolescents: The Bogalusa Heart Study. *J.Pediatr.* 150:12-17.

5. Hardman K., J.Marshall (2009) Second World-wide Survey of School Physical Education: Final Report. ICSSPE/CIEPSS, Berlin.

6. International Council of Sports Science and Physical Education (1999) The Berlin agenda for action for government ministers: 1st world summit of physical education. www.icsspe.org/index.php?m=13&n=78&o=41 (13 Feb. 2011).

7. International Council of Sports Science and Physical Education (2005) Magglingen commitment for physical education: 2nd world summit of physical education. www.icsspe.org/download/documente/declaration/Magglingen%20Commitment%20for%20Physical%20Education.pdf (1 Feb. 2011).

8. International Obesity Task Force (2009) Obesity: Understanding and challenging the global epidemic. 2009-2010 Report. www.iaso.org/site_media/uploads/IASO_Summary_Report_2009.pdf (13 Feb. 2011).

9. Jago R., R.G.McMurray, S.Bassin, L.Pyle, S.Bruceker, J.M.Jakicic, E.Moe, T.Murray, S.L.Volpe (2009) Modifying middle school physical education: Piloting strategies to increase physical activity. *Pediatr.Exerc.Sci.* 21:171-185.

10. Lund J.L., M.F.Kirk (2010) Performance-Based Assessment for Middle and High School Physical Education. Human Kinetics, Champaign, IL.

11. McKenzie T., D.Kahan (2008) Physical activity, public health, and elementary schools. *The Elem.School J.* 108:171-179.

12. Puhse U., M.Gerber (2005) International Comparison of Physical Education: Concepts, Problems, Prospects. Meyer & Meyer Sport (UK) Ltd. Oxford.

13. UNESCO (1978) International chapter of physical education and sport. http://portal.unesco.org/en/ev.phpURL_ID=13150&URL_DO=DO_TOPIC&URL_SECTION=201.html (3 Feb. 2011).

14. World Health Organization (2010) Global strategy on diet, physical activity and health: Childhood overweight and obesity. www.who.int/dietphysicalactivity/childhood/en/ (9 Feb. 2011).

Aggression and fouls in professional football

Hayrettin Gümüşdağ[1], İbrahim Yıldıran[2], Faruk Yamaner[1], Alparslan Kartal[1]

[1] Hitit University, School of Physical Education and Sports, Çorum; [2] Gazi University, School of Physical Education and Sports, Ankara, Turkey

Summary

Study aim: To assess the frequency, timing, zone and player category of fouls and of aggressive behaviour in professional football.
Material and methods: Video recordings of 17 matches played by one team out of 18 of the Turkish Football Super League with all other teams were analysed with the use of observational foul analysis form. The following criteria were considered: time, score of the match, zone, players' position and foul category. The fouls were analysed in 6 periods of a match, 15 min each. Foul location in the football field was analysed in four zones according to player's positions: Defence, Defence mid-zone, Offensive mid-zone and Attack.
Results: Eleven out of 17 analyzed matches 11 were won, 3 were lost and 3 were even. A total of 652 fouls were recorded, mean numbers of fouls per match amounting to 24.2, 87.0 and 41.7 in won, lost and even matches, respectively. Most of the fouls (50.8%) were committed by middle zone players mostly in the defensive and offensive middle zones (33.9%). Only 1.2% of all fouls were unintentional, 11% were intentional, hostile, the other ones were intentional, instrumental.
Conclusions: The fouls could be attributed to the social learning theory that values the environmental factor in the cognitive process of aggression. The presented results may be of help to football coaches and sport psychologists teaching players how to control aggression and how to play the game wit minimum harm while increasing their performance.

Keywords: Aggressive behaviour – Fouls – Football

Introduction

The boost in the progress of football has turned it into a potential market to the extent that in the contemporary global economy it is realised as an industry with enormous capital. The progress in football in the last decade resulted in e.g. increased physical contact between players. In view of the technological and scientific developments that often exceed the physiological limits in order to increase the players' performance, FIFA has taken a series of precautions to protect the players; FIFA states that football is a harsh game and the referee is to permit to continue the game even if the player-ball interferences are tough Nevertheless, behaviours like intending to interfere or interfering in a harmful manner need be punished.

Aggressiveness and fouls in football: Aggression is a behaviour intended to harm others; Baron von Richardson defined aggression as behaviour committed to harm or injure a living creature that tries to avoid it. The behaviour need not necessarily be physical; any oral behaviour that produces psycho-emotional harm to the victim can also be considered an aggression. Aggression in sports is the result of challenging struggle of players to prove their superiority over the opponents, which was already present in the human nature [5]. Bayern Munich player, Jupp Kapellmann, admitted that "*I am not quite unlike an animal; we are trying to survive by means of all substances. Everybody can attempt to destroy one another.*" Thus, fouls in sports can be defined as an intentional behaviour aimed at harming the opponent [7]. Violence is most prevalent in team contact sports, such as ice hockey, football, and rugby. While most occurrences of violence emanate from players, others, including coaches, parents, fans, and the media, also contribute to what has been described as an epidemic of violence in sports today [14].

Aggressive behaviours are classified in sport psychology as instrumental (tactical) and hostile. In both types the main idea is making harm either physically or psycho-emotionally [6]. Thus, the following foul categories can be discerned:

Author's address Dr Hayrettin Gümüşdağ, School of Physical Education and Sports, Hitit University, Çorum, Turkey

1. Unintentional foul – the player unconsciously hits or may harm the opponent;
2. Intentional foul (instrumental) – the player does not intend to harm the opponent but his behaviour may be harmful;
3. Intentional foul (hostile) – the behaviour is deliberate, aimed at injuring the opponent.

Fouls in football can be considered in relation to aggression theories with regard to the psychology of the players, and the reasons of the fouls [3].

Instinctive aggression theory: Freud, McDougall, Lorenz and others claimed that aggression was one of the instincts inherent in the human nature. In human beings, the frustration of death is compensated by aggressive behaviours, yet followed by re-emerging frustration. For this reason, Freud [8] views aggression of human beings as inevitable. Lorenz considered aggression as tolerable or non- tolerable depending on the degree of harm done. Thus, while war is considered to be an unacceptable way of exhibiting aggression, sports are considered to be just the opposite. The contemporary view supports the role of sports in human life as a way to discharge aggressive behaviours.

Frustration-aggression theory: According to psychologists, frustration hinders or stops a person from reaching an aim or target, and the greater frustration the more intense are the aggressive intuitions that may lead to aggression. For instance, a striker, who cannot pass a defence player, may intentionally hit him with his feet and elbow, or show a violent behaviour like Mike Tyson, who bit off his opponent's (E. Hoolyfield) ear. Therefore, frustration always causes aggression, and aggression is a result of frustration [8]. Frustration appears when one's efforts to reach a particular goal are blocked. In sports, frustration can be caused by questionable calls by officials, failure to make a specific play, injuries that interfere with optimum performance, heckling from spectators, or taunts by coaches or players [13].

Social learning theory: Social learning theory of aggression was developed by Bandura [1]; according to that author, rather than being inherited from the ancestors, aggressiveness is a feature that is solely learnt by environmental observation. Sociologists supported the view that aggressiveness develops as a result of socialisation of individuals. In contrast to other aggression theories that value aggression as a genetically programmed behaviour, social learning theory stresses the environmental factor in the process of learning aggressive behaviours. The social learning theory has received the most empirical verification and maintains that aggressive behaviour is learned through modelling and reinforced by rewards and punishments. Young athletes take sports heroes as role models and imitate their behaviour. Parents, coaches and team mates are also models that may demonstrate support for an aggressive style of play [13].

As suggested also by FIFA, fouls are the inevitable events in football. There are no foul-free football matches due to frequent physical contacts combined with aggressiveness. For this reason, it is crucial to figure out when, where, and by whom fouls are committed before the players learn how to control their aggression and to play football without harming each other while improving their performance. Therefore, the aim of this study was to analyse the fouls committed in the professional football matches in terms of frequency, timing, place, category, and player interactions, in order to determine the relationship of the fouls with aggressive behaviours from a theoretical perspective.

Material and Methods

Out of 18 teams of the Turkish Football Super League, one was randomly selected and 17 video recordings (by 18 cameras) of all matches of that team were analysed. An observational foul analysis form was designed using the following criteria: time, score of the match, zone, players' position, and foul category. In order to determine the timing of fouls, the matches were analysed in 6 periods, 15 min each. Foul location in the football field was analysed in four zones according to player's positions: Defence, De-fence mid-zone, Offensive mid-zone and Attack.

Analysis of the recordings was supervised by 2 football coaches and 2 football referees. The frequencies and rankings of events were analysed using the chi-square function or one-way ANOVA, that latter followed by Tukey's *post-hoc* test. The level of $p \leq 0.05$ was considered significant.

Results

Eleven out of 17 analysed matches 11 were won, 3 were lost and 3 were even. A total of 652 fouls were recorded, mean numbers of fouls per match amounting to 24.2, 87.0 and 41.7 in won, lost and even matches, respectively. The distribution of fouls by pitch zone and positions of players is shown in Table 1 and Fig. 1.

The numbers of fouls committed in 15-min intervals did not differ significantly between winners and losers; thus, they were combined and presented as percent frequencies in Fig. 2. A significant ($p<0.001$) opposite tendency in frequencies between winner/loser teams and tie matches can be noted.

Table 1. Distribution of fouls by zones and player positions

Players' position / Pitch zone	Own	Half-backs	Outer
Defence zone	78	64	4
Attack zone	57	46	6
Total	135	110	10
Defence mid-zone	75	117	25
Attack mid-zone	45	104	31
Total	120	221	56

Legend: Own – Defence players in the defence zone and attack players in the attack zone; Outer - Defence players in the attack zone and attack players in the defence zone

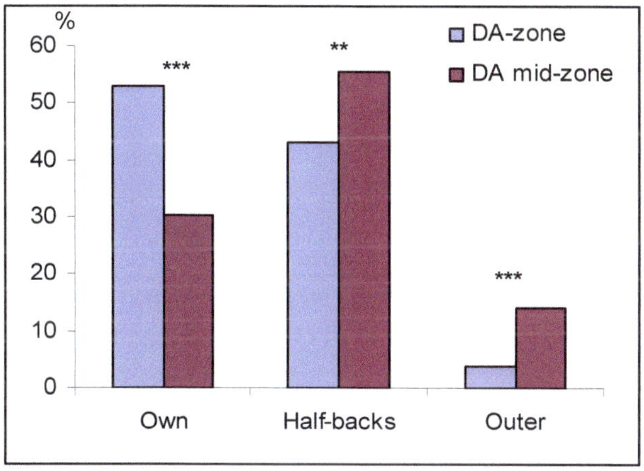

Fig. 1. Percent distribution of fouls by pitch zones and player positions

Legend: DA-zone – Defence or attack zone; DA mid-zone - Defence or attack mid-zone; For other explanations see Table 1; Significant differences between frequencies of fouls committed in the two kinds of zones: ** $p<0.01$; *** $p<0.001$

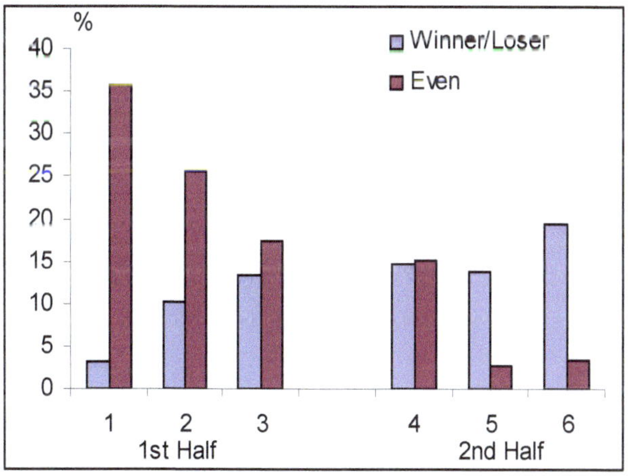

Fig. 2. Percent distribution of fouls by match result and 15-min time interval

Table 2. Distribution of fouls by match location and 15-min time intervals

Time interval / Matches	1st Half			2nd Half		
	1	2	3	4	5	6
Home matches	44	58	57	52	35*	61
Away matches	65	61	58	65	45	51

* Significantly ($p<0.01$) lower than in the time interval 2

Table 3. Distribution of fouls by categories and 15-min time intervals

Time interval / Foul category	1st Half			2nd Half		
	1	2	3	4	5	6
Unintentional	1	1	2	1	2	1
Intentional (instrumental)	105	104	105	103	61*	94
Intentional (hostile)	3	14	8	13	17	17

* Significantly ($p<0.05$) lower than in the time interval 2

Except for the significantly ($p<0.01$) lower frequency of fouls in middle part of the 2nd half compared with the 1st half of home matches, the frequencies were alike in both home and away matches (Table 2). When the fouls were analysed by categories, the unintentional ones constituted only 1.2% of all fouls recorded, and as much as 11.0% were intentional, hostile fouls, the remaining 87.8% being the intentional, instrumental ones. In that latter category, the frequency of fouls committed in middle part of the 2nd half was significantly ($p<0.01$) lower compared with the 1st half (Table 3).

Discussion

The presented results showed that most fouls were committed by players operating in their "natural" pitch zones, i.e. forwards in the attack zone (and attack mid-zone), full-backs in the defence zone (and defence mid-zone), and half-backs in the defence mid-zone. Yet, a fairly large proportion of fouls was attributed to half-backs in the attack zones. This finding is in contrast to the developing game systems and modern football concept that "defence starts by attack". Considering the fact that most of the fouls were committed in the defence and attack mid-zones, it may be concluded that the teams controlled the game from the mid-zone in order to prove their superiority over their opponents. It may be for this reason that they committed more fouls in an environment of struggle and aggression. The fouls that were committed by the mid-zone players, being intentional, instrumental fouls that were tactical in nature, can be explained with the social learning theories, yet to another extend it is possible to claim that the frustration and the tension that the players may have faced during the struggle and high physical contact in this zone may also have played a role in the abundance of fouls.

The fact that most fouls recorded in matches with a tie result were committed at the beginning of the match was striking. This might have been brought about by the strategically learned behaviour of the players so as to affect the destiny of the game by committing as much fouls as possible in the beginning of the game to intimidate the opponents and was reflected by an enormously high average foul rate of 86 fouls per match. Interestingly, the foul rate in matches won by the analysed team was over 4 times lower (19.9 fouls per match).

The results of this study suggested no significant difference between the victorious and defeated teams in foul frequencies (19.0 and 18.6 fouls per 14 matches, won and lost combined, respectively); that was in line with Gerisch and Sommer's study [3,4] and, besides, indicated no significant relationship between the amount of fouls committed by the victorious and defeated football teams. Despite the fact that the defeated teams were expected to behave in a more aggressive way and commit more fouls due to the increased frustration that defeat supposedly may have caused, this study could not support the frustration-aggression theory in professional football matches. However, the fact that there were slightly more fouls committed in the professional football matches that ended with equality may be explained with the frustration-aggression theory, as aggression occurs due to disappointment caused by a frustrated target [2].

Interestingly, no significant differences in the time-distributed numbers of fouls between matches played home or on opponents' grounds. Conventionally, the host teams would be expected to behave more aggressively and commit as many fouls as possible at the beginning of a match to get score advantage, as they would be inspired with their hall of fans and their tumultuous ovations. Yet, no such fact could be supported statistically.

However, this study showed that the host teams tended to commit more fouls in the last 15 min of the games than the visitors (20 and 15%, respectively; $p = 0.09$), probably in order to preserve the score or to be advantageous. The fact that the visitor teams tended to commit relatively more fouls in the 1st and 4th 15-min intervals, i.e. at the beginnings of the two halves of matches, they may have tried to cope with the ovations from the stadium and shown that they coveted the trophy (31 and 38%, respectively; $p = 0.09$; cf. Table 2).

Summing up, the analysis of fouls committed in professional football matches in terms of frequency, timing, place, category, and player interactions, was made to determine the relationship of the fouls with aggressive behaviours from a theoretical perspective. The fouls were classified into three categories (unintentional, intentional-instrumental, intentional-hostile), attributed to the instrumental, and hostile types of aggressive behaviours in sport psychology. In both types of aggression, the aim is to harm the targeted individual either physically and/or psycho-emotionally. Instrumental aggressive behaviours serve a specific aim – gaining advantage. Under such circumstances, the cognitive process of the individual is quite complex. The player learns how to use aggressive behaviours in order to balance the cost (punishment), and profit (ball advantage, score) in the right place and in the right time. With respect to the fact that the aggressive behaviours (fouls) are learnt in challenging match environments, they can be attributed to the social learning theory that values the environment factor in the process of learning aggressive behaviours. Wandzilak cites a number of intervention strategies, utilising Kohlberg's moral development model and social learning theories which were shown to produce improvement or modification of behaviour, moral reasoning and perception of sportsmanship [12]. Teachers and coaches should commit themselves to actively teaching positive sports-related values, and devise curricula that do so [11]. Across all types of aggression, it is given to people to be accepted for loss or be deemed excused. Therefore, sport rules of the game say not to hurt each other. Winning in an uncontrolled manner, in the sense of human behaviour, is detrimental [9]. In conclusion, the presented results may be of help to football coaches and sport psychologists teaching players how to control aggression and how to play the game wit minimum harm while increasing their performance.

References

1. Bandura A. (1973) Aggression: A Social Learning Analysis. Prentice-Hall, Englewood Cliffs, NJ.
2. Bird A.M., B.K.Cripe (1986) Aggression and Sport Psychology and Sport Behaviour. Times Mirror, Mosby.
3. Coakley, Jay J. (1982) Sport in Society, Issues and Controversies (2nd ed.). C.V.Mosby Co., St.Louis MO.
4. Gerisch G., D.Sommer (1988) Aggression Verhaltens im Fussball. *Leistungssport* 18(4):23-24.
5. Gerisch G., D.Sommer (1991) Fouls und Regelwidrigkeiten im Spitzenfußball. *Leistungssport* 21(3):28-30.
6. Gregor T. (1998) Agression in the personality of football players. *Acta Facultatis Educationis Physicae Universitatis Comenianae* 39:59-111.
7. Hellstedt J.C. (1988) Kids, parents and sport: some questions and answers. *The Physician and Sports Medicine* 16(4): 59-71. EJ 376 620.

8. Luxbacher J. (1986) Violence in sport: an examination of the theories of aggression, and how the coach can influence the degree of violence displayed in sport. *Coaching Rev.* 9:14-17.

9. Teipel D., G.Gerisch, M.Busse (1983) Evaluation of aggressive behaviour in football. *Int.J.Sport Psychol.* 14:228-242.

10. Tiryaki. Ş. (2000) Sports Psychology. Concepts, Theories and Practice. Eylül Kitap ve Yayımevi. Mersin, pp. 115-125.

11. Wandzilak T. (1985) Values development through physical education and athletics. *Quest* 37:176-185.

12. Wandzilak T., T.Carrroll, C.J.Ansorge (1988) Values development through physical activity: promoting sportsmanlike behaviors, perceptions and moral reasoning. *J.Teach.Phys.Educ.* 8:13-22.

13. Weiser K., P.Love (1988) Who owns your team? *Strategies* 2(1):5-8.

14. Wilbert M.L. (1988) A Sociological Perspective of Sport (3rd ed.) Macmillan Publishing Co., New York, p.166.

10

Associations between circulating adiponectin and selected plasma biochemical variables in physically active young men and women

Marzena Malara, Grażyna Lutosławska

Department of Biochemistry, University of Physical Education, Warsaw, Poland

Summary

Study aim: To evaluate the relationships between circulating adiponectin and FFA, and other biochemical variables (glycerol, glucose and insulin) in young, healthy non-obese men and women.
Material and methods: A group of 53 male and 54 female students participated in the study. The following compounds were determined in plasma: free fatty acids (FFA), glucose and glycerol (colorimetrically), and insulin and adiponectin (by immunoassay). Insulin resistance index (HOMA-IR) was calculated from fasting insulin and glucose concentrations.
Results: Mean plasma glucose was slightly lower ($p<0.01$), and plasma insulin and HOMA-IR markedly higher ($p<0.01 - 0.001$) in female than in male subjects. Percent body fat was positively correlated with plasma FFA in both groups ($p<0.01$), but with plasma glycerol ($p<0.001$) in female students only. Plasma adiponectin was negatively correlated with percent body fat ($p<0.02$), plasma glycerol ($p<0.001$) and FFA ($p<0.05$) in female subjects only.
Conclusions: Gender-related differences in body fat may affect the relationship between adiponectin and indices of lipid metabolism.

Key words: Young non-obese subjects – Adiponectin - Free fatty acids

Introduction

There is a wealth of studies indicating significant sexual dimorphism in neuroendocrine and metabolic responses to various physiological stressors. In women, both fasting and insulin-induced hypoglycaemia results in reduced counter-regulatory hormonal responses and lower endogenous glucose production as compared with men [11,14]. Marked sex-related differences were also noted in metabolic responses to prolonged dietary restriction, females being characterised by a greater body fat loss, more pronounced disturbances in sex hormone secretion and greater elevation of plasma cortisol levels than males [27].

Males and females also differ with respect to metabolic responses to exercise. In females, a single prolonged exercise results in greater lipolytic activity and FFA utilisation than in males [3,30]. In addition, during endurance exercise, female subjects utilise more intramuscular lipids than males [34]. Similarly, sex-related differences have been noticed in muscle responses to sprint exercise; women utilised much less glycogen as the energy source than men and their ATP recovery during a repeated bouts of sprint exercise was faster [16,17]. Moreover, males and females substantially differ with respect to the glucoregulatory responses to exercise. Following both intense exercise (14 min at 88% $\dot{V}O_2max$) and all-out 30 s test, hyperglycaemia in females is much greater than in males resulting in higher circulating insulin and, in consequence, in a more efficient glycogen resynthesis [26,38].

Due to greater body fat stores in lean females than in males, there is a pronounced sex-related difference in circulating adipokines that markedly affect metabolic processes [20]. Numerous studies focused recently on metabolic functions of adiponectin, a 30 kDa protein, synthesised and secreted almost exclusively by adipocytes with higher adiponectin gene expression and protein content in subcutaneous than in the visceral fat [41].

The most important role of adiponectin, i.e. the metabolic control of carbohydrate and lipid metabolism, has been well documented. Administration of adiponectin to mice alleviated diet-induced fatty liver [43] and in human serum the concentrations of adiponectin were positively

Author's address Dr Marzena Malara, Department of Biochemistry, University of Physical Education, 00-968 Warsaw 45, P.O.Box 55, Poland

correlated with those of circulating HDL-cholesterol and negatively with triacylglycerol [10,21].

Further studies revealed that adiponectin concentrations in plasma were inversely correlated with hepatic lipase activity, thus affecting HDL-cholesterol plasma levels [35]. Moreover, circulating adiponectin was found to be negatively correlated with markers of cholesterol synthesis and positively with those of cholesterol absorption [18]. It was further found to stimulate in vitro GLUT-4 translocation and glucose uptake into the muscle and to improve glucose utilisation and tolerance *in vivo* [8,31].

Circulating adiponectin is low in obese subjects, especially in the insulin-resistant ones; this is known to induce unfavourable lipoprotein profiles, insulin resistance and, in consequence, to increase the risk of atherosclerotic disease [23,36,40]. It is worth noting that adiponectin is under hormonal control in circulation but not in body fat. Both *in vitro* and *in vivo* studies revealed that adiponectin synthesis and its secretion from adipocytes was stimulated by insulin and leptin but inhibited by β-adrenoceptor agonists [9,12,13]. Moreover, an inverse relationship has been noted between circulating IL-6 and adiponectin, and between IL-6 and adiponectin m-RNA expression in adipose tissue in vitro, thus suggesting that endogenous pro-inflammatory cytokines may inhibit adiponectin synthesis [7]. In addition, adiponectin concentration in plasma increases in response to elevated plasma thyroid hormone concentrations; the biological significance of that remains, however, unknown [32].

Despite the abovementioned reports, not all factors affecting circulating adiponectin have been fully elucidated. For example, the association between circulating adiponectin and free fatty acids (FFA) remains controversial. Bernstein *et al.* [2] noted that inhibition of lipolysis and decreased plasma FFA bring about similar decrease in plasma adiponectin concentration. Also Krzyżanowska *et al.* [24] reported that acute elevations in plasma FFA levels were accompanied by higher circulating adiponectin. In contrast, Dullart *et al.* [15] found no effect of the changes in circulating adiponectin in response to fluctuations in FFA plasma concentration. Considering the gender-related differences in body fat content, it might be presumed that it affects the relationship between circulating adiponectin and FFA. Thus, this study aimed at assessing the relationship between circulating adiponectin and FFA, as well as between adiponectin and other biochemical variables (glycerol, glucose and insulin) in young, healthy non-obese men and women.

Material and Methods

Subjects: A group of 53 male and 54 female physical education students volunteered to participate in the study. All the participants were healthy, non-smokers, not taking regularly any vitamin and/or mineral supplements, not engaged in competitive sports. All subjects submitted their written consents after having been informed about study objective and protocol, the study being accepted by the local Ethics Committee.

Methodology: The following measurements were conducted: body mass and height using a standard anthropometer and medical scales, the accuracies amounting to 0.1 cm and 0.1 kg, respectively; the thickness of 3 skinfolds (abdominal, subscapular, triceps) was determined twice using Harpenden caliper (United Kingdom), average values being used for the calculation of body fat [33]. The subjects were requested to declare the volume of their weekly physical activities (h/week).

Blood was withdrawn into heparinised tubes from the antecubital vein in the preprandial state in the morning and centrifuged for 15 min at 4000 rpm, 40 C. Plasma was stored at -70^0 C until assayed. Free fatty acids (FFA), glucose and glycerol were determined in plasma colorimetrically using commercial kits (Randox Laboratories, U.K.), commercial immunoassay kits were used to determine insulin (BioSource, Belgium) and adiponectin (DRG, Germany). The within- and between-assay errors for insulin were 2.2 and 6.5%, respectively. The sensitivity of adiponectin determination was 2 ng/ml. Insulin resistance index (HOMA-IR) was evaluated by homeostasis assessment model from fasting insulin ($\mu IU \cdot ml^{-1}$) and glucose ($mmol \cdot L^{-1}$) concentrations (insulin × glucose/22.5) [29].

Data analysis: Shapiro-Wilk's test was used to assess the distributions; all variables except glucose proved skewed. Prior to computing the Pearson's correlation coefficients, all non-normally distributed variables were transformed to logarithms. Statistica 7.1 software (StatSoft, Inc. USA) was used in data analysis, the level of $p<0.05$ being considered significant.

Results

Somatic characteristics of the participants are presented in Table 1. Despite the significant ($p<0.001$) difference in body fat content, the reported weekly volumes of motor activities were in both groups alike. Regarding the biochemical variables (Table 2), mean plasma glucose concentration in female students was slightly but significantly ($p<0.01$) lower than in the male ones. In contrast, insulin levels in women were markedly higher than in men (by 31%; $p<0.001$). In consequence, insulin resistance index (HOMA-IR) in female participants was significantly higher than in the male ones (by 28%; $p<0.001$). There were no significant differences between men and women with respect to plasma FFA concentrations;

however, a tendency towards a higher plasma glycerol in women than in men was noted (by 12%; $p=0.06$). Mean plasma adiponectin concentration was significantly lower in women than in men (by 28%; $p<0.01$).

Table 1. Mean values (±SD) of somatic variables of young men and women

Variable / Group	Men n = 53	Women n = 54
Age (years)	22.4 ± 1.4	21.0 ± 1.2*
Body mass (kg)	81.1 ± 13.3	61.7 ± 7.6*
Body height (cm)	180.9 ± 5.9	169.4 ± 7.1*
Body fat content (%)	15.2 ± 4.2	22.8 ± 3.9*
LBM (%)	84.7 ± 4.5	77.1 ± 3.9*
Motor activity (h/week)	7.9 ± 2.2	7.4 ± 1.9

* Significantly ($p<0.001$) different from the respective value in men

Table 2. Mean values (±SD) of biochemical variables in plasma of young men and women

Variable / Group	Men n = 53	Women n = 54
Glucose (mmol/l)	4.8 ± 0.6	4.6 ± 0.6**
Insulin (μIU/ml)	5.5 ± 1.4	8.0 ± 3.6***
HOMA-IR	1.173 ± 0.421	1.635 ± 0.986***
Glycerol (μmol/l)	58.9 ± 27.4	67.3 ± 25.5 °
FFA (mmol/l)	0.362 ± 0.296	0.302 ± 0.190
Adiponectin (μg/ml)	30.8 ± 13.5	22.3 ± 13.0**

° Tends to differ from men ($p = 0.06$); Significantly different from the respective value in men: ** $p<0.01$; *** $p<0.001$

Table 3. Pearson's coefficients of correlation between percent body fat and biochemical variables in young men and women

Correlated variable / Group	Men n = 53	Women n = 54
Glucose (mmol/l)	0.050	0.118
Insulin (μIU/ml)	0.030	0.050
HOMA-IR	0.050	0.073
Glycerol (μmol/l)	0.150	0.450***
FFA (mmol/l)	0.386**	0.410**
Adiponectin (ng/ml)	-0.130	-0.370**

** $p<0.01$; *** $p<0.001$

Percent body fat was positively correlated with plasma FFA in both groups ($p<0.01$), but with plasma glycerol ($p<0.001$) in female students only (Table 3). Plasma adiponectin was negatively correlated with percent body fat ($p<0.02$; Table 3), plasma glycerol ($p<0.001$) and FFA ($p<0.05$) in female subjects only (Table 4).

Table 4. Pearson's coefficients of correlation between circulating adiponectin and other biochemical variables in young men and women

Correlated variable / Group	Men n = 53	Women n = 54
Glucose (mmol/l)	0.115	0.117
Insulin (μIU/ml)	0.160	0.114
HOMA-IR	0.135	0.128
Glycerol (μmol/l)	0.080	-0.440***
FFA (mmol/l)	-0.135	-0.283*

* $p<0.05$; *** $p<0.001$

Discussion

Our study confirmed other reports on a higher insulin resistance in female than in male subjects [1,39] and on higher plasma glycerol levels in women than in men due to lower density of α-adrenoceptors and higher that of β-adrenoceptors in adipose tissue of females than of males [42]. Additionally, our study revealed that in females both plasma glycerol and FFA were positively associated with percent of body fat – the major source of those compounds in plasma [5]. In young male subjects, their body fat (relative content) affected exclusively circulating FFA with no effect on plasma glycerol levels. However, the reason for the lack of associations between plasma glycerol and body fat could be only speculated. It is well known that under fasting conditions glycerol is taken up by the liver for gluconeogenesis [4]. On the other hand, there are data indicating more efficient *de novo* glucose production in male than in female subjects [19,22]. Thus, it seems feasible that plasma glycerol levels in men are to a greater extent affected by liver uptake than in women resulting in disappearance of a simple relationship with body fat stores.

Lower plasma adiponectin levels in women than in men reported in this study may be due not only to higher body fat stores but also to lower testosterone levels in females than in males [6,37] and, in addition, the relationship between plasma adiponectin and other biochemical variables was found in this study only in women. These findings do not rule out a contribution of adiponectin to the regulation of carbohydrate and lipid metabolism, mentioned in the introduction, or of body fat on circulating adiponectin in males, because detecting such effects may require a deeper multivariate analysis. Moreover,

Martin *et al.* [28] reported that the relationships of adiponectin with selected metabolic variables were weak in lean subjects but progressed with increasing adiposity and Lavoine *et al.* [25] suggested that the relationship between plasma adiponectin and FFA indirectly reflected an association between circulating adiponectin and body fat.

Summing up, our study revealed that in contrast to women, neither body fat nor circulating FFA affected plasma adiponectin levels in young, lean men. Thus, it seemed that the gender-related differences in body fat may affect the relationship between adiponectin and indices of lipid metabolism.

References

1. Basu R., Ch.D.Man, M.Campioni, A.Basu, G.Klee, G.Toffolo, C.Cobelli, R.A.Rozza (2006) Effect of age and sex on postprandial glucose metabolism. Differences in glucose turnover, insulin secretion, insulin action, and hepatic insulin extraction. *Diabetes* 55:2001-2014.

2. Bernstein E.L., P.Koutkia, K.Ljungquist, J.Breu, B.Canavan, S.Greenspoon (2004) Acute regulation of adiponectin by free fatty acids. *Metabolism* 53:790-793.

3. Boschmann M., M.Rosenbaum, R.L.Leibel, K.R.Segal (2002) Metabolic and hemodynamic responses to exercise in subcutaneous adipose tissue and skeletal muscle. *Int.J.Sports Med.* 23:537-543.

4. Bortz W.M., P.Paul, A.C.Haff, W.LHolmes (1972) Glycerol turnover and oxidation in man. *J.Clin.Invest.* 51:1537-1546.

5. Bouchard C., J-P.Després, P.Mauriège (2005) Genetic and nongenetic determinants of regional fat distribution. *Endocr.Rev.* 14:72-93.

6. Böttner A., J.Kratzsch, G.Müller, T.M.Kapellen, S.Blüher, E.Keller, S.Blüher, E.Keller, M.Blüher, W.Kiess (2004) Gender differences of adiponectin levels develop during the progression of puberty and are related to serum androgen levels. *J.Clin.Endocrinol.Metab.* 89:4053-4061.

7. Bruun J.M., A.S.Lihn, C.Verdich, S.B.Pedersen, S.Tourbo, A.Astrup, B.Richelsen (2003) Regulation of adiponectin by adipose tissue-derived cytokines: in vivo and in vitro investigations in humans. *Am.J.Physiol.Endocrinol.Metab.* 285:E527-E533.

8. Ceddia R.B., R.Somwar, A.Maida, X.Fang, G.Bikopoulos, G.Sweeney (2005) Globular adiponectin increases GLUT4 translocation and glucose uptake but reduces glycogen synthesis in rat skeletal muscle cells. *Diabetologia* 48:132-139.

9. Cong L., K.Chen, J.Li, P.Gao, Q.Li. S.Mi, X.Wu, A.Z.Zhao (2007) Regulation of adiponectin and leptin secretion and expression by insulin through a PI3K-PDE3B dependent mechanism in rat primary adipocytes. *Biochem.J.* 403:519-525.

10. Côté M., P.Mauriège, J.Bergeron, N.Alméras, A.Tremblay, I.Lemieux, J-P.Després (2005) Adiponectinemia in visceral obesity: impact on glucose tolerance and plasma lipoprotein and lipid levels in men. *J.Clin.Endocrinol.Metab.* 90:1434-1439.

11. Davis S.N., P.Galassetti, D.H.Wasserman, D.Tate (2000) Effects of gender on neuroendocrine and metabolic responses to exercise in normal men. *J.Clin.Endocrinol.Metab.* 85: 224-230.

12. Delporte M-L., T.Funahashi, M.Takahashi, Y.Matsuzawa, S.M.Brichard (2002) Pre-and post-translational negative effect of β-adrenoceptor agonist on adiponectin secretion: in vitro and in vivo studies. *Biochem.J.* 367:677-685.

13. Delporte M-L., S. A.El Mkadem, M.Quisquater, S.M.Brichard (2004) Leptin treatment increased plasma adiponectin but barely decreased plasma resisitin of ob/ob mice. *Am.J.Physiol. Endocrinol.Metab.* 287:E446-E453.

14. Diamond M.P., T.Jones, S.Caprio, L.Hallarman, M.C.Diamond, M.Addabbo, W.V.Tamborlane, R.S.Sherwin (1993) Gender influences counterregulatory hormone responses to hypoglycaemia. *Metabolism* 42:1568-1572.

15. Dullaart R.P.F., S.C.Riemens, J.R.Meinardi, B.H.R.Wolffenbuttel, W.J.Sluiter (2005) Plasma adiponectin is modestly decreased during 24-hour insulin infusion but not after inhibition of lipolysis by Acipimox. *Scand.J.Clin.Lab.Invest.* 65:523-532.

16. Esbjörnsson-Lijedahl M., C.J.Sundberg, B.Norman, E. Jansson (1999) Metabolic response in type I and type II muscle fibers during a 30-s cycle sprint in men and women. *J.Appl. Physiol.* 87:1326-1332.

17. Esbjörnsson-Lijedahl M, K.Bodin, E.Jansson (2002) Smaller muscle ATP reduction in women than in men by repeated bouts of sprint exercise. *J.Appl.Physiol.* 93:1075-1083.

18. Hallikainen M., M.Kolehmainen, U.Schwab, D.E.Laaksonen, L.Niskanen, R.Rauramaa, J.Pihlajamäki, M.Uusitupa, T.A.Miettinen, H.Gylling (2007) Serum adipokines are associated with cholesterol metabolism in the metabolic syndrome. *Clin.Chim.A.* 383:126-132.

19. Gustavsson C., K.Yassin, E.Wahlström, L.Cheung, J.Lindberg, K.Brismar, C-G.Östenson, G.Norstedt, P.Tollet-Egnell (2010) Sex-different hepatoglycogen content and glucose output in rats. *BMC Biochemistry* 11:38. (http://www.biochemistrycentralcom/

20. Hauner H. (2005) Secretory factors for human adipose tissue and their functional role. *Proc.Nutr.Soc.* 64:163-169.

21. Kazumi T., A.Kawaguchi, T.Hirano, G.Yoshino (2004) Serum adiponectin is associated with high-density lipoprotein cholesterol, triglycerides, and low-density lipoprotein particle size in young healthy men. *Metabolism* 53: 589-593.

22. Kley S., M.Hoening, J.Glushka, E.S.Jin, S.C.Burges, M. Waldron, E.T.Jordan, J.H.Prestegard, D.C.Ferguson, Sh.Wu, D.E.Olson (2009) The impact of obesity, sex, and diet on hepatic glucose production in cats. *Am.J.Physiol.Endocrinol.Metab.* 296:R936-R943.

23. Kowalska I., M.Straczkowski, A.Nikołajuk, A.Adamska, M.Karczewska-Kupczewska, E.Odziomek, I.Kinalska, M.Górska (2008) Insulin resistance, serum adiponectin, and proinflammatory markers in young subjects with the metabolic syndrome. *Metabolism* 57:1539-1544.

24. Krzyżanowska K., F.Mittermayer, W.Krugluger, M.Roden, G.Scherthaner, M.Woltz (2007) Adiponectin concentrations increase during acute FFA elevation in humans treated with rosiglitazone. *Horm.Metab.Res.* 39:769-772.

25. Lavoie F., F.Frisch, P.Brassard, F.Normand-Lauzière, D.Cyr, R.Gagnon, R.Drouin, J-P.Baillargeon, A.C.Carpentier (2009) Relationship between total and high molecular weight adiponectin levels and plasma nonestrified fatty acid tolerance during enhanced intravascular triacylglycerol lipolysis in men. *J.Clin.Endocrinol.Metab.* 94:998-1004.

26. Marliss E.B., S.H.Kreisman, A.Manzon, J.B.Halter, M. Vranic, Sh. J.Nessim (2000) Gender differences in glucoregulatory responses to intense exercise. *J.Appl.Physiol.* 88:457-466.

27. Martin B., M.Pearson, L.Kebejian, E.Golden, A.Keselman, M.Bender, O.Carlson, J.Egan, B.Ladenheim, J-L.Cadet, K.G. Becker, W.Wood, K.Duffy P.Vinayakumar, S.Maudsley, M.P. Mattson (2007) Sex-dependent metabolic, neuroendocrine, and cognitive responses to dietary energy restriction and excess. *Endocrinology* 148: 1318-1333.

28. Martin L.J., J.G.Woo, S.R.Daniels, E.Goodman, L.M.Dolan (2005) The relationship of adiponectin with insulin and lipids are strengthen with increasing adiposity. *J.Clin.Endocrinol. Metab.* 90: 4255-4259.

29. Matthews D.R., J.P.Hosker, A.S.Rudenski, B.A.Naylor, D.F.Treacher, R.C.Turner (1985) Homeostasis model assessment: insulin resistance and β-cell function from fasting plasma glucose and insulin concentrations in man. *Diabetologia* 28: 412-419.

30. Mittendorfer B., J.F.Horowitz, S.Klein (2002) Effect of gender on lipid kinetics during endurance exercise of moderate intensity in untrained subjects. *Am.J.Physiol.Endocrinol. Metab.* 283:E58-E65.

31. Nakashima Y., K.Inukai, K.Imai, Y.Ikegami, T.Awata, Sh.Katayama (2008) Involvement of low adiponectin levels in impaired glucose tolerance. *Metabolism* 57:1350-1354.

32. Nogueira A.Ch., L.L.Souza, A.Cabanelas, K.J.Oliveira, C.Cabanelas Pazos-Moura (2007) Effect of experimental hypo- and hyperthyroidism on serum adiponectin. *Metabolism* 56:6-11.

33. Piechaczek H. (1975) Piechaczek H. Estimation of total body fat by the densitometric and anthropometric methods. *Stud.Phys.Anthropol.* 2:33-46.

34. Roepstorff C., C.H. Steffensen, M. Madsen, B. Stallknecht, I.L. Kanstrup, E.A. Richter, B. Kiens (2002) Gender differences in substrate utilization during submaximal exercise in endurance-trained subjects. *Am. J. Physiol.* 282: E435-E447.

35. Schneider J.G., M.von Enyatten, S.Schiekofer, P.P.Nawroth, K.A.Dugi (2005) Low plasma adiponectin levels are associated with increased hepatic lipase activity in vivo. *Diabetes Care* 28:2181-2186.

36. Shimada K., T.Miyazaki, H.Daida (2004) Adiponectin and atherosclerotic disease. *Clin.Chim.A.* 344:1-12.

37. Smith J., M.Al-Amri, K.Cianflone (2006) Leptin and adiponectin in relation to body fat percentage, waist to hip ratio and the apoB/apoAI ratio in Asian Indian and Caucasian men and women. *BMC Nutrition and Metabolism* 3:18. (http://www.nutritionandmetabolism.com/

38. Vincent S., P.Berthon. H.Zouhal, E.Moussa, M.Catheline, D.Bentuè-Ferrer, A.Gratas-Delamarche (2003) Plasma glucose, insulin and catecholamine responses to a Wingate test in physically active women and men. *Eur.J.Appl.Physiol.* 91:15-21.

39. Vital P., E.Larietta, M.Hiriart (2006) Sexual dimorphism in insulin sensitivity and susceptibility to develop diabetes in rats. *J.Endocrinol.* 190:425-432.

40. Wasim H., N.M.Al-Daghrin, R.Chetty, P.G.McTernan, A.H.Barnett, S.Kumar (2006) Relationship of serum adiponectin and resistin to glucose intolerance and fat topography in south-Asians. *BMC Cardiovasc.Diabetol.* 5:10 (http://www.cardiab.com/

41. Więcek A, M.Adamczak, J.Chudek (2007) Adiponectin – an adipokine with unique metabolic properties. *Nephrol.Dial. Transplant.* 22:981-988.

42. Williams Ch. (2004) Lipid metabolism in women. *Proc. Nutr.Soc.* 63:153-160.

43. Xu A., Y.Wang, H.Keshaw, L.Yi Xu, K.S.L.Lam, G.J.S. Cooper (2003) The fat-derived hormone adiponectin alleviates alcoholic and nonalcoholic fatty liver disease in mice. *J.Clin. Invest.* 112:91-100.

Effects of age, gender and physical activity on plasma lipid profile

Joanna Okęcka-Szymańska, Elżbieta Hübner-Woźniak, Iwona Piątkowska, Marzena Malara

Department of Biochemistry, University of Physical Education, Warsaw, Poland

Summary

Study aim: To assess the effects of gender, age and engagement in physical activities of elderly subjects on their plasma lipid profiles.
Material and methods: Four groups of subjects, n = 11 each, participated in the study: young men (YM) and women (YW), aged 25 – 32 years, and sedentary, elderly men (EM) and women (EW), aged 58 – 66 years; additionally, a group of 7 women (AW), aged 60 – 65 years, who trained twice weekly (45-min sessions) for 8 months, was studied. The following concentrations of lipids in plasma were recorded: triacylglycerols (TG), total cholesterol (TC) and its fractions: HDLC and LDLC (computed), as well as the TC/HDLC ratio.
Results: Lipid profiles were, generally, less favourable in elderly than in younger subjects, high HDLC values noted in active, elderly women being an exception. In elderly subjects, men's profiles were closer to those of younger subjects than in elderly women and differed significantly ($p<0.001$) lower for TC and LDLC compared with EW group. Triacylglycerols were within normal limits in all groups except EW; LDLC values were mostly abnormally high, the percentages of subjects having normal values ranging from 0 (YM and EW) to 27% (YW).
Conclusions: The age dependent worsening of lipid profiles increased the risk of cardiovascular diseases in sedentary elderly subjects. On the other hand, the beneficial effects of motor activities on lipid profile observed in elderly women evidence the indispensability recommending of physical exercises to the elderly.

Key words: Men – Women – Lipid profile – Age – Physical activity

Introduction

Circulating lipoproteins contain triacylglycerols, cholesterol and its esters, and phospholipids, in addition to specific proteins. The high-density lipoproteins (HDL) carry cholesterol from peripheral cells to the liver, while low-density lipoproteins (LDL) carry cholesterol in the reverse direction. Due to those functions, increased levels of LDL augment the risk of cardiovascular diseases, while HDL is a vessel-protective agent preventing the formation of atherosclerotic changes [16]. Moreover, although an increased risk of cardiovascular diseases is associated with augmented levels of LDL and triacylglycerols, the latter induce that risk also independently of LDL [2].

Cardiovascular diseases, like ischaemic heart disease, infarction or cerebral stroke, affect mainly elderly and middle-aged subjects but the onset of those diseases takes place in the childhood [3,27]; increased LDL and decreased HDL are associated with arterial hypertension which precedes those diseases [23]. The prevalence of atherosclerosis was reported to be closely correlated with engagement in physical exercises which also significantly reduce plasma lipids, especially total cholesterol and LDL, and increase HDL [7,9]. It has been emphasised that a healthy lifestyle, i.e. restricted smoking and alcoholic drinks, well balanced diet and practicing motor activities, are prerequisites for a favourable plasma lipid profile and for preventing cardiovascular diseases [14].

A low level of LDL is known to reduce atherosclerotic changes and the prevalence of ischaemic heart disease, and a decreased risk of that latter disease resulting from the protective role of estrogens in pre-menopausal women was associated with significantly lower LDL and triacylglycerols, and higher HDL compared with men [12]. Those trends are, however, often reversed in post-menopausal women [4].

Concentrations of total cholesterol and its fractions in blood are known to depend on practicing motor activities [26]; HDL levels were reported to be significantly higher in athletes than in sedentary subjects [17,18]. However, no detailed reports on the intensity, volume and frequency of exercises necessary to induce positive

Author's address Prof. Elżbieta Hübner-Woźniak, Department of Biochemistry, University of Physical Education, Marymoncka 34, 00-968 Warsaw, Poland

changes in lipid profile, especially in elderly subjects. Thus, the aim of this study was to assess the effects of gender, age and engagement in physical activities of elderly subjects on their plasma lipid profiles.

Material and Methods

Subjects: Four groups of subjects, n = 11 each, participated in the study: young men (YM) and women (YW), aged 25 – 32 years, and sedentary, elderly men (EM) and women (EW), aged 58 – 66 years; additionally, a group of 7 women (AW), aged 60 – 65 years, who trained twice weekly for 8 months, was studied. Their training consisted of 45-min sessions which included gymnastics, dancing and flexibility exercises. None of the subjects smoked. All subjects submitted their written consents to participate in the study after having been familiarised with its scope and protocol. The study was approved by the local Ethics Committee.

Measurements: Body height, body mass and BMI were recorded by using standard anthropometer and medical scales, the accuracies amounting to 0.1 cm and 0.1 kg, respectively. Body fat content was assessed from skinfold thickness measurements (biceps, triceps, hip and subscapular; accuracy 0.1 cm) according to Durnin *et al.* [8]. Blood samples were withdrawn from the antecubital vein in the pre-prandial state in the morning into heparinised tubes and centrifuged. The collected plasma was stored frozen at -70°C until assayed. The following concentrations of lipids in plasma were recorded: triacylglycerols (TG), total cholesterol (TC) and its HDL fraction (HDLC) using commercial assay kits (Alpha Diagnostics, Poland). The LDL fraction (LDLC) was computed using Friedewald's equation [11]. In addition, the TC/HDLC ratio was computed and the frequencies of normal values of those components were recorded in all groups of subjects, normal values being taken from the 3rd Report of the Team of Experts of the National Cholesterol Education Program, USA [29].

Data analysis: Shapiro-Wilk's test was used to assess data normality. Student's *t*-test for independent data was used to assess the between-group differences for normally distributed variables and the Mann-Whitney's *U*-test for variables deviating from normal distribution. Body fat content and BMI data for sedentary groups were subjected to two-way ANOVA. The log-linear form of the chi-square function was used to assess the frequencies. The level of $p \leq 0.05$ was considered significant.

Results

The results are presented in Tables 1 – 3. Regarding the most meaningful indices, i.e. body fat content and BMI, both age and gender showed significant ($p<0.01$) differences in body fat content while for BMI a significant difference was found only for age ($p<0.05$; by ANOVA). Active, elderly women (Group AW) had significantly lower body fat content ($p<0.01$) and BMI ($p<0.05$) than their sedentary mates (Group EW; cf. Table 1).

Table 1. Mean values (±SD) of somatic data of subjects

Variable / Group	YM n =11	YW n = 11	EM n = 11	EW n = 11	AW n = 7
Age (years)	28.5 ± 4.1	32.0 ± 3.9	66.2 ± 5.1	67.5 ± 4.25	68.0 ± 6.5
Body height (cm)	177.9 ± 5.9	165.6 ± 4.8^{A}	172.4 ± 6.2^{A}	159.0 ± 7.14$^{B C}$	156.9 ± 4.3
Body mass (kg)	78.5 ± 11.5	60.3 ± 4.8^{A}	78.3 ± 10.9	72.4 ± 10.0^{B}	63.0 ± 6.4^{B}
BMI *	22.9 ± 7.0	22.0 ± 1.7	26.6 ± 1.6	28.6 ± 2.8	25.6 ± 2.1^{B}
Body fat content (%)**	17.6 ± 4.9	29.9 ± 2.4	28.5 ± 0.6	43.9 ± 5.2	34.3 ± 5.7^{B}

Legend: Sedentary subjects: M – Men; W – Women; Y – Young (25 – 32 years of age); E – Elderly (58 – 66 years of age); AW – Physically active women aged 60 – 65 years; Significantly ($p<0.01$) different from: ^{A} Group YM, ^{B} Group EW, ^{C} Group EM; * Significant ($p<0.05$) difference between older and younger subjects; ** Significant ($p<0.01$) between-age and between-gender differences

Lipid profiles of young men and women (Groups YM and YW) were practically identical (Table 2). The profiles of sedentary elderly men and women were nearly parallel to one another, the profile of men (EM) being closer to that of younger subjects than that of women and differed significantly from young men (YM) only in TG ($p<0.01$). The profile of elderly women (EW) differed significantly ($p<0.001$) from that of young women (YW) in all variables except HDLC and from their male mates in TC and LDLC. The profile of active elderly women (AW) was closest to that of young women, the TC and HDLC being significantly ($p<0.05$) higher. That latter value was significantly ($p<0.05$) highest compared with all other groups. As to the TC/HDLC ratio, significantly ($p<0.001$) highest values were noted in sedentary elderly subjects (Groups EM and EW).

Table 2. Mean values (±SD) of lipid profile components

Group Variable	YM n =11	YW n = 11	EM n = 11	EW n = 11	AW n = 7
TG (mmol/l)	0.78 ± 0.14[A]	0.69 ± 0.17***	1.35 ± 0.55	1.59 ± 0.65	0.72 ± 0.17**
TC (mmol/l)	4.88 ± 0.77	4.87 ± 0.59***	5.25 ± 0.77***	6.56 ± 0.83	6.04 ± 1.16* [B]
HDLC (mmol/l)	1.55 ± 0.72	1.53 ± 0.36	1.29 ± 0.21	1.52 ± 0.32	1.90 ± 0.24* [B]
LDLC (mmol/l)	2.98 ± 0.30	3.07 ± 0.62***	3.34 ± 0.63***	4.31 ± 0.80	3.81 ± 1.18
TC/HDLC	3.50 ± 0.97	3.39 ± 1.03***	4.20 ± 0.97	4.46 ± 1.12	3.25 ± 0.88***

Legend: TG – Triacylglycerols; TC – Total cholesterol; HDLC – HDL fraction of cholesterol; LDLC – LDL fraction of cholesterol; Significantly different from Group EW: * p<0.05; *** p<0.001); [A] Significantly (p<0.01) different from Group EM; [B] significantly different from Group YW; For other explanations see Table 1

Table 3. Frequencies of normal values of lipid constituents recorded in studied subjects

Group Variable	YM n =11		YW n = 11		EM n = 11		EW n = 11		AW n = 7	
	n	%	n	%	n	%	n	%	n	%
TG	11	100	11	100	10	91	7	64*	7	100
TC	6	55	8	73*	4	36	0	0*	1	14
HDLC	4	36	7	64	1	9*	6	55	6	86*
LDLC	0	0°	3	27°	2	18°	0	0°	1	14

* Significantly (p<0.01) different from all other groups; ° Significantly (p<0.05) different from Group YW; For other explanations see Tables 1 and 2
The reference (normal) values (mmol/l): TG – up to 1.7, TC – up to 5.2, HDLC – above 1.5, LDLC – up to 2.6 [29]

Regarding the frequencies of normal values of studied variables recorded in all groups (Table 3), the TG values were within normal limits in all groups except EW (p<0.05). Only 37% of TC values were within normal limits in all groups combined, 47% of HDLC and as few as 12% of LDLC values. Abnormally high total cholesterol predominated in elderly subjects.

Discussion

The here presented concentrations of triacylglycerols, and cholesterol and its fractions, are in agreement with those of other authors. Ardern *et al.* [1] found no gender-related differences in TG, TC, HDLC and LDLC concentrations and in the TC/LDLC ratio in subjects aged about 35 years. Also Habib *et al.* [13] found no gender-related differences in TC and LDLC in subjects aged about 50 years but women had lower concentrations of TG and higher of HDLC than men. Women aged 18 – 50 years had lower TG and LDLC, and higher HDLC concentrations than men [12]. In women aged 25 years, HDLC levels were higher than in men, although TG, TC and LDLC concentrations were alike [15]. On the other hand, HDLC levels in the post-menopausal women were reported to decrease due to reduced oestradiol secretion [28]. In this study, no such age-related differences were found in women but the frequency of normal HDLC values in women was significantly higher than in men. According to Collins [5], the post-menopausal period is characterised by increased concentrations of TG and LDLC and decreased HDLC compared with the pre-menopausal ones. That tallies with our data except HDLC, which was not significantly decreased.

In the study of De Nino et al. [6] on 178 women, lower TC values were found in young (20 – 35 years of age) than in the elderly (61 – 78 years of age) ones. The authors suggested that the age-related changes in the lipid profile were due to an increasing content of visceral fat. Although visceral fat was not specifically assessed in this study, the total body fat content was significantly (p<0.01) higher in elderly subjects compared with their younger mates. Similar findings were reported by e.g. Essig *et al.* [10] who found body fat content, TG, TC and LDLC to increase in men and women with age (61 – 70 vs. 21 – 30 years of age).

Regarding the gender-related differences, the concentrations of lipids in plasma of both younger groups (YM and YW) were alike but normal values of TC and LDLC were significantly less frequent in men than in women. In elderly subjects the situation was reversed, only the frequency of normal values of HDLC was in men lower than in women.

Elderly women engaged in regular motor activities were markedly superior to their sedentary mates in all components of lipid profile and body fat content and had highest concentration of HDLC among all studied groups. The effect of exercise could have been mediated by lower body fat content as TC and LDLC increased and HDLC decreased with increasing BMI, thus, indirectly, with body fat content [24]. That latter depends on genetic factors but the environmental ones are indispensable for the obesity to develop [21].

Sedentary lifestyle increases the risk of cardiovascular diseases; when the time spent on driving and watching TV exceeded 23 h/week that risk increased by 37% compared with those who spent on those activities less than 11 h/week [30]. It would be interesting to know what kinds or forms of exercise decrease that risk but such data are lacking. A minimum of exercising 2 h weekly was shown necessary to increase the level of HDLC, the frequency or intensity of exercises having no effect on lipid profile [19]. On the other hand, exercising frequency was shown to affect the lipid profile more than exercise volume or intensity, although that latter was also of importance; nevertheless, elderly subjects ought to exercise at low or moderate intensity in order to avoid possible injuries, heart attack, etc. [22]. Kraus *et al.* [20] studied 159 subjects aged 40 – 65 years and found that a high exercise volume was effective in improving lipid profile; the changes were more pronounced in those whose jogging distance amounted to 17 – 18 miles/week compared with those jogging 11 miles/week. A decreased TC/HDLC ratio was noted only in those who practiced running, not less than 150 min/week [25]. On the other hand, no significant changes in lipid profile was found in women aged over 60 years, who participated in controlled exercises for a year, despite a decrease in the TC/HDLC ratio [31]. It should be noted that in this study active, elderly women spent 90 min/week on exercising which was associated with decreases in TG and TC/HDLC ratio, and increased HDLC compared with their sedentary mates.

Summing up, sedentary elderly subjects, compared with their younger mates, exhibited a marked worsening of the plasma lipid profile which was indicative of an augmented risk of cardiovascular diseases. Gender-related differences in mean values of the studied lipids and lipoproteins were noted only in elderly subjects but values within normal ranges (except TG) were significantly more frequent in young women than in men. Lipid profile in elderly, physically active women was significantly better than in their sedentary mates, especially regarding the HDLC fraction. Thus, in order to reduce the risk of cardiovascular diseases, elderly subjects ought to be strongly advised to engage in motor activities.

References

1. Ardern C.I., P.T.Katzmarzyk, I.Janssen, A.S.Leon, J.H. Wilmore, J.S.Skinner, D.C.Rao, J.P.Despres, T.Rankinen, C. Bouchard (2004) Race and sex similarities in exercise-induced changes in blood lipids and fatness. *Med.Sci.Sports Exerc.* 36: 1610-1615.
2. Austin M.A. (1998) Plasma triglyceride as a risk factor for cardiovascular disease. *Can.J.Cardiol.* 14 (Suppl B):14B-17B.
3. Berenson G.S. (2002) Childhood risk factors predict adult risk associated with subclinical cardiovascular disease: the Bogalusa Heart Study. *Am.J.Cardiol.* 90:3L-7L.
4. Callejon D.R., D.R.Rios, S.A.Franceschini, M.R.Toloi (2009) Transdermal estradiol and lipid profile: effects on a specific group of Brazilian postmenopausal women. *Arq.Bras. Cardiol.* 93:571-575.
5. Collins P. (2008) HDL-C in post-menopausal women: an important therapeutic target. *Int.J.Cardiol.* 124:275-282.
6. De Nino W.F., A.Tchernof, I.J.Dionne, M.J.Toth, P.A.Ades, C.K.Sites, E.T.Poehlman (2001) Contribution of abdominal adiposity to age-related differences in insulin sensitivity and plasma lipids in healthy nonobese women. *Diabetes Care* 24: 925-932.
7. Devoe D., R.G.Israel, T.Lipsey, W.Voyles (2009) A long-duration (118-day) backpacking trip (2669 km) normalizes lipids without medication: a case study. *Wilderness Environ. Med.* 20:347-352.
8. Durnin J.V.G.A, J.Womersley (1974) Body fat assessed from total density and its estimation from skinfold thickness: measurements on 481 men and women aged from 16 to 72 years. *Br.J.Nutr.* 32:77-97.
9. Durstine J.L., P.W.Grandjean, P.G.Davis, M.A.Ferguson, N.L.Alderson, K.D.DuBose (2001) Blood lipid and lipoprotein. Adaptation to exercise. *Sports Med.* 31:1033-1062.
10. Essig F., D.Sinclair, J.Hare, J.Moreillon, D.Funk, A.M. Swank (2004) Cross-sectional analysis of cardiovascular factors for participants of a university faculty and staff wellness program. *J.Exerc.Physiol.* 7:37-43.
11. Friedewald W.T., R.J.Levy, D.S.Fredrickson (1972) Estimation of concentration of low density lipoprotein cholesterol in plasma without use of the preparative ultracentifuge. *Clin.Chem.* 18:449-506.
12. Garelnabi M., E.Veledar, J.Abramson, J.White-Welkley, N.Santanam, W.Weintraub, S.Parthasarathy (2010) Physical inactivity and cardiovascular risk: baseline observations from men and premenopausal women. *J.Clin.Lab.Anal.* 24:100-105.
13. Habib S.S., M.Aslam, W.Hameed (2005) Gender differences in lipids and lipoprotein(a) profiles in healthy individuals and patients with type 2 diabetes mellitus. *Pak.J.Physiol.* 1:15-19.
14. Hata Y., K.Nakajima (2000) Life-style and serum lipids and lipoproteins. *J.Atheroscler.Thromb.* 7:177-197.
15. Henderson G.C., R.M.Krauss, J.A.Fattor, N.Faghihnia, M.Luke-Zeitoun, G.A.Brooks (2010) Plasma triglyceride concentrations are rapidly reduced following individual bouts of endurance exercise in women. *Eur.J.Appl.Physiol.* 109:721-730.
16. Hertzberg G.R. (2004) Aerobic exercise, lipoproteins and cardiovascular disease: benefits and possible risk. *Can.J.Appl. Physiol.* 29:800-807.
17. Hübner-Woźniak E., M.Malara, J.Okęcka-Szymańska, K.Witek (2008) Cholesterol fractions, C-reactive protein and creatine kinase activity in plasma of female athletes. *Phys.Educ. Sport* 52:195-198.
18. Hübner-Woźniak E., M.Malara, Z.Prawecki (2007) Serum lipid profile in competitive athletes. *Phys.Educ.Sport* 51:81-84.
19. Kodama S., S.Tanaka, K.Saito, M.Shu, Y.Sone, F.Onitake, E.Suzuki, H.Shimano, S.Yamamoto, K.Kondo, Y.Ohasi, N.Yamada, H.Sone (2007) Effect of aerobic exercise training on serum levels of high-density lipoprotein cholesterol. *Arch.Intern.Med.* 167:999-1008.
20. Krauss W.E., J.A.Houmard, B.D.Duscha, K.J.Knetzger, M.B.Wharton, J.S.McCartney, C.W.Bales, S.Henes, G.P.Samsa, J.D.Otvos, K.R.Kulkarni, C.A.Slentz (2002) Effect of the amount and intensity of exercise on plasma lipoproteins. *N.Engl.J.Med.* 347:1483-1492.
21. Loos R.J.F., T.Rankinen (2005) Gene-diet interaction on body weight changes. *J.Am.Diet Assoc.* 105:S29-S34.

22. Mensink G.B.M., D.W.Heerstrass, S.E.Neppelenbroek, A.J.Schuit, B.M.Bellach (1997) Intensity, duration and frequency of physical activity and coronary risk factors. *Med.Sci. Sports Exerc.*29:1192-1198.

23. Misigoj-Duraković M., Z.Duraković (2009) The early prevention of metabolic syndromc by physical exercise. *Coll. Antropol.* 33:759-764.

24. Mora S., L.I-Min, J.E.Buring, P.M.Ridker (2006) Association of physical activity and body mass index with novel and traditional cardiovascular biomarkers in women. *JAMA* 295:1412-1419

25. Nybo L., E.Sundstrup, M.D.Jakobsen, M.Mohr, T.Hornstrup, L.Simonsen, J.Bulow, M.B.Randers, J.J.Nielsen, P.Aagaard, P.Krustrup (2010) High-intensity training versus traditional exercise interventions for promoting health. *Med.Sci. Sports Exerc.* 42:1951-1958.

26. Skoumas J., C.Pitsavos, D.B.Panagiotakos, C.Chrysohoou, A.Zeimbekis, I.Papaioannou, M.Toutouza, P.Toutouza, C.Stefanidis (2003) Physical activity, high density lipoprotein cholesterol and other lipids level, in men and women from the ATTICA study. *Lipids Health Dis.* 2:3-9.

27. Sporisević L., V.Krzelj, A.Bajraktarević, E.Jahić (2009) Evaluation of cardiovascular risk in school children. *Bosn.J. Basic Med.Sci.* 9:182-186.

28. Sultan N., M.Nawaz, A.Sultan, M.Fayaz, A.Baseer (2003) Effect of menopause on serum HDL-cholesterol level. *J.Ayub. Coll.Abbottabad* 15:24-26.

29. Third Report of the National Cholesterol Education Program (NCEP), Expert Panel on Detection, Evaluation and Treatment of High Blood Cholesterol in Adults (Adult Treatment Panel III), NIH Publication No. 02-5215. (2003) *Medycyna Praktyczna* 3:87-116.

30. Van Roie E., C.Delecluse, J.Opdenacker, K.De Bock, E.Kennis, F.Boen (2010) Effectiveness of a lifestyle physical activity versus a structural exercise intervention in older adults. *J.Aging Phys.Act.* 18:335-352.

31. Warren T.Y., V.Barry, S.P.Hooker, X.Sui, T.S.Church, S.N.Blair (2010) Sedentary behaviors increase risk of cardiovascular disease mortality in men. *Med.Sci.Sports Exerc.* 42: 879-885.

Relationships between competitive anxiety, social support and self-handicapping in youth sport

Agata Wężyk

Noffer Institute of Occupational Medicine, Łódź, Poland

Summary

Study aim: To assess the level of self-handicapping tendency, competitive anxiety (trait) and social support within groups of young male and female athletes, as well as to determine the relationships between those variables.
Material and methods: A group of 75 athletes (46 male football players and 29 female volleyball players) from Sport Mastery School in Łódź, aged 16 - 19 years, participated in the study. Three questionnaires were administered: Anticipative Strategy of Self-Esteem Protection Scale (ASO) to measure self-handicapping tendency, Social Support Scale (SWS) and Reactions to Competition (RnW), in order to measure the competition-related anxiety (trait).
Results: Female athletes attained significantly higher scores in ASO and RnW while male players perceived their social support higher than girls. No significant correlations between self-handicapping and anxiety were found. Most of the observed relationships between self-handicapping and social support were negative, like those between anxiety and social support.
Conclusions: It is advisable to work with young athletes on eliminating self-handicapping activities and replacing them with other, more efficient, ways of coping with anxiety. Social support (adequate to the athlete's needs) might be crucial in that proceeding. The hypothesis of relationship between sport competitive anxiety and self-handicapping was not confirmed, maybe due to the relatively small number of subjects.

Key words: Self-handicapping – Competitive anxiety – Social support – Team sports – Youth sport

Introduction

Two social psychologists E. Jones and S. Berglas in the late 70's introduced the concept of self-handicapping [3]. In the literature, this phenomenon is described as any kind of action, decision or behaviour that increases the chances of externalising (or justifying) failure or internalising success [16]. Such an action is a way to protect one's self-esteem, especially under highly stressful conditions, when being individually assessed or when the subject is not sure about the effect (failure/success) of own actions are highly likely. Obvious examples of such conditions are sports competitions. Jones and Berglas [3] pointed out that self-handicapping is widely demonstrated by athletes. Other researchers confirmed the presence of this phenomenon in sport [2,4,10,19,20,22]. However, no study that examined the relationships between the 3 variables presented in this paper could be found in the available literature.

Depending on the situation, there are two ways of maintaining positive self-image after completing the task. In case of failure, an individual blames the external conditions, while after gaining success, he/she claims that it was due to own merits. This is the phenomenon known as the attributions (cf. [1]). Self-handicapping is similar, but for the moment of action. It is applied prior to (or sometimes during) performing the task. Researchers indicate three forms of self-handicapping: behavioural, claimed and symbolic [7]. The first one includes active strategies like alcohol consumption or insufficient preparation to the task. Thus, an athlete may e.g. be late for training session, spend not enough time on exercising, put not enough effort in it [7,20] or – in case of sports like long-distance running – quite the contrary, engaging oneself in great effort, consequence of which is fatigue. It seems that it is easier to admit having not completed some part of the task ('*I have lost because I was not prepared*') than not being able to do something ('*I have lost because I have got no talent*').

Claimed self-handicaps are based on reporting certain weaknesses, such as shyness, feeling anxious, or telling about specific experience, that might excuse oneself

Author's address Agata Wężyk M.S., Department of Work Psychology, Noffer Institute of Occupational Medicine, Św. Teresy 8, 91-348 Łódź, Poland

of failure [7]. In sports, it might take the form of telling about one's negative feelings and stress (*'I feel so nervous/shaky, I feel sick, I am trembling with fear all the time, I have problems with concentration'*, etc.) or about former injuries (*'I am afraid of twisting my ankle again'*). It does not mean that athletes are never stressed or that all of them make excuses in that way. Nevertheless, such claims/messages might be a form of self-handicapping.

Symbolic self-handicapping consists of indicating external factors as possible causes of failure. Those may be, e.g., partner's lack of talent, worse performance or bad conditions during the task (competition) such as noise, insufficient light, high temperature [7]. This kind of self-handicapping brings about lowest costs since the subject does not actively reduce own chances for success (as it happens in case of behavioural self-handicaps) and does not deteriorate his/her image by admitting weaknesses (like in claimed self-handicaps). However, overusing such symbolic strategies may lead to earning a negative reputation [7].

Anxiety, classified as state or trait [7] is a multidimensional construct which was widely described also in sport psychology (cf. [23]). State anxiety is an *'immediate emotional state that is characterised by apprehension, fear, tension and an increase in physiological arousal'* and trait anxiety is a *'predisposition to perceive certain environmental situation as threatening, and to respond to these situations with increased state anxiety'* ([6], p. 93). In this study, the sport competition-related state anxiety was assessed [14]. Anxiety contains two components: somatic and cognitive. Somatic anxiety consists in physiological reactions such as increased heart rate, muscle tension or sweating. Cognitive anxiety is manifested in negative expectations about performing the task, unpleasant emotions, worrying or problems with concentration [9,17,23]. For athletes, one of the most im portant things is effective coping with anxiety, as it may seriously impair their performance [9,23].

There are two possible kinds of relationships between anxiety and self-handicapping. On one hand, anxiety usually appears in case of danger (cf. [14]). Sports competition could be seen as some kind of threat and is an anxiety-evoking situation (it poses a threat to one's self-esteem), thus self-handicapping may play a protective role [2]. On the other hand, when an athlete reports in-tense somatic anxiety (*'I have butterflies in my stomach, I feel sick, My hands are shaking, I can't breath'*) and/or cognitive anxiety (*'I can't concentrate, Thoughts are racing through my head'*), it may be a form of self-handicapping [19].

Another way of coping with anxiety is making use of the received social support. Two perspectives of social support can be discerned: structural (availability of social support, sources, density of social network) and functional (type of social interaction and exchanged resources). In this study, social support was assessed by a questionnaire based on Tardy's model [12]. It enables assessing 4 types of social support: emotional (showing interest, care, positive feelings), instrumental (any kind of material support: money, time), informational (advice, knowledge, information) and appraisal (motivating, appraising, acceptance, feedback about the performance) received from any given network. In sports, there are three essential sources of social support: team (or club) mates, coaches, and family and friends [15,21]. It seems that social support plays a vital role in one's functioning by protecting self-esteem [12,18] and that may be crucial in self-handicapping, which has similar function. It was, however, reported that the higher group consistency (that theoretically implies intense social support), the more likely is the use of self-handicapping strategies. It is explained in terms of excessive, unreasonable eagerness to meet the group's expectations [4,10].

The aim of this study was to assess the level of self-handicapping tendency, competitive anxiety (trait) and social support within groups of young male and female athletes, as well as to determine the relationships between those variables.

Material and Methods

The study was conducted at the turn of 2007 and 2008 in the Sport Mastery School in Łódź. Out of 120 students aged 16 – 19 years, 46 male football players and 29 female volleyball players (62,5% in total) completed the administered questionnaires. The study was conducted upon the consent of the headmaster and approval of the local Committee of Ethics. Three questionnaires were applied:

1 - Anticipative Strategy of Self Esteem Protection Scale (ASO) [7], based on the Jones' Self-handicapping Scale (SHS). The Polish version contained 25 items assessed on a scale from 1 (I don't agree at all) to 6 (I agree completely). Thus, the results could range 25 to 150 points and the higher the result, the higher one's self-handicapping tendency. Only the overall results were taken into consideration.

2 - Social Support Scale (SWS) [13] – consisting of 24 items assessed on 5-point scale (1 – yes, 2 – rather yes, 3 – sometimes yes, sometimes not, 4 -rather not, 5 – no). The questionnaire contained 4 subscales pertaining to various types of social support (informational, instrumental, emotional, appraisal). The participants got that test in triplicate and were asked to assess the social

support received from three sources: team/club mates, coaches, family (parents, siblings). All possible results (each type of support from each resource, as well as overall results regarding each sources and each type of support) were included in further analysis.

3 - Reactions to Competition Questionnaire (RnW) – based on Martens' SCAT; this enabled determining the level of competitive trait-anxiety. The questionnaire contained 3 subscales : somatic anxiety (9 items), worrying (7 items) and concentration distractions (5 items). All items were assess on a 4-point scale (1 – absolutely not, 2 - rather not, 3 – rather yes, 4 – absolutely yes). In further analysis, the subscale results and the overall result (indicating the level of competitive trait-anxiety) were subjected to analysis.

Results

As shown in Table 1, female subjects attained significantly ($p<0.001$) higher values in the self-handicapping tendency as well as in variables related to anxiety while male subjects attained higher results in support scales ($p<0.05 – 0.001$).

Table 1. Mean values (±SD) of examined variables recorded in male and female athletes aged 16 – 19 years

Variable / Group	Male n = 46	Female n = 29
Age (years)	17.5 ± 2.3	18.0 ± 1.1
Training experience (years)	7.6 ± 2.1	4.1 ± 2.3
Self-handicapping tendency	74.5 ± 10.5	92.1 ± 9.9***
Competitive anxiety (total)	40.8 ± 8.1	46.8 ± 9.5**
Somatic anxiety	15.3 ± 4.5	19.8 ± 5.3***
Social support (family)	107.3 ± 9.4	93.2 ± 16.9***
Social support (total)	279 ± 31	253 ± 36**
Informational support (total)	71.8 ± 7.7	64.6 ± 10.4**
Instrumental support (total)	67.7 ± 10.3	61.4 ± 10.4*
Emotional support (total)	75.2 ± 8.7	66.3 ± 10.1***

Significantly different from male athletes: * $p<0.05$; ** $p<0.01$; *** $p<0.001$

Correlation coefficients between self-handicapping tendency and anxiety variables are presented in Table 2. No significant correlations between self-handicapping tendency and anxiety were noted except self-handicapping tendency and concentration distractions in female subjects.

Inasmuch all the relationships between the self-handicapping tendency and social support variables were of similar magnitude and negative, only those related to family or coaches were significant ($p<0.05$) in the female group, all other ones being significant ($p<0.05$) in the male group only (Table 3). Competitive anxiety significantly ($p<0.05$) correlated with informational and total support from the family, the former correlating also with worrying ($p<0.01$). Quite unexpectedly, all those correlations were positive (Table 4).

Table 2. Relationships between self-handicapping tendency and anxiety variables in male and female athletes aged 16 – 19 years

Variable / Group	Male n = 46	Female n = 29
Competitive anxiety (total)	0.168	0.248
Somatic anxiety	0.020	0.100
Worrying	0.214	0.209
Concentration distractions	0.341*	0.197

* $p<0.05$

Table 3. Relationships between self-handicapping tendency and social support variables in male and female athletes aged 16 – 19 years

Source and type of support / Group		Female n = 29	Male n = 46
Family	Appraisal	-0.182	-0.298*
	Total	-0.273	-0.302*
Coaches	Instrumental	-0.205	-0.317*
	Informational	-0.410*	-0.250
	Instrumental	-0.397*	-0.237
Total	Appraisal	-0.430*	-0.127
	Emotional	-0.386*	-0.126
	Total	-0. 447*	0.250

* $p<0.05$; ** $p<0.01$

Table 4. Relationships between anxiety and family support in male athletes (n = 46) aged 16 – 19 years

Kind of support	Competitive anxiety (total)	Worrying
Informational	0.341*	0.396**
Total	0.297*	0.183

* $p<0.05$; ** $p<0.01$

In female athletes, anxiety variables were mostly significantly correlated with social support variables, all the significant ones being negative (Table 5). Worrying correlated with informational, emotional and total support from mates and informational support from family, while concentration distractions were related to informational support from mates and coaches, as well as to total informational and instrumental support.

Table 5. Relationships between anxiety and social support variables in female athletes (n = 29) aged 16 – 19 years

Source and type of support		Competitive anxiety (total)	Somatic anxiety	Worrying	Concentration distractions
Team/club mates	Informational	-0.582**	-0. 488**	-0.495**	-0.379*
	Instrumental	-0.379*	-0.438*	-0.203	-0.188
	Appraisal	-0.405*	-0.445*	-0.234	-0.224
	Emotional	-0.528**	-0.525**	-0.478**	-0.108
	Total support	-0.567**	-0. 564**	-0.430*	-0.262
Family	Informational	-0.235	-0.245	-0.441*	0.023
Coaches	Informational	-0.101	-0.043	0.079	-0.450**
Social support (total)	Informational	-0.431*	-0.362*	0.179	-0.578**
	Instrumental	-0.389*	-0.418*	-0.170	-0.332
	Emotional	-0.334*	-0.492*	-0.193	-0.286
	Total support	-0.470*	-0.482**	-0.219	-0.430*

* $p<0.05$; ** $p<0.01$

Discussion

Mean values obtained with the use of ASO scale in male and female subjects amounted to 74.5 and 92.1 points, respectively, or about 40 and 54% of the scale range, respectively. However, no reference values are available for that scale and no sport-related studies using the Polish version of that test exist. Therefore, it is impossible to discuss the presented results in relation to athletes or general population.

In this study, female athletes attained significantly higher results than the male ones which was not consistent with the paper of Hurt *et al.* [11] who reported that men were mostly more likely to self-handicap than women especially in terms of behavioural strategies. However, men differ from women with respect to the sources of self-esteem (intellectual vs. social tasks, respectively) and, due to that different situations may pose a threat to their self-image [7]. It seems that in sport competition (especially in team sports) certain social skills (e.g. communication, interactions and cooperation) are essential in addition to physical abilities. Moreover, sport competitions are still considered men's domain. Because of that stereotype, women can perceive such a situation as a greater threat for their self-esteem. To protect oneself from destructive criticism and unjust, harmful opinions (‘*You're not able to that - it's not for women*, *You're a total disaster'*), female athletes may engage in self-handicapping. They may prepare in advance specific excuses in case of failure, blaming certain changeable, external conditions (e.g. lack of proper warm-up, coming late for trainings, forgetting to bring the equipment). There might be also another, quite simple explanation for the observed difference in self-handicapping. When ASO scale was being developed, the research showed that women usually scored higher than men [7]. This may be e.g. because of a higher self-awareness of women compared with men. They usually have greater insight in themselves and their functioning.

Competitive anxiety proved also gender-specific. Male athletes demonstrated lower somatic (but not the cognitive) anxiety than women which was consistent with former research [17]. This supports the view that women are more likely to react with somatic symptoms in a difficult, stressful situation and, undoubtedly, sport competition is exactly such a situation.

Analysis of the social support scale revealed that male athletes rated the received support higher than the female ones. This might have been due to the specificity of the Sport Mastery School as other authors [15,21] did not report such differences. At the time of this study, female students attended the school just for 1½ years; they were in minority and most of them came to the school from different regions of Poland and so they received little family support.

Anxiety was reported to play a vital role in self-handicapping [7]. However, in this study, no significant correlations between those variables were found. The results obtained for female athletes may suggest a relationship between cognitive anxiety (concentration distractions) and self-handicapping but further research on a greater number of subjects would be needed to confirm that suggestion.

As far as the relationships between self-handicapping and social support are concerned, the analysis showed that male players who evaluated appraisal and total support from families, demonstrated lower tendency to self-handicap compared with their female mates. This is not astonishing, as the appraisal support is a known protector of self-esteem. Thus, athletes who get proper appraisal support have no need to self-handicap. On the other hand, the correlation only indicated an interrelationship between variables but not a causal relationship. It was suggested that people who self-handicap may engage themselves in conflicts and arguments [8]. This may be an alternative explanation for the results obtained in this study – the higher self-handicapping tendency, the less support an individual receives.

In the female group, social support from particular sources did not prove significant in self-handicapping. However, the total informational, emotional, instrumental and appraisal supports were negatively correlated with self-handicapping tendency. It could be speculated that support from one specific source was not sufficient, but a high total support would reduce the tendency to self-handicap in female subjects.

Unexpectedly, positive correlations between competitive anxiety and social support were found in male athletes. Those who evaluated higher informational and total support received from their families, attained higher results in the RnW test (total score and in subscale "Worrying"). This could have been due to excessive family's expectations about individual's sports career and, further, to excessive information and advice resulting in mixed perceptions including feeling of being overprotected. In sports, if the coach's roles are taken over by not always competent parents, an athlete may find himself in a harmful conflict (because of contradictory information from two important groups). Furthermore, social support inadequate (in terms of type or amount) to the situation or to one's needs might prove stressful [18].

Female athletes receiving high support (total informational, instrumental and emotional) were less likely to react with somatic anxiety to sport competitions. Moreover, the higher total informational support, the lower cognitive anxiety (concentration distractions). This is not surprising, as within informational support one receives knowledge and information helpful in further actions [12]. This may alleviate the anxiety in new, unfamiliar situations or uncertainty about coping with difficult situation, as well as to prevent distractions (a person has a plan, knows what to do and has no need to think about other things or look for other solutions).

Emotional support from team/club mates correlated negatively with competitive anxiety both somatic and cognitive (worrying). This type of support includes showing positive feelings (interest, trust, care, friendliness) towards a person and that enables acting free of concerns about disappointing others or loosing their interest. It was demonstrated [5] that the failure itself poses no threat for an individual, only its negative consequences. Social support was claimed to have a protective role and to reduce stress and anxiety [10]. Nevertheless, it is also true that people having low anxiety are more friendly, confident and easy-going, so it is easier for them to access and benefit from social support [14,15].

Summing up, the presented results are at least partly consistent with the literature reports but further research is needed especially on larger groups of athletes, including individual sports. It may be, however, concluded that young athletes ought to be given support adequate to their needs. This may result in better coping with competitive anxiety and lower likeliness to self-handicap.

References

1. Aronson E., T.Wilson, R.Akert (2010) Social Psychology. Prentice Hall, Upper Saddle River NJ.

2. Bailis D.S. (2001) Benefits of self-handicapping in sport: A field study of university athletes. *Can.J.Behav.Sci.* 4:213-228.

3. Berglas S., E.E.Jones (1978) Drug choice as a self-handicapping strategy in response to noncontingent success. *J.Personality Soc.Psychol.* 36:405-417.

4. Carron A., H.Prapavessis, J.R.Grove (1994) Group effects and self-handicapping. *J.Sport Exerc.Psychol.* 16:246-257.

5. Conroy D.E. (2003) Representational models associated with fear of failure in adolescents and young adults. *J.Pers.* 71: 757-784. DOI: 10.1111/1467-6494.7105003

6. Cox R. (1998) Sport Psychology. Concepts and Applications. WCB McGraw-Hill, Boston.

7. Doliński D., A.Szmajke (1994) Self-handicapping: advantages and disadvantages. PTP, Olsztyn.

8. Ferrari J.R., J.S.Harriot, M.Zimmerman (1999) The social support networks of procrastinators: Friends or family in times of trouble? *Pers.Ind.Differ.* 26:321-331.

9. Hanin Y. (2000) Emotions in Sport. Human Kinetics, Champaign IL.

10. Hausenblas H.A., A.V.Carron (1996) Group cohesion and self-handicapping in female and male athletes . *J.Sport Exerc.Psychol.* 18:132-143.

11. Hirt E.R., R.K.Deppe, L.J.Gordon (1991) Self-reported versus behavioral self-handicapping: empirical evidence for theoretical distinction. *J.Personality Soc.Psychol.* 61:981-991.

12. Kmiecik-Baran K. (1995) Social Support Scale: Its content and psychometric parameters. *Psych.Rev.* 38:201-214.

13. Lavallee L., F.Flint (1996) The relationship of stress, competitive anxiety, mood state, and social support to athletic injury. *J.Athl.Training* 31:296-299.

14. Lazarus, R., S.Folkman (1984) Stress, Appraisal, and Coping. Springer Pub. Co., New York

15. Leahy T., F.Cheung (1995) Social support among Hong-Kong athletes. In: H.F.Fu, M.Ng (eds.) Sport Psychology: Perspectives and Practices Toward 21st Century. Hong-Kong Baptist University, Hong-Kong.

16. Leary M.R. (1996) Self-Presentation: Impression Management and Interpersonal Behavior. Westview Press, Boulder CO.

17. Martens R., R.S.Vealey, D.Burton (1990) Competitive Anxiety in Sport. Human Kinetics, Champaign IL.

18. Pommersbach J. (1988) Social support and illness. *Psychol.Rev.* 30:503-525.

19. Prapavessis H., J.R.Grove, R.Maddison, N.Zillman (2003) Self-handicapping tendencies, coping and anxiety responses among athletes. *Psychol.Sport Exerc.* 4:357-375. DOI: 10.1016/S1469-0292(02)00020-1

20. Rhodewalt F., A.T.Saltzman, J.Wittmer (1984) Self-handicapping among competitive athletes: The role of self-esteem protection. *Basic Appl.Soc.Psychol.* 5:197-209.

21. Rosenfeld L.B., J.M.Richman, C.J.Hardy (1989) Examining social support networks among athletes: Description and relationship to stress. *Sport Psychol.* 3:23-33.

22. Treasure D.C., K.K.Kuczka (2005) Self-handicapping in competitive sport: influence of the motivational climate, self-efficacy and perceived importance. *Psychol.Sport Exerc.* 6:539-550. DOI: 10.1016/j.psychsport.2004.03.007

23. Wann D. (1996) Sport Psychology. Prentice Hall, Boston MA.

Acknowledgements

Thanks are due to Prof. M. Krawczyński for making available Polish version of the Competition Questionnaire

Omega-3 fatty acids and exercise: a review of their combined effects on body composition and physical performance

Gül Tiryaki-Sönmez[1], Brad Schoenfeld[1], Serife Vatansever-Ozen[2]

[1]Lehman College, Department of Health Sciences, The City University of New York, Bronx, NY, USA; [2]Abant Izzet Baysal University, School of Physical Education and Sport, Department of Training Science, Bolu,Turkey

Summary

Omega-3 (n-3) fatty acids, and the long-chain n-3 derivatives eicosapentaenoic acid (EPA) and docosahexaenoic acid (DHA) in particular, have been extensively researched for their nutritive effects. Among their many purported benefits, n-3 acids have been implicated as positive mediators of cardiovascular health and body composition. It has therefore been speculated that supplementation may enhance the beneficial effects of physical activity, potentiating greater reductions in body fat and improvements in exercise performance. This paper has three objectives: first, to assess the theoretical basis for a synergistic ef-fect when n-3 supplementation is combined with exercise; second, to review the literature as to specific findings on the subject and third, to make relevant conclusions and recommendations for future research.

Key words: Omega-3 fatty acids – Body composition – Physical performance

Introduction

Omega-3 (n-3) fatty acids, and the long-chain n-3 derivatives eicosapentaenoic acid (EPA) and docosahexaenoic acid (DHA) in particular, have been extensively researched for their nutritive effects. However, despite evidence dating back to the 1930's that n-3 acids are essential for normal growth and dermal function, only in the past several decades have they received just attention for their role as health-promoting agents [32]. Among their many purported benefits, n-3 acids have been implicated as positive mediators of cardiovascular health and body composition.

Initial interest in the cardiovascular benefits of EPA and DHA was aroused by the finding that the Greenland Eskimos and other populations who consume diets rich in these fatty acids have exceedingly low incidences of cardiovascular diseases [20,85]. A large number of both experimental and epidemiological studies have since been conducted to examine the effect of consuming fish oil, which contains high amount of n-3 acids, on cardiovascular health, with a majority showing an inverse correlation on morbidity and mortality [1,33,40,51,63,68]. The cardioprotective effects of n-3 acids are attributed to improvements in various cardiovascular risk factors including a reduction in blood platelet aggregation [45,58], decreased inflammation [29,88], enhanced endothelial function [21], positive changes in blood lipids [9,28,30], and decreased blood pressure [55,60].

The n-3 consumption has also been associated with favourable alterations in body composition. Animal studies have consistently shown a reduced adiposity and an increase in lean tissue growth when dietary n-3 derivatives are substituted for saturated fats [27,50,54], monounsaturated fats [71], and omega-6 (n-6) fatty acids [16, 34,56] on a calorie-for-calorie basis. To date, controlled experiments examining the effect of differing dietary fatty acid compositions on body composition in human subjects are conflicting. Some human trials [15,38,49,78], but not all [22,36], have reported reductions in fat mass with n-3 consumption compared to other oils. Interestingly, DeLany *et al.* [18] found that omega-3s were preferentially metabolised by the body after ingestion in comparison to other fatty acids, noting a high linear relation between oxidation and the number of double bonds.

Given the purported benefits of n-3 on the cardiovascular system and fat metabolism, it has been speculated that supplementation may enhance the beneficial effects of physical activity, potentiating greater reductions in body fat and improvements in exercise performance.

Author's address Prof. Gül Tiryaki Sönmez, Lehman College, The City University of New York, Department of Health Sciences, 250 Bedford Park Blv. West, Bronx, NY 10468, USA

Thus, the purpose of this paper will be threefold: first, to assess the theoretical basis for a synergistic effect when n-3 supplementation is combined with exercise; second, to review the literature as to specific findings on the subject, and, third, to make relevant conclusions and recommendations for future research.

Theoretical Basis for n-3 Supplementation in Combination with Exercise

Biochemically, n-3 acids are a class of essential polyunsaturated fatty acids that have the first carbon-carbon double bond in the third position from the methyl end of the fatty acid (the n-3 position) and additional double bonds depending on the molecule. Numerous longer chain n-3 fatty acids exist in nature, the most studied of which include the 20 carbon chain EPA with 5 double bonds (known as 20:5) and the 22 carbon chain DHA with 6 double bonds (22:6). EPA and DHA are found in various cold water fish including salmon, mackerel, sardines, and herring. The shortest chain form of n-3 is α-linolenic acid (ALA), which contains 18 carbon atoms and 3 double bonds (18:3). ALA is found in various plant sources such as flaxseeds, soybeans, and walnuts. Human beings can convert ALA into longer chain derivatives through the delta-desaturase enzymatic pathways [47]. However, conversion is largely inefficient, with only 5% of ALA reportedly converted to EPA and less than 0.5% to DHA [59]. This is significant because the longer chain derivatives are purported to have the greatest biological effects in human beings.

With respect to exercise, one potential mechanism whereby n-3 supplementation may enhance benefits is *via* increased lipolysis and β-oxidation. Specifically, n-3 fatty acids are claimed to act as metabolic fuel partitioners [13], upregulating lipid oxidative enzymes and downregulating lipogenic gene expression [35,62]. This is due, at least in part, to the ability of n-3 acids to bind and activate the various peroxisome proliferator-activated receptor (PPAR) isoforms [42,48,67]. PPARs are members of the nuclear receptor superfamily and include PPAR-α, PPAR-γ, and PPAR-δ [24]. The n-3 acids have a particular affinity to act as ligands for the PPAR-α isoform, which is located in the cell nucleus of many body tissues, predominantly those that exhibit high oxidative rates of fatty acids such as the liver, heart, kidney, and muscle [19]. PPAR-α was shown to play an integral role in the management of glucose and fatty acid homeostasis [72], inducing the expression of several gene encoding proteins involved in lipid transport and oxidation including hepatic carnitine acyltransferase, and hepatic and skeletal muscle peroxisomal acyl-CoA oxidase [14]. Hypothetically, increased PPAR-α activity should enable a greater reliance on fat for fuel during exercise while sparing muscle glycogen, and improving both body composition and exercise per-formance. Moreover, n-3 acids may indirectly influence lipid oxidation by suppressing the generation of acetyl-CoA carboxylase [84], which catalyses synthesis of the lipogenic co-enzyme A derivative malonyl-CoA [12]. Malo-nyl-CoA serves as a fatty acid precursor primarily by impairing the activity of the enzyme carnitine palmitoyl-transferase [87], responsible for facilitating the transport of existing fatty acids back into the mitochondrial matrix where they can be oxidised for fuel. By suppressing ma-lonyl CoA, n-3 acids indirectly increase the levels of carnitine palmitoyltransferase, thereby favouring the entry of fatty acids into the mitochondria. This, conceivably, would further enhance the availability of fatty acid substrate for β-oxidation during exercise.

Another mechanism, whereby n-3 acids may confer a positive effect on exercise, is by improving fatty acid delivery to exercising muscles *via* an increased blood flow [31]. Blood flow improvements are believed to be due to an n-3 mediated suppression of n-6 eicosanoid production. Specifically, n-3 and n-6 acids compete for δ-6 desaturase, i.e. for further elongation and desaturation [32]; a high n-6/n-3 ratio can lead to elevated levels of pro-inflammatory prostaglandins and thromboxanes [33,79]. Given that these eicosanoids are pro-aggregatory vasoconstrictors, excessive amounts can lead to reductions in vascular blood flow [64]. Supplementing with n-3 can potentially help to inhibit inflammatory eicosa-noid production, as well as interacting with cyclooxygenase in a manner that reduces platelet aggregation, increases dilation of blood vessels, and improves circulatory response [33,46,80]. Indeed, Walser *et al.* [80] demonstrated that 6 weeks of supplementation with DHA (2.0 g/day) and EPA (3.0 g/day) enhanced exercise-induced increases in brachial artery diameter and blood flow during 90 s of low-intensity handgrip exercise.

Supplementation with n-3 acids may facilitate additional blood flow improvements in exercise by helping to prevent a reduction in red blood cell (RBC) deformability. Exercise has been shown to cause stiffening of erythrocytes [23] which, in turn, can impede circulatory responses [73]. These reductions in RBC deformability have been attributed to an increased peroxidation of lipid membranes resulting from exercise-induced free radical production [74]. A number of studies suggest that n-3 derivatives help to increase the deformability of RBCs [11,76] which would theoretically heighten oxygen and nutrient delivery to exercising muscles and thereby enhance performance.

Table 1. Findings of studies with omega-3 fatty acids ingestion

Effects of omega-3 fatty acids on cardiovascular health	
Low morbidity and mortality	[1,33,40,51,63,67]
Reduction in blood platelet aggregation	[45,58]
Decreased inflammation	[29,88]
Enhanced endothelial function	[21]
Positive changes in blood lipids	[9,28,30]
Increased blood flow	[31,33,46]
Decreased blood pressure	[55,60]
Effects of omega-3 fatty acids on body composition	
Reduced adiposity and increased lean body tissue	[27,38,49,50,53, 54,78]
Decreased appetite	[53]
Effects of omega-3 fatty acids during exercise	
Increased brachial artery diameter	[80]
Loss of body fat	[17,31,81]
Attenuated red blood cell deformability	[26]
Decreased submaximal O_2 uptake and heart rate	[8,57]
Delayed muscle soreness	[75]
Increased exercise-induced protein synthesis	[49,65,70]

Studies Investigating n-3 Acids and Exercise

Despite a wealth of research on the health-related benefits of n-3 acids, studies investigating the effects of combining n-3 supplementation and exercise are limited. The following is a review of the current literature as to studies specifically addressing changes in body composition and exercise performance. To date, only 4 studies could be located that directly evaluated changes in body composition associated with the combined effects of n-3 supplementation and exercise but the results were not uniform.

Warner *et al.* [81] randomly assigned 34 hyperlipidemic subjects to one of 4 groups: fish oil plus exercise, fish oil, corn oil, and control [81]. The exercise group performed aerobic training 3 days a week for 45 – 50 min at 75 – 80% of maximal heart rate. Supplementation amounted to 50 ml of either fish oil or corn oil daily. After 12 weeks, only the fish oil plus exercise group lost a significant amount of body fat. However, the study was limited by the lack of an exercise-only control group, making it difficult to ascertain whether results were due to the combination of fish oil and training *versus* the training protocol alone.

In a controlled study, Brilla and Landerholm [7] assigned healthy, previously sedentary male subjects (19 – 34 years of age; body fat content 15 – 22%) to one of 4 groups: fish, exercise, fish and exercise, and control. The exercising subjects performed three, one-hour aerobic sessions per week. Total omega-3 fatty acid intake in the groups consuming fish was calculated at 4 g/day. After 10 weeks, no significant differences in body composition were noted between any of the groups studied. The fairly low initial body fat levels in participants, however, may have limited the results.

Hill *et al.* [31] assigned 65 overweight (BMI > 25), previously sedentary subjects (24 males, 41 females) with hypertension and/or hyperlipidemia to one of 4 groups: fish oil, fish oil plus exercise, sunflower oil (a source of n-6 fatty acids), or sunflower oil plus exercise. Exercise consisted of walking at 75% of age-predicted maximal heart rate for 45 min three days a week. After 12 weeks, 6 g of fish oil plus exercise resulted in a significantly greater reduction in body fat compared to an equal dose of sunflower oil plus exercise (1.2% and 0.1%, respectively).

Most recently, DeFina *et al.* (2010) conducted a placebo-controlled, randomised trial where 128 overweight and obese subjects (BMI≥26 and <40) were assigned to receive either capsules containing 3.0 g of EPA and 0.6 g of DHA or placebo [17]. Both groups underwent dietary counselling and were provided with calorie-controlled nutritional regimens. In addition, participants received health club memberships and were instructed to perform aerobic exercise at 50 – 85% $\dot{V}O_2max$, 150 min a week, in combination with 20 – 30 min of total-body strength training exercise performed twice weekly. Adherence to the protocol was monitored by the completion of dietary recalls and exercise diaries. After 24 weeks, subjects in both groups lost slightly more than 5% of their body mass with no significant between-group differences reported. The study was limited by self-reported energy intake and expenditure information, which has been shown to be unreliable, particularly in overweight and obese individuals [4,69].

As with the research on body composition, the number of studies directly examining the effects of n-3 supplementation on exercise performance is also limited. Guezennec *et al.* [26] examined the effects of fish oil supplementation on RBC deformability in 14 trained male subjects (19 – 38 years of age) over 6 weeks. Subjects were divided into two groups: a supplement group that consumed 6 g/day of fish oil and a control group that consumed a “standard diet” rich in saturated fats. The participants performed two, one-hour cycling bouts at 70% $\dot{V}O_2max$, pre- and post-study. One test was performed at sea level and the other in a hypobaric chamber at a simulated altitude of 3000 m. The results showed that fish oil supplementation significantly attenuated RBC deformability under hypoxic conditions compared to controls. In contrast to those findings, Oostenbrug et al. [52] recruited 24 trained male cyclists (aged 19 – 42 years) to investigate the effects of 3 weeks of fish oil supplementation (6 g/day) on RBC deformability. At the end of the supplementation period, subjects performed a one-hour bicycle time trial and were evaluated for RBC characteristics. Results showed no significant difference in RBC characteristics nor were any improvements in aerobic endurance performance noted. However, the three-week protocol may not have been long enough to realise an ergogenic effect.

Peoples *et al.* [57] investigated the effect of fish oil supplementation on oxygen consumption during exercise. Using a double-blind, parallel design, 16 well-trained male cyclists were randomly assigned to consume either 8 g/day of fish oil (n = 9; age 23.2 ± 1.2 years) or 8 g/day of olive oil, a source of omega-9 fatty acids (n = 7; age 27.1 ± 2.7 years) for 8 weeks. Subjects were tested on a cycle ergometer for peak oxygen consumption and sustained submaximal exercise at 55% of peak workload both before and after supplementation. At the end of the study, those of the fish oil group had significantly lowered heart rates during incremental workloads to exhaustion as well as displaying lowered steady-state submaximal exercise heart rates, whole-body oxygen consumption, and rate pressure product. However, fish oil supplementation had no significant impact on peak oxygen consumption, a finding consistent with some [52,61] but not all [39] studies.

Yates *et al.* [86] studied lipid profiles and the use of n-3 acids in professional football players. A total of 36 active national football players were randomly assigned to 2 groups: the first group (n = 20) was provided fish oil capsules (2200 mg of mixed DHA, EPA, and 360 mg of other omega-3 acids), and the second group (n = 16) served as controls during a 60-day trial. Serum LDL, HDL, and other subfractions were measured. Compliance, side effects, and seafood consumption data were also collected. Supplementation with n-3 significantly improved the lipid profile of active players randomised to treatment. It was suggested that n-3 supplementation should be considered as a method to improve modifiable cardiovascular risk lipid factors in professional football players.

Finally, Buckley *et al.* [8] evaluated the effects of n-3 on endurance performance and recovery in 25 elite Australian Rules football players. In a double-blind design, subjects were randomly assigned to either 6 g/day of DHA or sunflower oil over the course of a 5-week training period. The subjects performed two separate treadmill trials to exhaustion at a speed equivalent to their average running speed for a 2200-m time-trial, pre- and post-study. The trials were separated by 5-min intermissions. Time to exhaustion (TTE) for Trial 1 was used to assess endurance performance while TTE for Trial 2 was used to assess exercise recovery. Results showed that while heart rate during submaximal exercise was reduced in the fish oil group, no differences were noted between groups in exercise performance or recovery.

Concluding Remarks

At this time, research is largely inconclusive as to the potential synergistic benefits when n-3 is supplemented in conjunction with exercise. There is some evidence that n-3 can modestly enhance lipolysis and β-oxidation during exercise and thereby improve fat loss. There also is modest evidence that n-3 supplementation may help to improve various aspects of exercise performance. However, limitations in study design make it difficult to draw firm conclusions on these topics.

Other areas related to the combined effects of n-3 supplementation and exercise still remain to be explored. For example, given the antagonistic effect of n-3 acids on pro-inflammatory eicosanoids [10], supplementation may help to alleviate exercise-related delayed-onset muscle soreness (DOMS), which can indirectly benefit exercise performance. Positive effects on DOMS may be augmented by the ability of n-3 acids to increase blood flow, thereby aiding in a more rapid nutrient delivery post-exercise. Some studies have shown a beneficial effect [75] while others have not [41]. Further studies are warranted to assess whether n-3 acids may, in fact, produce analgesic effects.

Another area for potential study is the effect of n-3 supplementation on exercise-induced protein metabolism. A number of studies show that n-3 supplementation results in greater accretion of muscle proteins in both animals [3,5,25] and human beings [19,65,70]. Increased protein synthesis may be secondary to n-3 mediated increases in cell membrane fluidity [2]. Cell membranes are vital for regulating the passage of nutrients, hormones and chemical signals into and out of cells. When cell membranes are fluid, they become more permeable, allowing substances and secondary messenger molecules associated with protein synthesis to readily penetrate the cytoplasm [5,25,37]. The n-3 may also enhance mTOR/p70s6k signalling [70], a pathway believed to act as a master network regulating skeletal muscle growth [6,77]. In addition, there is some evidence that n-3 supplementation may decrease proteolysis by downregulating the ubiquitin-proteasome pathway [82,83], which in conjunction with heightened protein synthesis would result in an even greater accretion of muscle proteins. However, none of these studies were carried out in conjunction with physical activity, making it impossible to draw any conclusions to exercising conditions. Further research is needed to examine whether n-3 supplementation may potentiate gains in lean muscle mass when combined with regimented exercise.

Finally, it is possible that n-3 may improve weight loss during exercise by helping to regulate appetite. Parra *et al.* [53] showed that diets rich in n-3 modulate postprandial satiety in overweight and obese volunteers during weight loss. Given that exercise has been shown to result in better short-term appetite control [43], it would be interesting to assess whether n-3 supplementation might have a synergistic effect on improving post-workout satiety when combined with regimented exercise. If so, this could have significant implications for long-term weight management.

In conclusion, the potential synergism between n-3 supplementation and exercise provides an exciting area for research. Future studies should seek to build on the current body of literature with more stringent controls in study design. Moreover, studies to-date have focused solely on cardiovascular exercise, but it would be interesting to investigate whether n-3 may confer beneficial effects when combined with resistance training. It should be also noted that a high consumption of n-3 can lead to immunosuppression and prolong bleeding time [44,66]. Thus, attempts should be made to establish optimal n-3 dosages to maximise the risk/reward ratio of supplementation.

References

1. Albert C.M., H.Campos, M.J.Stampfer, P.M.Ridker, J.E. Manson, W.C.Willett, J.Ma (2002) Blood levels of long-chain n–3 fatty acids and the risk of sudden death. *N.Engl.J.Med.* 346:1113–1118.

2. Alexander J.W (1998) Immunonutrition: the role of omega-3 fatty acids. *Nutrition* 14:627-633.

3. Alexander J.W., H.Saito, O.Trocki, C.K.Ogle (1986) The importance of lipid type in the diet after burn injury. *Ann.Surg.* 204:1-8.

4. Bandini L.G., D.A.Schoeller, H.N.Cyr, W.H.Dietz (1990) Validity of reported energy intake in obese and non-obese adolescents. *Am.J.Clin.Nutr.* 52: 421-425.

5. Bergeron K., P.Julien, T.A.Davis, A.Myre, M.C.Thivierge (2007). Long-chain n-3 fatty acids enhance neonatal insulin-regulated protein metabolism in piglets by differentially altering muscle lipid composition. *J.Lipid.Res.* 48:2396-2410.

6. Bodine, S.C., T.N.Stitt, M.Gonzalez, W.O.Kline, G.L. Stover, R.Bauerlein, E.Zlotchenko, A.Scrimgeour, J.C.Lawrence, D.J.Glass, G.D.Yancopoulos (2001) Akt/mTOR pathway is a crucial regulator of skeletal muscle hypertrophy and can prevent muscle atrophy in vivo. *Nat.Cell.Biol.* 3:1014–1019.

7. Brilla L.R., T.E.Landerholm (1990) Effect of fish oil supplementation and exercise on serum lipids and aerobic fitness. *J.Sport Med.Phys.Fitn.* 30:173-180.

8. Buckley J.D., S.Burgess, K.J.Murphy, P.R.Howe (2009) DHA-rich fish oil lowers heart rate during submaximal exercise in elite Australian Rules footballers. *J.Sci.Med.Sport* 12:503-507.

9. Calabresi L., N.Villa, M.Canavesi, C.R.Sirtori, R.W.James, F.Bernini, G.Franceschini (2004) An omega-3 polyunsaturated fatty acid concentrate increases plasma high-density lipoprotein 2 cholesterol and paraoxonase levels in patients with familial combined hyperlipidemia. *Metabolism* 53:153-158.

10. Calder P.C. (2006) n-3 polyunsaturated fatty acids, inflammation, and inflammatory diseases. *Am.J.Clin.Nutr.* 83: 1505S-1519S.

11. Cartwright I. J., A.G.Pockley, J.H.Galloway, M.Greaves, F.E.Preston (1985) The effects of dietary ω-3 polyunsaturated fatty acids on erythrocyte membrane phospholipids, erythrocyte deformability and blood viscosity in healthy volunteers. *Atherosclerosis* 55:267-281.

12. Clarke S.D. (2000) Polyunsaturated fatty acid regulation of gene transcription: a mechanism to improve energy balance and insulin resistance. *Br.J.Nutr.* 83:S59-S66.

13. Clarke S.D. (2001) Polyunsaturated fatty acid regulation of gene transcription: a molecular mechanism to improve the metabolic syndrome. *J.Nutr.* 131:1129-1132.

14. Clarke S.D., D.Jump (1997) Polyunsaturated fatty acids regulate lipogenic and peroxisomal gene expression by independent mechanisms. Prostaglandins Leukot.Essent.Fatty *Acids* 57:65-69.

15. Couet C., P.Delarue, J.M.Autoine, F.Lamisse (1997) Effect of dietary fish oil on body fat mass and basal fat oxidation in healthy adults. *Int.J.Obes.Relat.Metab.Disord.* 21:637-43.

16. Cunnane S.C., K.R.McAdoo, D.F.Horrobin (1986) n-3 Essential fatty acids decrease weight gain in genetically obese mice. *Br.J.Nutr.* 56:87-95.

17. Defina, L.F., L.G.Marcoux,, S.M.Devers, J.S.Cleaver, B.L.Willis (2011) Effects of omega-3 supplementation in combination with diet and exercise on weight loss and body composition. *Am J Clin Nutr.* 93:455-462.

18. DeLany J.P., M.M.Windhauser, C.M.Champagne, G.A. Bray (2000) Differential oxidation of individual dietary fatty acids in humans. *Am.J.Clin.Nutr.* 72:905-911.

19. Diep Q.N., R.M.Touyz, E.L.Schiffrin (2000) Docosahexaenoic acid, a peroxisome proliferator-activated receptor-alpha ligand, induces apoptosis in vascular smooth muscle cells by stimulation of p38 mitogen-activated protein kinase. *Hypertension* 36:851-855.

20. Dyerberg, J., H.O.Bang, E.Stofferson, S.Moncada, J.R. Vane (1978) Eicosapentaenoic acid and prevention of thrombosis and atherosclerosis. *Lancet* 2:117-119.

21. Fleischhauer F.J., W.D.Yan, T.A.Fischell (1993) Fish oil improves endothelium-dependent coronary vasodilation in heart transplant recipients. *J.Am.Coll.Cardiol.* 21:982-989.

22. Fontani G., F.Corradeschi, A.Felici, F.Alfatti, R.Bugarini, A.I.Fiaschi, D.Cerretani, G.Montorfano, A.M.Rizzo, B.Berra (2005) Blood profiles, body fat and mood state in healthy subjects on different diets supplemented with omega-3 polyunsaturated fatty acids. *Eur.J.Clin.Invest.* 35:499–507.

23. Galea G., R.J.L.Davidson (1985) Hemorrheology of marathon running. *Int.J.Sports.Med.* 6:136-138.

24. Gani O.A. (2008) Are fish oil omega-3 long-chain fatty acids and their derivatives peroxisome proliferator-activated receptor agonists? *Cardiovasc.Diabetol.* 20(7):6.

25. Gingras A.A., P.J.White, P.Y.Chouinard, P.Julien, T.A. Davis, L.Dombrowski, Y.Couture, P.Dubreuil, A.Myre, K.Bergeron, A.Marette, M.C.Thivierge (2007) Long-chain omega-3 fatty acids regulate bovine whole-body protein metabolism by promoting muscle insulin signalling to the Akt-mTOR-S6K1 pathway and insulin sensitivity. *J.Physiol.* 579:269-284.

26. Guezennec C.Y., J.F.Nadaud, P.Satabin, F.Leger, P.Lafargue (1989) Influence of polyunsaturated fatty acid diet on the hemorrheological response to physical exercise in hypoxia. *Int.J.Sports Med.* 10:286-291.

27. Hainault I., M.Carolotti, E.Hajduch, C.Guichard, M.Lavau (1993) Fish oil in a high lard diet prevents obesity, hyperlipidemia, and adipocyte insulin resistance in rats. *Ann.NY.Acad.Sci.* 683: 98-101.

28. Harris W.S. (1989) Fish oils and plasma lipid and lipoprotein metabolism in humans: a critical review. *J.Lipid Res.* 30:785-807.

29. Heller A, T.Koch, K.Schmeck, K.Van Ackem (1998) Lipid mediators in inflammatory disorders. *Drugs* 55:487-496.

30. Herrmann W., J.Biermann, G.M.Kostner (1995) Comparison of effects of N-3 to N-6 fatty acids on serum level of lipoprotein(a) in patients with coronary artery disease. *Am.J. Cardiol.* 76:459–462.

31. Hill A.M., J.D.Buckley, K.J.Murphy, P.R.C.Howe (2007) Combining fish-oil supplements with regular aerobic exercise improves body composition and cardiovascular disease risk factors. *Am.J.Clin.Nutr.* 85:1267-1274.

32. Holman R.T. (1998) The slow discovery of the importance of omega 3 essential fatty acids in human health. *J.Nutr.* 128:427S-433S.

33. Hu, F.B., L.Bronner, W.C.Willett, M.J.Stampfer, K.M.Rexrode, C.M.Albert, J.E.Manson (2002) Fish and omega-3 fatty acid intake and risk of coronary heart disease in women. *JAMA* 287:1815-1821.

34. Jones P.J. (1989) Effect of fatty acid composition of dietary fat on energy balance and expenditure in hamsters. *Can.J. Physiol.Pharmacol.* 67:994-998.

35. Jump D.B., S.D.Clarke, A.Thelen, M.Liimatta (1994) Coordinate regulation of glycolytic and lipogenic gene expression by polyunsaturated fatty acids. *J.Lipid Res.* 35:1076-1084.

36. Krebs J.D., L.M.Browning, N.K.McLean, J.L.Rothwell, G.D.Mishra, C.S.Moore, S.A.Jebb (2006) Additive benefits of long-chain n-3 polyunsaturated fatty acids and weight-loss in the management of cardiovascular disease risk in overweight hyperinsulinaemic women. *Int.J.Obes.* 30:1535-1544.

37. Kummerow F.A. (1983) Modification of cell membrane composition by dietary lipids and its implications for atherosclerosis. *Ann.NY.Acad.Sci.* 414:29-43.

38. Kunešová M., R.Braunerová, P.Hlavatý, E.Tvrzická, B. Stanková, J.Skrha, J.Hilgertová, M.Hill, J.Kopecký, M.Wagenknecht, V.Hainer, M.Matoulek, J.Parízková, A.Zák, S.Svacina (2006) The influence of n-3 polyunsaturated fatty acids and very low calorie diet during a short-term weight reducing regimen on weight loss and serum fatty acid composition in severely obese women. *Physiol.Res.* 55:63-72.

39. Leaf D.A., C.R.Rauch (1988) Omega-3 supplementation and estimated VO_2 max: a double blind randomized controlled trial in athletes. *Ann.Sport Med.* 4:37-40.

40. Lemaitre R.N., I.B.King, D.Mozaffarian, L.H.Kuller, R.P. Tracy, D.S.Siscovick (2003) n-3 Polyunsaturated fatty acids, fatal ischemic heart disease, and nonfatal myocardial infarction in older adults: the Cardiovascular Health Study. *Am.J. Clin.Nutr.* 77:319-325.

41. Lenn J., T.Uhl, C.Mattacola, G.Boissonneault, J.Yates, W.Ibrahim, G.Bruckner (2002) The effects of fish oil and isoflavones on delayed onset muscle soreness. *Med.Sci.Sport Exerc.* 34:1605-1613.

42. Lin Q., S.E.Ruuska, N.S.Shaw, D.Dong, N.Noy (1999) Ligand selectivity of the peroxisome proliferator-activated receptor alpha. *Biochemistry* 5(38):185-190.

43. Martins C., L.Morgan, H.Truby (2008) A review of the effects of exercise on appetite regulation: an obesity perspective. *Int.J.Obes.* 32:1337-1347.

44. Meydani S.N., S.Endres, M.M.Woods, B.R.Goldin, C.Soo, A.Morrill-Labrode, C.A.Dinarello, S.L.Gorbach (1991) Oral (n-3) fatty acid supplementation suppresses cytokine production and lymphocyte proliferation: comparison between young and older women. *J.Nutr.* 121:547-555.

45. Mori T.A., L.J.Beilin, V.Burke, J.Morris, J.Ritchie (1997) Interactions between dietary fat, fish, and fish oils and their effects on platelet function in men at risk of cardiovascular disease. *Arterioscler.Thromb.Vasc.Biol.* 17:279–286.

46. Mori T.A., G.F.Watts, V.Burke, E.Hilme, I.B.Puddey, I.J.Beilin (2000) Differential effects of eicosapentaenoic acid and docosahexaenoic acid on vascular reactivity of the forearm microcirculation in hyperlipidemic, overweight men. *Circulation* 102:1264-1269.

47. Nakamura, M.T., T.Y.Nara (2004) Structure, function and dietary regulation of Δ6, Δ5 and Δ9 desaturases. *Ann.Rev.Nutr.* 24:345-376.

48. Neschen S., K.Morino, J.Dong, Y.Wang-Fischer, G.W. Cline, A.J.Romanelli, J.C.Rossbacher, I.K.Moore, W.Regittnig, D.S.Munoz, J.H.Kim, G.L.Shulman (2007) n-3 Fatty acids preserve insulin sensitivity in vivo in a peroxisome proliferator-activated receptor-alpha-dependent manner. *Diabetes* 56: 1034-1041.

49. Noreen E.E., M.J.Sass, M.L.Crowe, V.A.Pabon, J.Brandauer, L.K.Averill (2010) Effects of supplemental fish oil on resting metabolic rate, body composition, and salivary cortisol in healthy adults. *J.Int.Soc.Sports Nutr.* 8:7-31.

50. Okuno M, K.Kajiwara, S.Imai, T.Kobayashi, N.Honma, T.Maki, K.Suruga, T.Goda, S.Takase, Y.Muto, H.Moriwaki (1997) Perilla oil prevents the excessive growth of visceral adipose tissue in rats by down-regulating adipocyte differentiation. *J.Nutr.* 127:1752-1757.

51. Oomen C.M., E.J.Feskens, L.Räsänen, F.Fidanza, A.M. Nissinen, A.Menotti, D.Kromhout (2002) Fish consumption and coronary heart disease mortality in Finland, Italy, and The Netherlands. *Am.J.Epidemiol.* 151:999-1006.

52. Oostenbrug G.S., R.P.Mensink, M.R.Hardeman, T.De Vries, F.Brouns, G.Hornstra (1997) Exercise performance, red blood cell deformability, and lipid peroxidation: effects of fish oil and vitamin E. *J.Appl.Physiol.* 83:746–752.

53. Parra D., A.Ramel, N.Bandarra, M.Kiely, A.Martínez, I.Thorsdottir (2008) A diet rich in long chain omega-3 fatty acids modulates satiety in overweight and obese volunteers during weight loss. *Appetite* 51.676-680.

54. Parrish C.C., D.A.Pathy, A.Angel (1990) Dietary fish oils limit adipose tissue hypertrophy in rats. *Metabolism* 39: 217-219.

55. Paschos G.K., F.Magkos, D.B.Panagiotakos, V.Votteas, A.Zampelas (2007) Dietary supplementation with flaxseed oil lowers blood pressure in dyslipidaemic patients. *Eur.J.Clin.Nutr.* 61:1201-1206.

56. Pellizzon M., A.Buison, F.Ordiz Jr, L.Santa Ana, K.L.Jen (2002) Effects of dietary fatty acids and exercise on body-weight regulation and metabolism in rats. *Obes.Res.* 10:947-955.

57. Peoples G.E., P.L.McLennan, P.R.Howe, H.Groeller (2008) Fish oil reduces heart rate and oxygen consumption during exercise. *J.Cardiovasc.Pharm.* 52:540-547.

58. Phang M., A.J.Sinclair, L.F.Lincz, M.L.Garg (2010) Gender-specific inhibition of platelet aggregation following omega-3 fatty acid supplementation. *Nutr.Metab.Cardiovasc.* DOI:10.1016/j.numecd.2010.04.012.

59. Plourde M., S.C.Cunnane (2007) Extremely limited synthesis of long chain polyunsaturates in adults: implications for their dietary essentiality and use as supplements. *Appl.Physiol. Nutr.Metab.* 32:619-634.

60. Prasad K. (2009) Flaxseed and cardiovascular health. *J.Cardiovasc.Pharmacol.* 54:369-377.

61. Raastad T., A.T.Hostmark, S.B.Stromme (1997) Omega-3 fatty acid supplementation does not improve maximal aerobic power, anaerobic threshold and running performance in well trained soccer players. *Scand.J.Med.Sci.Spor.* 7:25-31.

62. Raclot T., R.Groscolas, D.Langin, P.Ferre (1997) Site-specific regulation of gene expression by n-3 polyunsaturated fatty acids in rat white adipose tissues. *J.Lipid Res.* 38:1963-1972.

63. Rissanen T., S.Voutilainen, K.Nyyssonen, T.A.Lakka, J.T.Salonen (2000) Fish oil-derived fatty acids, docosahexaenoic acid and docosapentaenoic acid, and the risk of acute coronary events: the Kuopio Ischaemic Heart Disease Risk Factor Study. *Circulation* 102:2677-2679.

64. Robinson J.G., N.J.Stone (2006) Antiatherosclerotic and antithrombotic effects of omega-3 fatty acids. *Am.J.Cardiol.* 98:39i-49i.

65. Ryan A.M., J.V.Reynolds, L.Healy, M.Byrne, J.Moore, N.Brannelly, A.McHug, D.McCormack, P.Flood (2009) Enteral nutrition enriched with eicosapentaenoic acid (EPA) preserves lean body mass following esophageal cancer surgery: results of a double-blinded randomized controlled trial. *Ann. Surg.* 249:355-363.

66. Saynor R., V.Derel, T.Gillott (1984) The long-term effect of dietary supplementation with fish lipid concentrate on serum lipids, bleeding time, platelets and angina. *Atherosclerosis* 50:3-10.

67. Schacky, von C. (2007) n-3 PUFA in CVD: influence of cytokine polymorphism. *Proc.Nutr.Soc.* 66:166-170.

68. Schacky, von C., P.Angerer, W.Kothny, K.Theisen, H. Mudra, (1999) The effect of dietary omega-3 fatty acids on coronary atherosclerosis. A randomized, double-blind, placebo-controlled trial. *Ann.Intern.Med.* 130:554–562.

69. Schoeller D.A. (1995) Limitations in the assessment of dietary energy intake by self-report. *Metabolism* 44:18-22

70. Smith G.I., P.Atherton, D.N.Reeds, B.S.Mohammed, D.Rankin, M.J.Rennie, B.Mittendorfer (2010) Dietary omega-3 fatty acid supplementation increases the rate of muscle protein synthesis in older adults: a randomized controlled trial. *Am.J.Clin.Nutr.* (e-publ.).

71. Su W., P.J.Jones (1993) Dietary fatty acid composition influences energy accretion in rats. *J.Nutr.* 123(:2109-2114.

72. Sugden M.C., K.Bulmer, G.F.Gibbons, B.L.Knight, M.J.Holness (2002) Peroxisome-proliferator-activated receptor-alpha (PPARalpha) deficiency leads to dysregulation of hepatic lipid and carbohydrate metabolism by fatty acids and insulin. *Biochem.J.* 1(364 Pt 2):361-368.

73. Suzukawa M., M.Abbey, P.R.Howe, P.J.Nestel (1995) Effects of fish oil fatty acids on low density lipoprotein size, oxidizability, and uptake by macrophages. *J.Lipid Res.* 36:473-484.

74. Szygula Z. (1990) Erythrocytic system under the influence of physical exercise and training. *Sports Med.* 10:181-197.

75. Tartibian B., B.H.Maleki, A.Abbasi (2009) The effects of ingestion of omega-3 fatty acids on perceived pain and external symptoms of delayed onset muscle soreness in untrained men. *Clin.J.Sport Med.* 19:115-119.

76. Terano T., A.Hirai, T.Hamazaki, S.Kobayashi, T.Fujita, Y.Tamura, A.Kumagai (1983) Effect of oral administration of highly purified eicosapentaenoic acid on platelet function, blood viscosity and red cell deformability in healthy human subjects. *Atherosclerosis* 46:321-331.

77. Thomas, G., M.N.Hall (1997) TOR signaling and control of cell growth. *Curr.Opin.Cell Biol.* 9:782-787.

78. Thorsdottir I., H.Tomasson, I.Gunnarsdottir, E.Gisladottir, M.Kiely, M.D.Parra, N.M.Bandarra, G.Schaafsma, J.A. Martinez (2007) Randomized trial of weight-loss diets for young adults varying in fish and fish oil content. *Int.J.Obesity (London)* 31:1560-1566.

79. Trebble T.M., S.A.Wootton, E.A.Miles (2003) Prostaglandin E_2 production and T-cell function after fish-oil supplementation: response to antioxidant co-supplementation. *Am.J.Clin.Nutr.* 78:376-382.

80. Walser B., R.M.Giordano, C.L.Stebbins (2006) Supplementation with omega-3 polyunsaturated fatty acids augments brachial artery dilation and blood flow during forearm contraction. *Eur.J.Appl.Physiol.* 97:347-354.

81. Warner J.G., I.H Ullrich, M.J Albrink, R.A.Yeater (1989) Combined effects of aerobic exercise and omega-3 fatty acids in hyperlipidemic persons. *Med.Sci.Sport Exerc.* 21:498-505.

82. Whitehouse A.S., H.J.Smith, J.L.Drake, M.J.Tisdale (2001) Mechanism of attenuation of skeletal muscle protein catabolism in cancer cachexia by eicosapentaenoic acid. *Cancer Res.* 61:3604-3609.

83. Whitehouse A.S., M.J.Tisdale (2001) Downregulation of ubiquitin-dependent proteolysis by eicosapentaenoic acid in acute starvation. *Biochem.Biophys.Res.* 285:598-602.

84. Willumsen N., J.Skorve, S.Hexeberg, A.C.Rustan, R.K. Berge (1993) The hypotriglyceridemic effect of eicosapentaenoic acid in rats is reflected in increased mitochondrial fatty acid oxidation followed by diminished lipogenesis. *Lipids* 28: 683-690.

85. Yamori, Y., Y.Nara, N.Iritani, R.J.Workman, T.Inagami (1985) Comparison of serum phospholipid fatty acids among fishing and farming Japanese populations and American islanders. *J.Nutr.Sci.Vitaminol. (Tokyo)* 31:417-422.

86. Yates A., J.Norwig, J.C.Maroon, J.Bost, J.M.Bradley, M.Duca, D.A.Wecht, R.Grove, A.Iso, I.Cobb, N.Ross, M.Borden (2009). Evaluation of Lipid Profiles and the Use of Omega-3 Essential Fatty Acid in Professional Football Players. *Sports Health a Multidisciplinary Approach* 1:21-30.

87. Zammit V.A. (1999) The malonyl-CoA-long-chain acyl-CoA axis in the maintenance of mammalian cell function. *Biochem.J.* 1(343 Pt 3):505-515.

88. Zhao G., T.D.Etherton, K.R.Martin, S.G.West, P.J.Gillies, P.M.Kris-Etherton (2004) Dietary alpha-linolenic acid reduces inflammatory and lipid cardiovascular risk factors in hypercholesterolemic men and women. *J.Nutr.* 134:2991–2997.

Acknowledgment: Thanks are due to Dr Andrea Boyar for her assistance with this review

Sport and other motor activities of Warsaw students

Elżbieta Biernat

Warsaw School of Economics, Warsaw, Poland

Summary

Study aim: To assess the engagement of students of Warsaw university schools in sports and in recreational motor activities.

Material and methods: A cohort (n = 1100) of students attending B.S. or M.S. courses at 6 university schools in Warsaw were studied by applying questionnaire techniques. The questions pertained to participation in competitive sports and in recreational motor activities throughout the last year.

Results: 8% of all students participated in competitive sports, 5% were members of college athletic clubs. Over 90% of students declared practicing leisure motor activities regularly (53%), seasonally (29%) or occasionally (11%). Most differences were related to the study year, 2nd year students being more active than their 4th year mates.

Conclusions: Higher engagement of 2nd than of 4th year students in motor activities may result from obligatory, curricular physical education activities. Academic communities ought to undertake substantial effort towards shaping continuous health-directed habits of students.

Key words: Competitive sport – Motor activity - Sport for all – Students

Introduction

Popularising sports and the related attitudes and behavioural patterns is an important element of social culture. Because of their future roles in the society, including culture shaping, students ought to assume and cultivate the health-directed lifestyle, motor activities being an essential part of it [1]. An engagement in sport activities during the university studies shapes the attitudes towards motor activities [7,9] and enhances maintaining such habits in the adult age [8].

When talking of engagement in sports, it is understood in Poland as competitive sport [8], i.e. usually a club membership and participation in competitions, while in many European countries also diverse leisure motor activities are called sports [7]. Thus, population statistics contain competitive athletes together with those practicing recreational sports [3,4,14] and in this study both categories were considered. Apart from that, the activities in the "Sport for All" movement [4] were studied and presented. The aim of the study was to assess the engagement of students of Warsaw university schools in competitive sports sport for all and in recreational motor activities.

Material and Methods

Subjects: Two-stage randomising was used to select the cohort of students. First, 6 university schools were selected and then student groups (Year 2 – B.S. students and Year 4 – M.S. students) within those schools. The questionnaires were distributed at the curricular foreign language courses (Year 2) or at other lectures (Year 4), the rate of refusing to participate not exceeding 3 – 5%. A total of 511 male and 589 female students from the following schools consented to participate: Warsaw University (n = 201), Warsaw University of Technology (n = 204), University of Physical Education (n = 124), Warsaw University of Life Sciences (n = 201), Warsaw School of Economics (n = 200) and Military College of Technology (n = 170).

Methodology: The study was conducted from 2006 to 2008, always in March and November, for in those months the temperatures and precipitation were alike and, besides, in those months no increased motor activities could be expected. Standardised questionnaires were applied by direct interviews by specially trained and supervised interviewers. The questions pertained to the kind of sports practiced, numbers of training sessions

Author's address Dr Elżbieta Biernat, CWFiS, Warsaw School of Economics, al. Niepodległości 162, 02-554 Warsaw, Poland

per week, type of club and participation in competitions, types and frequency of leisure motor activities, etc.

Leisure motor activities were defined as recreational, i.e. voluntary, free-time undertaking selected sports like runs, cycling, swimming, gymnastics, etc. Regular activities meant practicing them at least once weekly for at least 5 months in a year. Seasonal activities meant practicing them many times but during summer or winter seasons only, or for e.g. weight losing. Incidental activities meant occasional practicing them 10 – 20 times a year. Sport for all meant regular engagement in competitive or recreational sports.

The SPSS 14 for Windows software was used in data analysis. Log-linear approach [14] was applied to the analysis of frequencies, the level of $p \leq 0.05$ being considered significant.

Results

The results are presented in Tables 1 – 3. Only 8.0% of all students practiced competitive sports; this included those who practiced it once (1.1%), twice (3.5%) and more than twice (3.5%) weekly, the percentage of exercising once weekly being significantly ($p<0.001$) lower from the other ones. No significant differences between genders or study years were noted.

About 16% of all students were members of various sport clubs (Table 1), significantly ($p<0.01$) more men than women (9.6 and 6.3%, respectively), the most popular ones being university clubs and fitness clubs (mainly female students). The so-called other clubs focused on dance, martial sports, horse riding, etc.

Table 1. Percentages of male and female members of sport clubs in the last year

Club type		Men n = 511	Women n = 589
Competitive sports		0.6	0.5
Fitness		0.6*	2.7 °
University		6.8 ^*	2.5 °
Other		1.6	0.5
	Total	9.6*	6.3

* Significantly ($p<0.01$) different from the respective value in women; ^ Significantly ($p<0.001$) different from other club types; ° Significantly ($p<0.01$) different from competitive sports and other clubs

As many as 92.6% of all students declared participating in leisure motor activities. No significant differences between genders or study years were noted in that respect. However, regular activities were practiced by 41 – 64.7% of students, significantly ($p<0.001$) more among those on the 2nd years of study than on the 4th but the situation was reversed in case of seasonal or occasional activities. Male students significantly ($p<0.001$) more frequently declared practicing leisure activities seasonally than did the female ones (Table 2). Significant differences were shown only for category-related contrasts, not for groups.

Table 2. Percentages of male and female students practicing leisure motor activities

Group	4th year M	4th year F	2nd year M	2nd year F
Total (n)	283	320	228	269
Regular	41.0	45.9	62.3	64.7
Seasonal	38.5	26.3	25.0	24.5
Occasional	13.4	16.9	6.1	6.7
Category	Year of study		Gender	
	4th year	2nd year	M	F
Total (n)	603	497	511	589
Regular	43.6*	63.6	50.5	54.5
Seasonal	32.0*	24.7	32.5*	25.5
Occasional	15.3*	6.4	10.2	12.2

Significantly ($p<0.001$) different from the other category

No significant gender-related differences were noted in percentages of students classified as engaged in the sport for all. On the other hand, the respective percentage of 2nd year students was significantly ($p<0.001$) higher compared with their 4th year mates (63.6 and 43.6%, respectively).

Table 3. Percentages of male and female students engaged in competitive sports

Sport / Gender	Men n = 50	Women n = 39
Fitness	4	38*
Volleyball	14	13
Combat sports	20	8
Other sports	62	41

* Significantly ($p<0.001$) different from the percentage of men

No significant gender-related differences were found in the numbers of those engaged in competitive sports (Table 3). Fitness was an exception as significantly ($p<0.001$) more female than male students practiced it. The category "other sports" included basketball, dance, swimming, sport roller skating, football, tennis and squash.

Table 4. Percentages of male and female students engaged in recreational sports

Sport \ Group	4th year M n = 263	4th year F n = 285	2nd year M n = 213	2nd year F n = 258
Swimming	33.2	48.2*	36.2	49.8*
Cycling	53.4	46.8	51.2	47.9
Fitness	0.4	40.8*	0.5	33.9*
Body building	27.1	10.6*	24.9	9.3*
Skiing	11.5	14.1	12.2	19.1*
Jogging	14.5	13.0	20.2	13.6
Football	22.9	0.4*	36.6°	1.2*
Volleyball	10.3	12.7	19.7°	16.3
Tennis	8.8	4.2*	7.5	7.0
Basketball	14.9	1.1*	18.3	3.1*

Significantly ($p<0.01$) different: * From the respective male group; ° From the respective 4th year group

Among the most popular recreational sports were swimming and cycling (men and women), fitness (women), body building and football (men). Significant differences in the declared frequencies were noted between genders or between study years as shown in Table 4.

Discussion

One of the principal objectives of university schools is to prepare students for functioning in the society, and for an active reception of and participation in (broadly speaking) culture, including physical culture. However, when inspecting physical education (PE) curricula of various university schools, obligatory PE courses last one year (Warsaw School of Economics, Warsaw University of Life Sciences) or one to 3 years, depending on the faculty (Warsaw University, Warsaw University of Technology), and for other university schools in Warsaw are only optional. In that latter case, students may participate in optional courses organised by the school or by various student associations.

As follows from the presented data, sport for all, viewed according to the tendencies in the European Union, seems to be a stable element of daily life for about half of the respondents. It should be emphasised that only those students were classified into that category who declared regular participation in competitive and/or recreational sports at least once weekly for at least 5 months in a year. The sport for all category did not include those who declared only seasonal or occasional activities.

The report of the Bridging the East-West Health Gap [5] project contained an alarming information that as many as 70% of Polish subjects practiced no physical activities. The results of other project, Eurobarometer, presented in 2004 [6] and 2010 [7], showed that nearly half of Polish population never engaged in sports or physical exercises and only about one-fourth practice regular (at least once weekly) motor activities. Sport activities were regularly undertaken predominantly by schoolchildren and students but only 36% of them met the recommended amount of motor activities [2].

In view of those reports, the participation of Warsaw students in regular sport activities may be rated as high. It ought to be remembered, however, that students are particularly aware of civilisation-related risks due to their education and prospective social positions. This supports the view that broadening knowledge enhances the health-directed behaviours, including motor activities [4,13].

The fairly high percentage of sport-practicing students, especially the 2nd year ones, might have been due to obligatory or optional PE courses; since that percentage of 4th year students was by about one-third lower, the pressure on maintaining a high level of physical education awareness by university students could be rated as evidently insufficient. That fact has a great impact on the quantitative and qualitative engagement in motor activities in later adulthood, affecting both professional and family functioning.

That socially focused question ought to be seriously considered by university managements, especially in view of their efforts to improve educational functioning, and steps should be taken to improve the accessibility of sport objects, their equipment and attractiveness.

References

1. Bourdieu P., J-C.Passeron (1970) La reproduction. Eléments pour une théorie du système d'enseignement. http://fr.wikipedia.org/wiki/La_Reproduction (08.02.2011).

2. Centers for Disease Control and Prevention. Youth Risk Behavior Surveillance - United States, 2005. Surveillance Summaries, MMWR, 2006, vol. 55 (SS-5): 1-108.

3. Definition of Sport (2010) www.google.pl/search?hl=pl&q=Definition+of+sport.+The+European+Sport+for+All+Charter+%28Council+of+Europe%2C+1980%29+divided+sport+into+four+broad+categories&lr=&aq=o&oq.

4. Dishman R.K., J.F.Sallis (1994) Determinants and interventions for physical activity and exercise. In: C.Bouchard (ed.), Physical Activity, Fitness and Health. Human Kinetics Publishers, Champaign IL, pp. 214-238.

5. Drygas W., A.Skiba, W.Bielcki, P.Puška (2001) Assessment of physical activity of inhabitants of six European countries. "Bridging East–West Health Gap" project. *Medicina Sportiva* 5(Suppl. 2):119-128.

6. European Commission (2004) Sport and Physical Activity, Special Eurobarometer 72.3. http://ec.europa.eu/public_opinion/archives/ebs/ebs_213_report_en.pdf.

7. European Commission (2010) The citizens of the European Union and Sport, Special Eurobarometer 213/62.0. http://ec.europa.eu/public_opinion/archives/ebs/ebs_334_en.pdf.

8. Gratton C. (ed.; 1999) COMPASS, UK Sports Council, British Sports Council, Italian National Olympic Committee, pp. 13-14.

9. Kraut A.S., S.Melamed, D.Gofer, P.Froom (2003) Effect of school age sports on leisure time physical activity in adults. The CORDIS Study. *Med.Sci.Sports Exerc.* 35:2038-2042.

10. McElroy M. (2002) Resistance to exercise: A social analysis of inactivity. Human Kinetics, Champaign IL.

11. Mussino A. (2010) Conceptual and operational problems in measuring participation in sport. www.stat.fi/isi99/proceedings/arkisto/varasto/muss0846.pdf .

12. Shepard R.J. (2004) A reed for more experimental studies of physical activity during childhood. Special communications: Letters to the Editor-in-Chief. *Med.Sci.Sports Exerc.* 36: 915.

13. Stephens T., C.J.Caspersen (1994) The demography of physical activity. In: C.Bouchard, R.J.Shephard, T.Stephens (eds.) Physical Activity, Fitness and Health. Human Kinetics Publishers, Champaign IL, pp. 204-213.

14. Stupnicki R. (2008) Analysis and Presentation of Questionnaire Data. University of Physical Education Editions, Warsaw, Poland.

Effects of 8-week training on aerobic capacity and swimming performance of boys aged 12 years

Ryszard Zarzeczny [1], Mariusz Kuberski [1], Agnieszka Deska [1], Dorota Zarzeczna [1], Katarzyna Rydz [1], Anna Lewandowska [2], Tomasz Bałchanowski [3], Janusz Bosiacki [3]

[1] Institute of Physical Culture and Tourism, Jan Długosz University, Częstochowa; [2] Primary School No. 36, Częstochowa; [3] Primary School No. 48, Częstochowa, Poland

Summary

Study aim: To assess the effects of 8-week endurance training in swimming on work capacity of boys aged 12 years.
Material and methods: The following groups of schoolboys aged 12 years were studied: untrained control (UC; n = 14) and those training swimming for two years. The latter ones were subjected to 8-week training in classical style (CS; n = 10) or free style (FS; n = 13). In all boys maximal oxygen uptake ($\dot{V}O_2max$) was determined, and the CS and FS groups were subjected to 6 tests: swimming at 50 and 400 m distances (time recorded) and to 12-min swimming (distance recorded), all by free and classical styles pre- and post-training. From swimming times at 50 and 400 m distances the so-called critical swimming speed (CSS) was computed: CSS = (400 – 50) / ($t_{400} - t_{50}$).
Results: No training-induced improvement in $\dot{V}O_2max$ was noted in any group. Yet, boys subjected to classical style training significantly ($p<0.05$) improved their free-style swimming velocity at CSS and at the 400 m distance by about 6%, and their heart rate following the 12-min test in classical style decreased by nearly 16% ($p<0.001$) compared with the pre-training values.
Conclusions: The 8-week training in given swimming style does not negatively affect the performance in other style than the trained one. This may be of importance in competitive training.

Key words: Swimming – Critical velocity – Physical training – Work capacity – Boys

Introduction

Anaerobic threshold, a widely used indicator of anaerobic capacity (AC) [5], has been considered more sensitive to changes in AC than maximal oxygen uptake ($\dot{V}O_2max$) [3]. Thus, anaerobic threshold, apart from reflecting the AC level, has been used in setting the training intensity which, at or slightly above the anaerobic threshold, is considered an efficient training stimulus in adults leading to augment their AC [7].

Toubekis *et al.* [10], who studied young male swimmers (mean age 12.9 years), reported a significant relationship between the so-called critical swimming speed (CSS), determined from swimming times at distances 50, 100, 200 and 400 m, and swimming speed at the lactate threshold; they suggested that CSS could be determined from two distances only – 50 and 400 m. The aim of this study was to assess the effects of 8-week training in clas-sical and free-style swimming at CSS-intensity on the performance of 12-year old boys.

Material and Methods

Subjects: Two groups of boys aged 12 years were studied: untrained control group (UC; n = 14), consisting of boys who attended only the curricular physical education classes and practiced no sports, and swimming group consisting of members of school sport clubs who practiced swimming for two years. They were assigned into two subgroups: submitted to 8-week training in classical style (CS; n = 10) or in free style (FS; n = 13). All parents submitted their signed consents to participation of their sons in the study which was approved by the local Committee of Ethics.

Methodology: All boys were subjected to the Åstrand-Ryhming's cycle ergometer test before and just after the training period. Test results served to indirectly assess the boys' maximum oxygen uptake using the equation: $Y = 1.444 + 0.522 \cdot \dot{V}O_2max$ (from a nomogram) [11]. The swimmers were additionally subjected to 6 tests: swimming at 50 and 400 m distances (time recorded) and

Author's address Prof. Ryszard Zarzeczny, Institute of Physical Culture and Tourism, Jan Długosz University, Armii Krajowej 13/15, 42-200 Częstochowa, Poland

to 12-min swimming (distance recorded), all by free and classical styles [4]. Heart rate (HR) was recorded immediately following every test. From swimming times at 50 and 400 m distances the so-called critical swimming speed (CSS) was computed: CSS = (400 – 50) / ($t_{400} - t_{50}$).

Both subgroups of swimmers trained 3 days a week, every 60-min session consisting of standard warm-up (10 min), 3 bouts of swimming at CSS, 10 min each, separated by 5-min intermissions for discussing technical errors, and relaxation (10 min).

Data analysis: The results were subjected to one- or two-way ANOVA with repeated measures followed by the Newman-Keuls' *post-hoc* test. The level of $p \leq 0.05$ was considered significant.

Results

As shown in Table 1, some significant differences were noted in body height and mass of boys over the 8-week period. Interestingly, $\dot{V}O_2max$ (maximal oxygen uptake), both absolute and relative, tended to decrease in all groups.

Table 1. Mean values (±SD) of body height and mass, and maximal oxygen uptake ($\dot{V}O_2max$) of boys aged 12 years, and of individual changes (Δ) following 8-week period (sedentary or training)

Group	Control (n = 14)		Free style (n = 13)		Classical style (n = 10)	
Variable	Pre	Δ	Pre	Δ	Pre	Δ
Body height (cm)	154.6 ± 9.7	1.8 ± 6.7**	159.5 ± 8.3	1.2 ± 1.1*	156.1 ± 9.2	2.6 ±1.3***
Body mass (kg)	49.2 ± 14.7	0.5 ± 1.7	49.7 ± 8.3	1.3 ± 2.1*	46.4 ± 13.3	0.5 ± 1.8
$\dot{V}O_2max$ (l/min)	2.32 ± 0.11	-0.08 ± 0.11*	2.41 ± 0.14	0.01 ± 0.13	2.41 ± 0.17	-0.07 ± 0.24
(ml/min/kg)	50.8 ± 14.2	-1.70 ± 1.93**	48.9 ± 7.6	-0.42 ± 3.16	54.9 ± 12.2	-1.74 ± 6.50

* $p<0.05$; ** $p<0.01$; *** $p<0.001$

Table 2. Mean values (±SD) of free-style swimming velocities and post-exercise heart rates, and of the respective individual changes (Δ) following 8-week period (sedentary or training), in boys aged 12 years

Group	Free style (n = 13)		Classical style (n = 10)	
Variable	Pre	Δ	Pre	Δ
CSS (m/s)	0.89 ± 0.12	0.01 ± 0.07	0.83 ± 0.14	0.05 ± 0.07*
50 m (m/s)	1.31 ± 0.14	-0.01 ± 0.06	1.24 ± 0.21	0.01 ± 0.08
HR_{post} (bpm)	160.7 ± 13.1	-5.7 ± 23.2	147.6 ± 23.5	23.4 ± 24.2
400 m (m/s)	0.93 ± 0.12	0.01 ± 0.06	0.86 ± 0.14	0.05 ± 0.07*
HR_{post} (bpm)	182.6 ± 13.7	-12.4 ± 18.6*	174.0 ± 24.8	3.0 ± 26.6

* $p<0.05$

Table 3. Mean values (±SD) of classical style swimming velocities and post-exercise heart rates, and of the respective individual changes (Δ) following 8-week period (sedentary or training), in boys aged 12 years

Group	Free style (n = 13)		Classical style (n = 10)	
Variable	Pre	Δ	Pre	Δ
CSS (m/s)	0.78 ± 0.09	-0.02 ± 0.04	0.75 ± 0.08	0.01 ± 0.05
50 m (m/s)	0.95 ± 0.12	0.03 ± 0.10	0.94 ± 0.12	0.04 ± 0.04
HR_{post} (bpm)	165.9 ± 15.0	-0.9 ± 21.5	139.2 ± 29.6	50.0 ± 36.2***
400 m (m/s)	0.80 ± 0.09	-0.02 ± 0.03	0.77 ± 0.09	0.01 ± 0.05
HR_{post} (bpm)	168.0 ± 10.6	6.1 ± 18.1	174.6 ± 14.6	-7.2 ± 19.1

* $p<0.05$; ** $p<0.01$; *** $p<0.001$

Table 4. Mean values (±SD) of distances covered in 12-min swimming tests and post-exercise heart rates, and of the respective individual changes (Δ) following an 8-week period (sedentary or training), in boys aged 12 years

Group Variable	Free style (n = 13) Pre	 Δ	Classical style (n = 10) Pre	 Δ
12-min FS-Test (m)	642.5 ± 109.0	-32.9 ± 76.0	575.6 ± 71.7	-4.1 ± 35.1
HR_{post} (bpm)	168.0 ± 23.1	-16.2 ± 26.3	176.0 ± 16.4	-14.0 ± 15.2
12-min CS-Test (m)	526.2 ± 93.3	4.6 ± 54.6	513.9 ± 62.0	30.8 ± 40.0
HR_{post} (bpm)	156.9 ± 13.2	-7.4 ± 15.7	183.4 ± 14.9 ##	-28.6 ± 23.2***

*** Significant increment (p<0.001); ## Significantly (p<0.01) different from the respective value in free-style group

Only few significant between-group differences were noted in the studied variables (Tables 1 – 4); boys subjected to classical style training significantly (p<0.05) improved their free-style swimming velocity at CSS and at the 400-m distance by about 6% (Table 2), and their heart rate following the 12-min test in classical style decreased by nearly 16% (p<0.001) compared with the pre-training values. Moreover, their heart rate following that latter test was significantly (p<0.01 higher pre-training than in FS group (Table 4).

Discussion

Endurance training brings about many adaptive changes in adults reflected in an increased $\dot{V}O_2max$ and in the anaerobic threshold [5]. A 10-week swimming training applied to young men increased their $\dot{V}O_2max$ in swimming tests but not in treadmill tests [6]. Those effects were attributed to differences in the environmental (position, water/land environment) and cardio-respiratory conditions and to a specific adaptation to those conditions in the training process. Those reports were not fully confirmed by the presented results which showed no improvement in swimming performance of 12-year old boys subjected to 8-week training at steady swimming speed, equivalent to the critical one (CSS), in free and classical styles; yet, that 8-week training in given style did not affect swimming performance in the test in other, untrained style.

Our results are difficult to explain unequivocally. Endurance training induces increases in $\dot{V}O_2max$ ranging 15 – 30% in adults [9] but in children such changes are none or do not exceed 6% [1]. Such small relative changes in children may be attributed to an inadequate training stimulus [1] or to insufficient motivation for regular training [8]. A random monitoring of heart rate during training (140 – 160 bpm) and immediately after having completed the 12-min swimming tests showed that the postulated [1] intensity of 80% of HRmax, necessary to increase aerobic capacity, had not been attained. It ought to be emphasised that the boys were voluntary, ambitious members of school sport clubs and the study was explained to them as part of between-club competition, thus a reduced motivation seemed rather unlikely. Still, the relatively short training period (8 weeks) might have been one of the factors responsible for the low improvement.

Training-induced effects are known to be expressed more strongly when the same kind of exercise (e.g. running) was applied throughout the training and to determining $\dot{V}O_2max$, compared with mixed exercises, both in adults and in children [1]. In this study, two swimming styles were applied for 8-week training due to the difference in energy expenditures – 0.79 and 1.29 kJ/m for the free and classical styles, respectively [2]. This, combined with the fact that the performance depends (physiologically and biomechanically) on the functional capacity and movement technique [5], led to the presumption that boys training classical style swimming would improve their performance. Such improvement was actually noted in boys training classical style swimming but only in the 400-m test performed in free style. The 8-week training in given swimming style did not negatively affect the performance in other style than the trained one; thus, the results seem to point to a general improvement in physical fitness and not in swimming technique. This may be of importance in competitive training.

References

1. Baquet G., E.Van Praagh, S.Berthoin (2003) Endurance training and aerobic fitness in young people. *Sports Med.* 33: 1127-1143.

2. Caputo F., M.F.M. de Oliveira, B.S.Denadai, C.C.Greco (2006) Intrinsic factors of the locomotion energy cost during swimming. *Rev.Bras.Med.Esporte* 12:356e-360e.

3. Faude O., W.Kindermann, T.Meyer (2009) Lactate threshold concepts: how valid are they. *Sports Med.* 39:469-490.

4. Hoeger W.W.K., S.A.Hoeger (2009) Principles and Labs for Fitness and Wellness (10th ed.), Wadsworth, Cengage Learning, Belmont CA.

5. Joyner M.J., E.F.Coyle (2008) Endurance exercise performance: the physiology of champions. *J.Physiol.* 586:35-44.

6. Magel J.R., G.F.Foglia, W.D.McArdle, B.Gutin, G.S.Pechar, F.I.Katch (1975) Specificity of swim training on maximum oxygen uptake. *J.Appl.Physiol.* 38:151-155.

7. Midgley A.W, L.R.McNaughton, A.M.Jones (2007) Training to enhance the physiological determinants of long-distance running performance: can valid recommendations be given to runners and coaches based on current scientific knowledge? *Sports Med.* 37:857-880.

8. Rowland T.W., A.Boyajian (1995) Aerobic response to endurance exercise training in children. *Pediatrics* 96:654-658.

9. Saltin B., J.Henriksson, E.Nygaard, P.Andersen, E.Jansson (1977) Fiber types and metabolic potentials of skeletal muscles in sedentary man and endurance runners. *Ann.N.Y. Acad.Sci.* 301:3-29.

10. Toubekis A.G., A.P.Tsami, S.P.Tokmakidis (2006) Critical velocity and lactate threshold in young swimmers. *Int.J. Sports Med.* 27:117-123.

11. Woynarowska B. (1980) The validity of indirect estimations of maximal oxygen uptake in children 11-12 years of age. *Eur.J.Appl.Physiol.* 43:19-23.

Acknowledgement:
Thanks are due to the Faculty of Pedagogy, Jan Długosz University, for financial support

The index of insulin resistance (FIRI) is not associated with plasma homocysteine levels in young, non-obese healthy men and women

Anna Czajkowska[1], Grażyna Lutosławska[2], Krzysztof Mazurek[3], Jadwiga Ambroszkiewicz[4], Piotr Żmijewski[5]

[1] Department of Physiology, [2] Department of Biochemistry, [3] Department of Sports Medicine, University of Physical Education, Warsaw, Poland, [4] Department of Newborn Screening, Institute of Mother and Child, Warsaw, Poland, [5]Department of Physiology, Institute of Sport, Warsaw, Poland

Summary

Study aim: To evaluate plasma homocysteine (Hcy), insulin and glucose levels in blood and the insulin resistance index (FIRI) in young, healthy non-obese men and women.
Material and methods: A total of 152 young, healthy, non-obese (BMI<30) men (n = 81) and women (n = 71) participated in the study. The following substances were assayed in blood using commercial kits: total plasma homocysteine by fluorescence polarisation immunoassay, plasma glucose – by the oxidase method, and insulin by radioimmunoassay using monoclonal antibodies. From the latter two, the index of insulin resistance (FIRI) was computed.
Results: Mean plasma homocysteine concentration in men was significantly ($p<0.001$) higher than in women (10.3 ± 3.0 and 8.4 ± 2.4 µmol/l, respectively) and that of FIRI was significantly ($p<0.001$) lower than in women (1.310 ± 0.483 and 1.437 ± 0.420, respectively). Neither in men nor in women were plasma homocysteine concentrations correlated with FIRI.
Conclusions: Although no association between circulating homocysteine and FIRI was found in young, non-obese men and women, the existence of such association in Type 2 diabetes cannot be ruled out.

Key words: Homocysteine – Insulin resistance index – Non-obese subjects

Introduction

Homocysteine (Hcy), a non-protein sulphur containing amino acid, is formed during the metabolism of dietary methionine. Under physiological conditions, Hcy is either trans-sulphurated into cysteine in a reaction catalysed by cystathionine β-synthase (CBS), or remethylated back to methionine in two reactions: folate-independent, catalysed by methionine synthase (MS), or folate-dependent, catalysed by betaine-homocysteine S-methyltransferase (BHMT), the methylenetetrahydrofolate reductase (MTHFR) playing the key role [30].

Plasma Hcy concentrations are controlled by a variety of genetic and environmental factors. It is well documented that in humans and animals, mutations in the gene encoding enzymes of Hcy metabolism, result in hyperhomocysteinaemia [4,15]. Similarly, deficiency of B-vitamins, high coffee consumption and smoking bring about elevated plasma Hcy levels [22]. In contrast, B-vitamins and folate supplementation has a potential to decrease circulating Hcy [17].

Epidemiological data and evidence from observational studies indicated that hyperhomocysteinaemia brings about several metabolic disorders, like e.g. atherosclerosis, thrombosis and endothelial dysfunction [27]. Moreover, elevated plasma Hcy levels were reported to adversely affect the pregnancy outcome, bone turnover, cognitive functions in the elderly, and recently also liver function [2,5,14,16].

There is also a wealth of studies focused on the relationship between circulating homocysteine (Hcy) and insulin resistance. However, a consensus on this association remains elusive. In Type 2 diabetic subjects, insulin resistance was identified as an independent determinant of plasma Hcy levels [8]. In addition, a population-based study on healthy, non-obese middle aged men and women, indicated that increased plasma Hcy concentrations are associated with insulin resistance [1,9]. On the other hand, no relationship between insulin resistance and circulating Hcy has been found in middle-aged men and women and in premenopausal women aged 17 – 43 years [13,26]. Moreover, the inverse

Author's address Dr Anna Czajkowska, Department of Physiology, University of Physical Education, 00-968 Warsaw 45, P.O.Box 55, Poland

relationship between plasma Hcy concentrations and insulin resistance was noted in men and women of mean age of 51 years [24].

It should be emphasised that all the cited studies focused on middle-aged subjects or on subjects characterised by highly differentiated age. However, no data concerning the relationship between plasma Hcy levels and insulin resistance in young individuals were found in the available literature. Thus, our study aimed at the evaluation of the association between plasma Hcy levels and insulin, as well as between circulating Hcy and the calculated insulin resistance index (FIRI) in college-age, healthy, non-obese men and women.

Material and Methods

Subjects: The participants were recruited by advertisements posted in student dormitories and by spreading oral information. A total of 83 college-aged men and 80 women volunteered to participate in the study. All subjects were healthy, non-smokers, not taking any regular medication and non-obese (BMI<30). All subjects qualified for the study submitted their written consents to participate in the study which was approved by the local Ethics Committee. Two men and 4 women were excluded due to insulin and glucose plasma levels exceeding relevant physiological limits, which suggested non-fasting condition, and 5 other women due to obesity (BMI>30). In consequence, data analysis was performed for 81 men and 71 women. In all subjects body mass and height were measured using standard medical scales and anthropometer; body fat content was determined using the bioelectrical impedance technique (BC 418 MA equipment, Tanita Co., Japan). Inter- and intra-assay coefficients of variation for body fat measurements did not exceed 2 %.

Methodology: Blood was withdrawn between 8:00 – 8:30 a.m. after overnight fasting from the antecubital vein into heparinised plastic tubes and immediately centrifuged for 15 min at 4000 rpm, 4^{0}C. The collected plasma was stored at -70^{0}C until assayed. Plasma glucose was determined using the oxidase method (commercial kits of Randox Laboratories, U.K.), inter and intra-assay coefficients of variation not exceeding 5%. Total plasma homocysteine was determined using fluorescence polarisation immunoassay (FPIA) (commercial kits of Abbot, USA), inter and intra-assay coefficients of variation not exceeding 5.2%. Insulin was radioimmunoassayed using monoclonal antibodies (commercial kits of BioSource, Belgium), inter and intra-assay coefficients of variation equal to 2.2 and 6.5%, respectively. All assays were run in duplicates. Insulin resistance was evaluated by homeostasis model assessment (FIRI) calculated from fasting insulin and glucose concentrations (insulin [μIU/ml] × glucose [mmol/L]/25) [7].

Data analysis: All variables proved normally distributed by the Shapiro-Wilk's test. Student's *t*-test for independent data was used to assess the between-group differences. Pearson's correlations between plasma Hcy and other biochemical variables were computed. Statistica 7.1 (Statsoft, USA) software was used in data analysis, the level of $p \leq 0.05$ being considered significant

Results

The results of the study are presented in Table 1. Plasma Hcy and glucose levels in men were significantly higher than in women ($p<0.001$ and $p<0.05$, respectively), in case of plasma insulin the situation was reversed ($p<0.001$). Mean FIRI value was significantly lower in men than in women ($p<0.001$). Neither in men nor in women was circulating Hcy correlated with insulin, glucose or FIRI values.

Table 1. Mean values (±SD) of anthropometric and biochemical variables in young non-obese men and women

	Men (n = 81)	Women (n = 71)
Age (years)	19.8 ± 0.8	19.9 ± 1.1
Body height (cm)	180.6 ± 6.1	167.3 ± 5.3
Body mass (kg)	76.6 ± 8.9	59.0 ± 7.1
BMI	23.5 ± 2.5	21.1 ± 2.2
Body fat content (%)	12.4 ± 4.5	22.1 ± 4.3
Glucose (mmol/l)	4.7 ± 0.5	4.5 ± 0.4*
Insulin (μU/ml)	6.9 ± 0.8	8.1 ± 2.4***
FIRI	1.310 ± 0.483	1.437 ± 0.420***
Homocysteine (μmol/l)	10.3 ± 3.0	8.4 ± 2.4***

Significantly different from the respective value in men: * $p<0.05$; *** $p<0.001$

Discussion

The higher Hcy levels in male than in female subjects found by us were in agreement with other data [19] and close to those reported by others for subjects of similar age [3]. The gender-related differences in plasma Hcy concentrations have not been explained; however, a higher remethylation rate of Hcy to methionine in women than in men might be, at least partially, responsible [10]. In addition, the contribution of sex hormones to the regulation of plasma Hcy concentration was discussed but, until now, the data are contradictory indicating an inverse or no correlation between plasma Hcy and female sex hormones [12,20].

No relationship between circulating Hcy and insulin resistance index (FIRI) was found in this study which was at variance with other reports [1,9] in which, however, the subjects had higher BMI values suggesting a higher body fat content than in our participants. Considering the positive relationship between plasma Hcy and body fat content, and between body fat content and insulin resistance [11,28], an indirect relationship between insulin resistance and circulating Hcy could not be ruled out. Such an assumption is supported by data which indicate that elevated plasma Hcy levels in Type 2 diabetic patients are due to insulin-induced decrease in glomerular filtration, but not to hyperinsulinemia *per se* [21]. In addition, the pharmacological improvement in insulin action does not necessarily mean decreased plasma Hcy levels [6]. Thus, it seems feasible that elevated plasma Hcy concentrations observed in hyperinsulinemic subjects do not reflect a direct relationship between insulin action and plasma Hcy concentration and correlations occur in case of complications of Type 2 diabetes. Moreover, it should be stressed that insulin *per se* has a potential to decrease plasma Hcy levels due to activation of Hcy metabolising enzymes – cystationine β-synthase (CBS), and betaine-homocysteine S-methyltransferase (BHMT) in the liver [29]. Therefore, hyperinsulinemia would directly lead to decreased circulating Hcy. On the other hand, high levels of circulating Hcy may induce insulin resistance since Hcy was found to disrupt the insulin-signalling pathway and to depress adiponectin while inducing the resistin synthesis *in vitro* and *in vivo* [18,23,25].

In conclusion, it seems that there is no association between circulating homocysteine and insulin resistance index – FIRI, at least in young, healthy non-obese men and women. However, such a relationship may develop with increasing body fat, in Type 2 diabetes and/or hyperhomocystinaemia.

References

1. Björck J., M.Hellgren, L.Rästam, U.Lindblad (2006) Associations between serum insulin and homocysteine in Swedish population – a potential link between metabolic syndrome and hyperhomocysteinemia: The Skaraborg project. *Metabolism* 55:1007-1013.

2. Cetinkaya A., B.Kantarceken, M.A.Buyukbese, M.Celik, F.I.Tolun (2007) Serum homocysteine levels in patients with non-alkoholic fatty liver disease. *Eur.J.Gen.Med.* 4:19-24.

3. Chou S.T., L.E.Ko, P.S.Lim, J.L.Huang, C.S.Yang (2000) Effect of age and sex on plasma total homocyateine in Taiwanese subjects. *Chin.J.Physiol.* 31:159-164.

4. Chwatko G., G.H.Boers , K.A.Strauss, D.M.Shih, H.Jakubowski (2007) Mutations in methylenetetrahydrofolate reductase or cystationine β-synthase gene, or a high-methionine diet, increases homocysteine thiolactone levels in humans and mice. *FASEB* 21:1707-1713.

5. Daly S., A.Cotter, A.E.Molloy, J.Scott (2005) Homocysteine and folic acid: implications for pregnancy. *Sem.Vas.Med.* 5:190-200.

6. Derosa G., A.D'Angelo, E.Fogari, S.Salvadeo, A.Gravina, I.Ferrari (2007) Effects of nateglinide and glibenclamide on prothrombotic factors in naïve type 2 diabetic patients treated with metformin: A 1-year, double–blind, randomized clinical trial. *Internal Med.* 47:1837-1846.

7. Duncan M.H., M.M.Singh, P.H.Wise, G.Carter, J.A.Alaghband-Zadeh (1995) A simple measure of insulin resistance. *Lancet* 346:120-121.

8. Emoto M., H.Kanda, T.Shoji, T.Kawagishi, M.Komatsu, K.Mori (2001). Impact of insulin resistance and nephropathy on homocysteine in type 2 diabetes. *Diabetes Care* 24:533-538.

9. Fonseca V.A., L.M.Fink, P.A.Kern (2003) Insulin sensitivity and plasma homocysteine concentrations in non-diabetic obese and normal weight subjects. *Atherosclerosis* 167:105-109.

10. Fukagawa N.K., J.M.Marin, A.Wurthman, A.H.Prue, D.Ebenstein, B.O'Rourke (2000) Sex-related differences in methionine metabolism and plasma homocysteine concentrations. *Am.J.Clin.Nutr.* 72:22-29.

11. Gallistl S., K.Sudi, H.Mangge, W.Erwa, M.Borkenstein (2000) Insulin is independent correlate of plasma homocysteine levels in obese children and adolescents. *Diabetes Care* 23:1348-1352.

12. Giltay E.J., E.K.Hoogeeven, J.M.Elbers, L.J.Gooren, H.Asscheman, C.D.Stehouwer (1998) Effects of sex steroids on plasma total homocysteine levels: a study in transsexual males and females. *J.Clin.Endocrinol.Metab.* 83:550-553.

13. Godsland I.F., J.R.Rosankiewicz, A.J.Proudler, D.G.Johnston (2001) Plasma total homocysteine concentrations are unrelated to insulin sensitivity and components of the metabolic syndrome in healthy men. *J.Clin.Endocrinol.Metab.* 86:719-723.

14. Herrmann M., T.Widmann, G.Colaianni, S.Colucci, A.Zallone, W.Herrmann (2005) Increased osteoclast activity in the presence of increased homocysteine concentrations. *Clin.Chem.* 51:2348-2353.

15. Ilhan N., M.Kucuksu, D.Kaman, N.Ilhan, Y.Ozbay (2008) The 677 C/T MTHFR polymorphism is associated with essential hypertension, coronary artery disease, and higher homocysteine levels. *Arch.Med.Res.* 39:125-130.

16. Kim J., M.N.Park, E.Kim, C.Han, S.A.Jo, I.Jo (2007) Plasma homocysteine is associated with the risk of mild cognitive impairment in elderly Korean population. *J.Nutr.* 137:2093-2097.

17. Konstantinova S.V., S.E.Vollset, P.Berstad, P.M.Ueland, C.H.A.Drevon, H.Refsum (2007) Dietary predictors of plasma total homocysteine in the Hordaland Homocysteine study. *Br.J. Nutr.* 98:201-210.

18. Li Y., C.Jiang, G.Xu, N.Wang, Y.Zhu, C.Tang (2008) Homocysteine upregulates resistin production from adipocytes in vivo and in vitro. *Diabetes* 57:817-827.

19. Lim H.S., Y.R.Heo (2002) Plasma total homocysteine, folate, vitamin B_{12} in Korean adults. *J.Nutr.Sci.Vitaminol.* 48: 290-297.

20. Nakhai-Pour H.R., D.E.Grobbee, M.Muller, M.Emmelot-Vonk, Y.T. van der Schouw (2006) Serum sex hormone and plasma homocysteine levels in middle-aged and elderly men. *Eur.J.Endocrinol.* 155:887-893.

21. Ndrepepa G., A.Kastrati, S.Braun, W.Koch, K.Kölling, J.Mehilli (2008) Circulating homocysteine levels in patients with type 2 diabetes mellitus. *Nutr.Metab.Cardiovasc.Dis.* 18: 66-73.

22. Nygard O., H.Refsum, P.M.Ueland, S.E.Vollset (1998) Major life-style determinants of plasma total homocysteine distribution: the Hordaland Homocysteine Study. *Am.J.Clin. Nutr.* 67:263-270.

23. Patterson S., P.R.Flatt, L.Brennan, P.Newsholme (2006) Detrimental actions of metabolic syndrome risk factor, homocysteine, on pancreatic β-cell glucose metabolism and insulin secretion. *J.Endocrinol.* 189:301-310.

24. Rosolovă H., J.Šimon, O.Mayer, J.Racek, T.Dierzé (2002) Unexpected inverse relationship between insulin resistance and serum homocysteine in healthy subjects. *Physiol.Res* 51:93-98.

25. Song Z., Z.Zhou, I.Deaciuc, T.Chen, C.J.McClain (2008) Inhibition of adiponectin production by homocysteine: a potential mechanism for alcoholic liver disease. *Hepatology* 47: 867-879.

26. Tanrikulu-Kiliç F., S.Bekpinar , Y.Űnlűçerci, Y.Orhan (2006) Insulin resistance is not related to plasma homocysteine concentration in healthy premenopausal women. *Physiol.Res.* 55:285-290.

27. Troughton J.A,, J.V.Woodside, I.S.Young, D.Arveiler, D.Amouyel, J.Ferriérs (2007) Homocysteine and coronary heart disease risk in the PRIME study. *Atherosclerosis* 191:90-97.

28. Tulloch-Reid M.K,, R.L.Hanson, N.G.Sebring, J.C.Reynolds, A.Premkumar, D.J.Genovese (2004) Both subcutaneous and visceral adipose tissue correlate highly with insulin resistance in African Americans. *Obes.Res.* 12:1352-1359.

29. Wijekoon E.P., M.E.Brosnan, J.T.Brosnan (2007) Homocysteine metabolism in diabetes. *Biochem.Soc.Trans.* 35:1175-1179.

30. Williams K.T., K.LShalinske (2007) New insight into regulation of methyl group and homocysteine metabolism. *J.Nutr.* 137:311-314.

17

Muscle torques of lower leg rotators in untrained subjects

Mariusz Hrycyna[1], Jacek Zieliński [2]

[1] The Halina Konopacka University of Physical Education and Tourism, Pruszków; [2] University of Physical Education, Warsaw, Poland

Summary

Study aim: To determine the relationships between muscle torques of lower leg rotators and rotation angle, and angular position at the knee joint.
Material and methods: A group of 171 untrained male subjects aged 19 – 25 years were studied. A specially designed measuring set was used. Muscle torques were determined at -30, 0 and 45° of lower leg rotation, angular positions at the knee joint being 30 or 90°.
Results: Rotation angle and angular position at the knee joint, as well as the declared laterality, significantly affected muscle torques of lower leg rotators. Highest muscle torques amounted to 55.2 ± 5.6 Nm (lower leg pronation) and 42.6 ± 7.4 Nm (lower leg supination).
Conclusions: The results may contribute to a deeper evaluation of human locomotor apparatus and to reduce the destructive forces acting on the knee joint in athletes and to improve monitoring the functions of reconstructed knee joint in rehabilitees.

Key words: Muscle torques – Knee joint – Rotation

Introduction

Muscle mechanics, including the maximum attainable muscle torques have been extensively studied [1,11] due to the need to determine the fitness of athletes which is crucial for achieving high sport results [6,14]. Determining motion ranges and muscle torques is essential for assessing the functional status of the locomotor system not only in sports but in e.g. rehabilitation monitoring [2,12,13]. Those procedures may also be useful in analysing movement techniques, including the elimination of movements potentially hazardous for the joints.

With respect to the knee joint, most studies pertained to the functions of flexors and extensors, the rotators being of marginal interest. Considering the fact that knee joint is the most prone to injuries [8], it seems that all kinds of muscles deserve thorough investigation. Thus, the aim of this paper was to determine muscle torques of lower leg rotators in relation to the angular position at the knee joint and to the rotation angle, especially to its extreme values, at which the knee joint is most prone to injuries. Further, the pronation-to-supination relation of rotator muscle torques and the effects of the declared manipulative domination of lower extremities seemed of importance.

Material and Methods

Subjects: A group of 171 untrained male university students aged 19 – 25 years were studied. They were not engaged in competitive sports and experienced no serious knee injuries. They declared to be right- or left-legged (n = 141 and 30, respectively) and were subsequently classified according to the dominating leg. The study was approved by the local Committee of Ethics.

Methodology: A specially designed measuring stand (Fig. 2) was used to measure muscle torques of lower leg rotators; special attention was put on rigidly stabilising the trunk, thigh and foot. The thigh was stabilised at two points in order to eliminate rotations at the hip joint. The trunk and hip were stabilised with clamping rings and belts, two clamping rings and a belt were applied to the foot to prevent any movement at the ankle joint.

The following axial positions at the knee joint were used, based on literature [7] and pilot trials: 30° of inward position (Fig. 1 left; one measurement in outward rotation), 0° (two measurements – inward and outward rotations) and 45° of outward position (one measurement in inward rotation); all at two angular positions at the knee joint flexion: 30 and 90° (straight leg – 0°).

Author's address Dr Mariusz Hrycyna, The Halina Konopacka University of Physical Education and Tourism, Staszica 1, 05-800 Pruszków, Poland

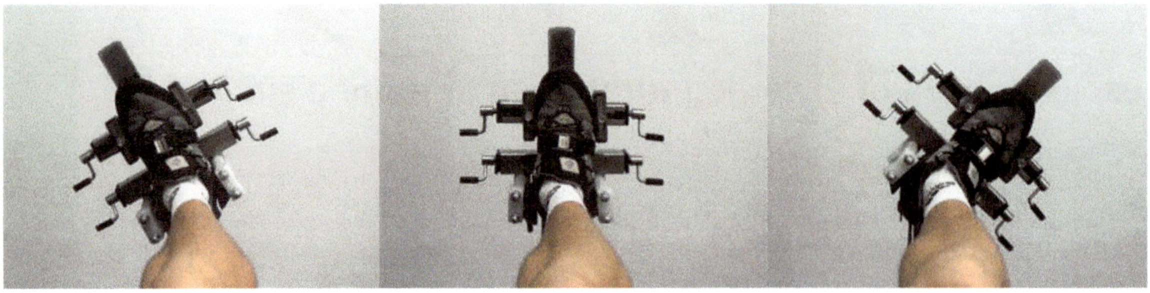

Fig. 1. Angular positions at the knee joint (-30, 0 and 45°, respectively)

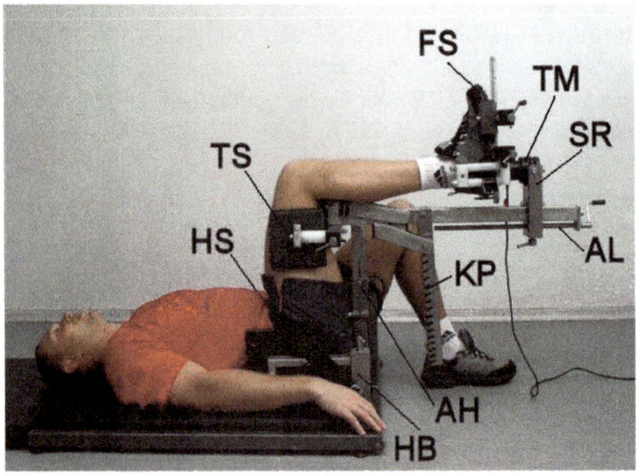

Fig. 2. Measuring stand for determining muscle torques of lower leg rotators

Legend: HS – Hip stabilisers; TS – Thigh stabilisers; FS – Foot stabilisers; TM – Torque meter; SR – Shank rotation adjustment; AL – Station arm length adjustment; KP – Knee angular position adjustment; AH – Station arm height adjustment; HB – Hip belt

The results, after having been classified into the dominating or non-dominating legs as declared by the sub-jects, were subjected to two-way ANOVA followed by the *post-hoc* Student's *t*-test for dependent data. The level of $p \leq 0.05$ was considered significant.

Results

The results are presented in Table 1 and in Figs. 3 and 4. In Table 1 are shown mean values (±SD) of anthropometric variables recorded for the dominating leg and for the difference between dominating and non-dominating legs.

Highest rotator muscle torques were recorded for the dominating leg at outward position 45° (pronation) in both knee positions, i.e. 30 and 90°, the torques amounting to 55.2 ± 5.6 and 52.4 ± 6.0 Nm, respectively. In the centred position (0°) lowest values were noted, the differences between inward and outward rotations being highly variable. Highest absolute difference amounted to 28 Nm, i.e. about 50% of the maximum mean value. Detailed values recorded for other pronation and supination rotation angles are shown in Fig. 3.

Table 1. Mean values (±SD) of anthropometric variables recorded for the dominating leg and for the difference between dominating and non-dominating legs in young, untrained male subjects (n = 171)

Variable	Means ±SD	
Age (years)	21.4 ± 1.9	
Body height (cm)	179.3 ± 5.8	
Body mass (kg)	77.8 ± 6.0	
	Dominating leg	Difference
Thigh length (cm)	42.4 ± 2.3	0.00 ± 0.07
Thigh girth (cm)	56.8 ± 3.7	-0.05 ± 0.54
Lower leg length (cm)	43.3 ± 2.2	0.00 ± 0.07
Calf girth (cm)	37.3 ± 2.1	0.04 ± 0.48
Knee width (cm)	10.0 ± 0.5	-0.01 ± 0.08

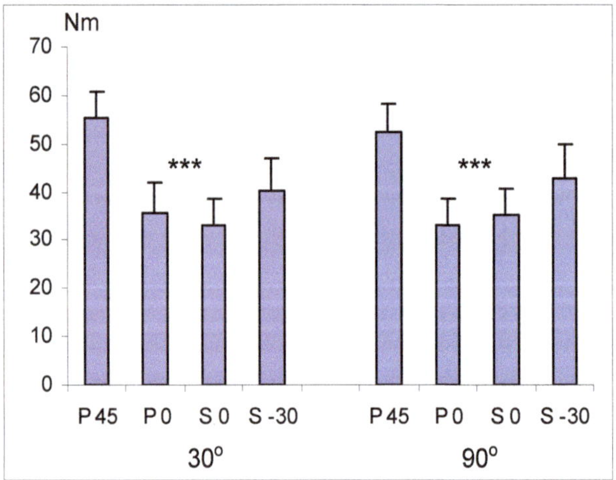

Fig. 3. Mean values (±SD) of muscle torques of lower leg rotators of the dominating leg at two angular flexions at the knee joint (30 and 90°) recorded in young, untrained male subjects (n = 171)

Legend: P – Pronation; S – Supination; The accompanying numbers are rotation angles; All values recorded at 30° significantly ($p<0.001$) differ from the respective ones at 90°; *** Significant ($p<0.001$) difference between inward (S) and outward (P) rotations at 0°

ANOVA revealed significant interaction between knee flexion angle and inward/outward rotations, thus all corresponding means were compared and proved significantly ($p<0.001$) different. Correlations of muscle torques with body mass were significant but low and ranged from r = 0.26 to 0.37.

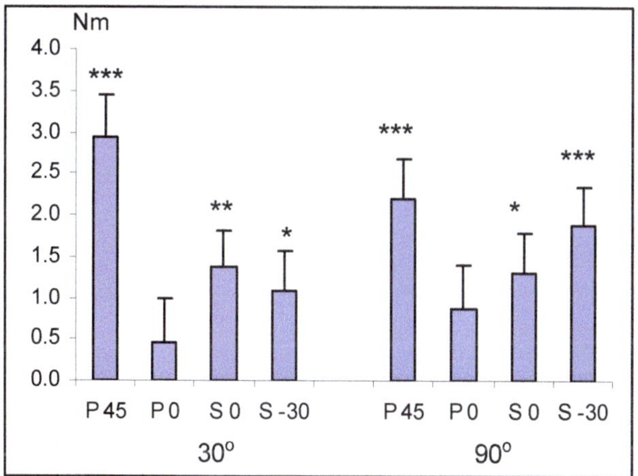

Fig. 4. Mean values (±SE) of differences between the dominating and non-dominating legs

Significant value: * $p<0.05$; ** $p<0.01$; *** $p<0.001$; For explanations of other symbols see Fig. 3

Mean differences between values for the dominating and non-dominating legs are shown in Fig. 4. The non-dominating leg was, on average, by 1 - Nm weaker from the dominant one in all cases except outward position (pronation) in both knee flexion positions. Those values were relatively alike, only those for outward position at 45° significantly differed from those at 0° ($p<0.001$ for 30° and $p<0.05$ for 90°).

Discussion

The effects of angular position at given joint on muscle torques were reported [5,9], thus the existence of optimum flexion angle at the knee joint for maximum muscle torque of lower leg rotators could be assumed. Inasmuch only few angular positions were examined in this study, highest rotator muscle torques were recorded for 45° of outward torsion and inward rotation, and for 30° of inward torsion and outward rotation, both at two flexion positions of the knee joint – 30 and 90°. This is in agreement with other reports stating that flexion angle affects the length of adjoining muscles and, thus, the power output [9]. Specifically, angular flexion at the hip joint had no significant effect on muscle torques of knee extensors in contrast to knee flexors. For the latter, highest values were recorded for 90° at the hip joint and 45° at the knee joint; highest values for knee extensors were recorded for knee angle equal to 75° [9]. Also other authors [15] reported that angular position at the hip joint (0 or 90°) had no effect on muscle torques of knee extensors in women, the knee angle amounting to 90°. Since most of the lower leg rotators are biarticular, their principal function being knee flexion, changes in angular position at the hip joint affect muscle length and their torques.

Muscle torques of knee flexors or extensors are severalfold higher than those of lower leg rotators. At knee position equal to 90°, muscle torques of knee extensors and flexors average 281 and 190 Nm, respectively [4], and of rotators – about 52 Nm. That big difference is due to different muscle functions; leg movements in the sagittal plane are under the load of the entire body mass while lower leg rotations are under the load of the mass of lower leg and foot which amounts to about 7% of total body mass [3]. Lower leg rotators are thus chiefly responsible for an active stabilisation of the knee joint and protect ligaments, especially the cruciate one, from damages. Muscle torques in inward rotation were by about 20% lower than in the inward lower leg rotation which could be due to differences in the numbers of muscles engaged in those movements.

Some authors [10] found no significant correlation between muscle torques of knee flexors and extensors and body mass, others [4] confirmed that for extensors only, the correlation coefficient for flexors amounting to 0.44. The respective correlation coefficients for rotator muscles found in this study, not exceeding the value of 0.37, were relatively high considering the fact that the loads in lower leg rotation amount to only 7% of body mass. It was also demonstrated that leg lateralisation had a significant effect on rotator muscle torques.

In conclusion, the results may contribute to a deeper evaluation of human locomotor apparatus and to reduce the destructive forces acting on the knee joint in athletes (e.g. in football or handball). The results may also contribute to improve monitoring the functions of the knee joint in rehabilitees since shaping the thigh girth or recovery from deep sensory disorders are not sufficient in preventing future injuries of that joint.

References

1 Anderson D.E., M.L.Madigan, M.A.Nussbaum (2007) Maximum voluntary joint torque as a function of joint angle and angular velocity: model development and application to the lower limb. *J.Biomech.* 40:3105-3113.

2. Beynnon B.D., B.C.Fleming, R.J.Johnson, C.E.Nichols, P.A.Renstrom, M.H.Pope (1995) Anterior cruciate ligament strain behavior during rehabilitation exercises in vivo. *Am.J. Sports Med.* 23: 24-34.

3. Braun W., O.Fischer (1889) Über den Schwerpunkt des Menschlichen Körpers mit Rücksicht auf die Ausrüstung der deutschen Infanteristen, Abhl.Koenigl.Sachs.Ges.Wiss. 15:H2.

4. Buśko K. (1997) Topography of muscle torques In men and women. *Biol.Sport* 14:32-36.

5. Hill A.V. (1922) The maximum work and mechanical efficiency of human muscles, and their most economical speed. *J.Physiol.* 14:19-41.

6. Janiak J., J.Eliasz, J.Gajewski (1997) Maximal static strength of lower limbs and the parameters of the vertical jump. *Biol.Sport* 14:65-70.

7. Kapandji I.A. (1970) Annotated Diagrams of the Mechanics of the Human Joints. The Physiology of the Joints. E&S Livingstone, Edinburgh and London.

8. Kwiatkowski K., J.Zielinski, R.Pitrus, J.Płominski (1997) Changes in axial rotation and muscle torque at the knee joint with damaged anterior cruciate ligament. *Biol.Sport* 14:307-311.

9. Ostrowska E., C.Urbanik, A.Mastalerz, D.Iwanska, A.Madej (1999) Influence of angular position in hip joint on isometric muscle torque values of knee flexors and extensors. *A.Bioeng. Biomech.* (Proc. 4th Polish Conference „Biomechanics 99") 1:353-356.

10. Pietraszewski B., J.Zawadzki, J.Pietraszewska, A.Burakiewicz (1997) Body composition and muscle torques of lower limbs. *Biol.Sport* 14:104-107.

11. Surakka J., A.Virtanen, S.Aunola, K.Maentaka, H.Pekkarinen (2005) Reliability of knee muscle strength and fatigue measurements. *Biol.Sport* 22:301-313.

12. Ścigała K. (1997) Biomechanics of the knee joint instability. *Biol.Sport* 14:266-270.

13. Szulc P., J.Mączynski, B.Marecki (1997) Comparison of various techniques of measuring elbow joint angles. *Biol.Sport* 14:139-143.

14. Trzaskoma Z., P.Lipinski (1997) Maximal power and maximal strength of lower limbs of athletes aged 16-18 years. *Biol.Sport* 14:156-161.

15. Wit A., A.Kosmol, A.Kudera, M.Wychowanski (1999) Knee muscle function assessment. *A.Bioeng.Biomech.* (Proc. 4th Polish Conference „Biomechanics 99") 1:559-567.

18

Psychological gender of women taking up typically masculine sports activity

Joanna Burdzicka-Wołowik

Department of Psychology, The Jozef Pilsudski University of Physical Education in Warsaw, Faculty of Physical Education and Sport in Biala Podlaska, Poland

Summary

Study aim: To examine which gender scheme is used by women who take up stereotypically masculine sports activity and to obtain an answer to the question of whether these subjects achieve higher results on the masculinity scale and lower results in femininity than women who practise other sports and women who do not take up any sports activity. Do women who practise masculine sports achieve a higher sports class and self-evaluate their results better if they identify with a masculine image?
Material and methods: 90 women participated in the research: 30 sportswomen who practise masculine sports (judo, boxing, wrestling); 30 women training in gymnastics, swimming and basketball; and 30 women not taking up any sports activity. The research utilized the inventory of psychological gender assessment (IPP) by Kuczynska and a questionnaire prepared by the author.
Results: The analysis of the results revealed that individuals taking up sports activity are to a large extent androgynic, while as far as masculine sports are concerned, a masculine gender scheme dominates. Women practising masculine sports gain significantly higher masculinity indices and lower femininity indices when compared to the remaining subjects. Simultaneously it was not proved whether individuals with a higher intensity of masculinity achieved a higher sports class or whether they self-evaluated their sports skills better.
Conclusions: Women that take part in sport activities considered by society as masculine, identify themselves with masculine and androgynic gender schema.

Key words: Psychological gender – Women – Masculine sport – Sports activity

Introduction

Until recently gender had been treated as an obvious construct in which a woman is feminine and a man is masculine. Human intuition enables us to differentiate women from men, which is facilitated by build, haircut, or clothes. The most frequent definition of gender we can encounter is the collection of features that allow for the creation of female and male gametes, fertilisation, and raising offspring. Biological gender is determined by two chromosomes, X and Y. Genetic differences determine the physiology, morphology, and anatomy of an individual. Additionally, attention is paid to the fact that biological gender may determine psychological gender, revealing itself in interests and social behaviour, and thus in a definite masculine or feminine type of features of an individual.

Contemporary science enables us to distinguish several types of gender, i.e., chromosomal, gonadal, hormonal, internal and external genital, phenotypic, metabolic, as well as social and mental gender. The latter two, owing to the needs of this work, will be presented in more detail. Biological gender enables an individual to reproduce; however, gender is not only reproduction. Any belief in what a woman is allowed to do and what a man is allowed to do is not the result of biological gender but rather from an opinion that a man and a woman are completely different individuals [16]. In the literature of psychology and sexology more and more space is devoted to the issue of psychological gender. Psychology deals with imitation and identification in the area of an individual's identification with gender, while sexology deals with the connection that individuals feel with their gender. Psychological gender is defined as the collection of mental features connected with gender created from early childhood, as well as the participation of an individual in social activity. Psychological gender determines the undertaken activity and constructive behaviour. The issue of gender identity was shown by Bem in her gender schema theory [2]. According to the theory, while assimilating contents from society we acquire information connected

Author's address Joanna Burdzicka-Wołowik, Department of Psychology, Faculty of Physical Education and Sport, Akademicka 2, 21-500 Biała Podlaska, Poland

with gender, and then we store it accordingly and create a cognitive gender scheme. These schemes determine facts that we perceive and remember. While learning the contents of the aforementioned schemes we get to know the distinguishing features of our gender. We learn what is feminine and what is masculine but we also examine different applications of the same attribute. We assess ourselves according to the scheme and behave in accordance with the scheme of masculinity or femininity. The profile of an individual is based on the attributes used, and on the preferred behaviour and gender. The research by Bem [2] showed that sexually defined individuals cluster information easily in the categories of masculinity or femininity. Approximately forty years ago it was believed that psychological gender could be presented as a continuum with two poles: masculinity and femininity. According to the author of this theory these are not two poles of the same continuum but two separate dimensions of personality, which allows for possessing both masculine and feminine features and creating an androgynic individual [5,6]. The undertaken research and theoretical assumptions made it possible to select four types of individuals: sexually defined individuals (compliance of psychological and biological gender, i.e., feminine women and masculine men), androgynic individuals (with a similar intensity of masculine and feminine features), sexually non-defined individuals (a weak intensity of masculine and feminine features), and transversely defined individuals (masculine women and feminine men). Owing to the fact that the basis for the typology is constituted by the connection of biological gender and mental features with stereotypes in a particular culture, the conventionality of the individuals with compliant biological and psychological gender and non-conventionality of the androgynic individuals is assumed. On the basis of theoretical assumptions and published results of the research by Bem [2,14], it can be concluded that sexually defined individuals undertake activity compliant with gender scheme more frequently than androgynic individuals. Moreover, when obliged to behave in a way not proper for their gender scheme, they feel irritated and their verbal behaviour is more compliant with gender scheme than in the case of androgynic individuals. Additionally, sexually defined individuals diversify people according to physical attractiveness and reveal considerable liveliness in contacts with attractive people. Bem [2] also revealed that androgynic humans are not socially influenced and have higher possibilities of constructive behaviour; thus, this gender type was accepted as an optimal model.

There occur apparent differences in the undertaken activity, as well as sports activity, between individuals of both genders. In numerous societies the superiority of a man over a woman is accepted; thus, dominance was recognised as a typically masculine feature. We distinguish the following four spheres in which men play the main roles: society in general, social roles, politics and business, and inter-group relations, e.g., international relations. Stereotypes encourage people to undertake particular activity. A liberal, altruistic, and empathic woman satisfies her needs in family, whereas a dominant, strong, and sometimes bossy man finds his place in leadership positions [16]. A woman's fears are connected with the lack of family, partner, and children. There occurs a strong need for contact with surroundings and social relations. A woman's personality does not often match the model of successful people. According to common opinion, the ideal of success is a masculine scheme. However, women exist who decided to oppose this view and they took up an activity that is not adequate to their gender, i.e., sport [7]. Every day a larger and larger percentage of women take up activities requiring physical contact, e.g., wrestling, physical effort (e.g., in weight-lifting), or fighting (e.g., in boxing). These women have to learn how to oppose criticism [10,11,15] and how to take up activities leading to success. The aforementioned fact may appear to be positive, since, as my research presented at the International Conference "Contemporary Problems in Women's Sport" proved, such activity among the female part of society leads to the fact that women shape type-B personality in this way. They become better adapted to coping in society, more emotionally balanced and open to the world. With a growing number of women in masculine sports, social acceptance of such activity of women grows; together with the growing acceptance, a particular sport ceases to be perceived as solely masculine.

The aim of the study was to identify which gender scheme is used by women who take up stereotypically masculine sports activity. Do these women achieve higher results in masculinity scale and lower results in femininity than women practising other sports or women not taking up any sports activity? Is there a statistically significant difference as far as a femininity and masculinity index is concerned between women training in typically masculine sports and women training in sports that are socially accepted as feminine, e.g., gymnastics and swimming? Is there any connection between the intensity of masculine features in respondents from group 1 (training a masculine sport) and the sports class as well as the self-evaluation of their sports skills and achievements?

Material and Methods

The research was carried out in 2010-2011 during sports camps. Ninety women divided into three research groups participated in the research. The first group (n=30) included female boxers (n=15), judokas (n=7), and wrestlers (n=8), i.e., athletes practicing sports that are perceived by society as typically masculine. Among them there were 13 athletes in the so-called master sports class, 16 athletes with lower classes, and only 1 athlete without any sports class. The second group included respondents (n=30) taking up neutral sports activity. They were highly qualified swimmers (n=9), gymnasts (n=10), and basketball players (n=11). This group included 26 athletes with master sports class, 1 athlete with the first class, and 3 athletes without any sports class. The third group included women (n=30) who do not deal with sport at all. They were students at the State School of Higher Education in Biala Podlaska who were studying at the faculties not connected with sport. Two groups of students were randomly selected and afterwards those students who do not participate in sports activity were chosen in these groups. All the examined women were adults with an average age of 20.9 ± 3.0 years. The oldest women were athletes practicing neutral sports whose average age was 21.2 ± 3.2 years, while the youngest ones practicing masculine sports, 20.5 ± 2.7 years.

In the research the following methods were used:

- Inventory of psychological gender assessment (IPP), by Alicja Kuczynska. This method enables the researcher to define one of the four types of psychological gender. It may be used for individual and group research. The inventory of psychological gender is built from 35 items, including 15 items concerning stereotypical femininity (femininity scale), 15 concerning stereotypical masculinity (masculinity scale), and 5 concerning neutral statements that characterise men and women to a similar extent. The sheet includes instructions according to which a respondent marks the extent to which the statement describes him or her. Answers should be given by marking one of five possible values beginning from "I'm not like that" (1) through intermediary answers to "I'm exactly like that" (5).

- A personal questionnaire created by the author, which makes it possible to collect basic data about the respondents. The questionnaire included 15 questions concerning age, level of education, place of living, sports experience, and sports class of the respondents. Additionally, it included questions concerning successes and the self-evaluation of sports results and skills in the 5-grade scale, where 1 means very low and 5 means very high.

The obtained results were then analysed statistically using the SPSS 17.0 software. The results were compared by using one-way analysis of variance (ANOVA) followed by the Duncan's test (*post hoc*). Pearson's correlation was used to assess relationships between the studied variables in group of women practicing masculine sports. In all analyses the level of $\alpha = 0.05$ was considered significant.

Results

On the basis of the research results it can be observed that the highest percentage of all the respondents included women using an androgynic gender scheme (46.7%). Women achieving a high result both in masculinity and in femininity constituted nearly a half of the respondents. The second-biggest group included feminine women, who constituted nearly one-quarter of the respondents (24.4%). Individuals defined transversely, i.e., masculine women, took the third position (22.2%). The smallest group included respondents who had a low level of both masculine and feminine features (sexually non-defined people) (6.7%).

While comparing types of gender identity in the three examined groups, the highest index of androgyny was revealed among women taking up physical activity which is associated exclusively with men (group 2), while the lowest number of individuals describing themselves as ones who possess both masculine and feminine features was found in the group of women not taking up any sports activity. Due to the type of the research question, it is worth highlighting that the biggest number of masculine women was found in the group of respondents who train sports stereotypically associated with a male part of the society on an everyday basis. The lowest percentage of women who identify with a masculine gender scheme occurred in the group of women not practising any sport. In this group feminine women constituted as much as 60%. It is worth highlighting that women identifying with typically feminine features were not found in the group of women training such sports as judo, boxing, and wrestling (group 1). The description of the respondents seems interesting since the largest number of women identifying with a masculine gender scheme can be found in the group of women practising stereotypically masculine sports while in the group of women practising other sports the biggest percentage is comprised of androgynic individuals. However, as far as women who don't take up any sports activity are concerned, the highest level of correlation between a psychological and biological gender is revealed. Therefore, it may be pointed out that in the examined group of women practising various sports, the biggest number is comprised of androgynic and masculine individuals, whereas the lowest number by feminine women. An analogous situation can be observed in the group of women not taking up any sports activity. The largest group includes women identifying with stereotypically feminine features and the lowest number of ladies expressed the concept of their personality as masculine (Figure 1).

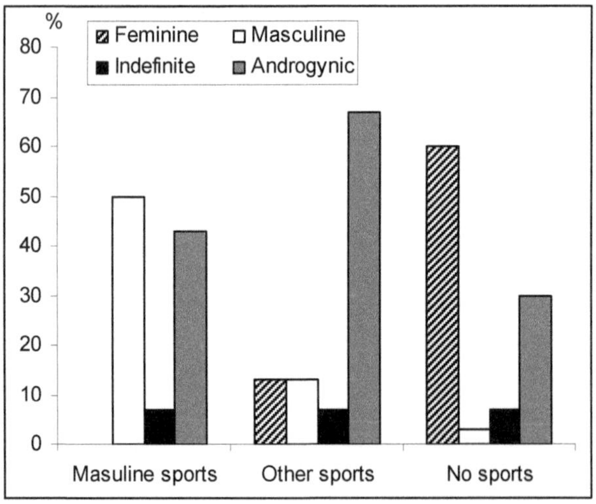

Fig.1. The types (%) of gender identity among women training masculine, other or not practicing any sports (n = 30 in each group)

The analysis of variance ANOVA (variables had a normal distribution) revealed that there exist highly significant differences in the intensity of masculinity ($F_{2, 87} = 22.2$; $p<0.001$) and femininity index ($F_{2, 87} = 11.9$; $p<0.001$) in the subjects. Women taking up masculine sports activity have a significantly lower femininity index than women training in other sports and a highly significantly lower index than women not practising any sports who have the highest femininity index (59.5±5.1; Table 1). As far as masculinity index is concerned, the situation is similar, i.e., women taking up masculine sports activity have a significantly higher masculinity index than the remaining groups ($p<0.01$). Additionally, women not taking up sports activity have a significantly lower masculinity index than the remaining ones.

Table 1. Mean values (±SD) and ranges of femininity and masculinity indices recorded in women training a masculine sport (MS; n = 30), other sports (OS; n = 30) and in women not taking up any sports activity (NS; n = 30)

Variable	MS	OS	NS
Femininity index	52.0±7.0 (38÷67)	55.6±5.6* (46÷66)	59.5±5.1** # (47÷68)
Masculinity index	57.5±6.2 (47÷70)	53.4±6.9* (38÷65)	47.1±5.0** ## (37÷57)

Significantly different from MS group: * $p<0.05$; ** $p<0.01$;
Significantly different from OS group: # $p<0.05$; ## $p<0.01$;

In a further part of the analysis, it was checked whether differences exist in the intensity of masculine and feminine features between those women training masculine sports and those women practising sports that are perceived by society as more feminine (only gymnasts and swimmers were taken into account, n = 19). Significant differences between the groups were observed, regarding the femininity index ($F_{1, 47} = 5.09$; $p<0.05$) and the masculinity index ($F_{1, 47} = 6.29$; $p<0.05$). Indeed, as compared with women training typical masculinity disciplines, those involved in feminine sports have higher values of femininity scale (52.0±7.0 and 56.3±5.6, respectively) and lower values of masculinity scale (57.7±6.2 and 52.5±7.6, respectively).

In the group of women training in masculine sports, no significant correlation was found between the intensity of masculinity and other features such as a sports class, self-evaluation of one's own skills, evaluation of sports achievements, and number of successes.

Discussion

It was observed in the research that the highest percentage of all respondents is comprised of androgynic individuals. It is the most desirable scheme of gender identity. In order to function efficiently in a society and to fulfil their roles, contemporary humans must possess features of their own gender as well as features of the opposite gender. An androgynic woman is factual, assertive and rational at work, and empathic and sensitive at home. The domination of androgynic respondents is visible in two groups that are connected with sports activity. Most probably the participation in sport makes an individual more androgynic and masculinises her gender identity. When a woman enters the sphere of sport, she creates numerous masculine features and learns masculine behaviours, as opposed to men, who only master them [13,11]. Therefore, it may be predicted that a woman's sports career depends on the creation of both masculine and feminine features [8,18]. Cashmor also noted that sportswomen must create many masculine features in order to achieve more [4]. An androgynic sportswoman is flexible and can adapt to changeable, frequently stressful situations [1,3,12]. The lowest percentage of androgynic individuals was revealed in the group of women not taking up any sports activity. Sport makes a woman learn masculine behaviours and create features non-compliant with the femininity stereotype [17]. Being able to use a masculine repertoire of behaviours becomes a factor determining effective sports activity [12]. Masculine features facilitate achieving success in sport.

In the literature of the subject, claims concerning a wide spectrum of behaviours of a contemporary woman can be found. Sports activity is not limited to the stereotypical feminine model on condition that there is no pressure from the surroundings. Research by Terelak and Siołkowska [20] did not confirm the assumption concerning a more frequent occurrence of androgynic and masculine women among sportswomen than non-training women and did not allow for the conclusion that one type is the dominating one among women not practising sport [20]. The results of the research do not correspond to the aforementioned conclusions. The research revealed that a correlation between biological gender and sports activity exists. In fact, among women dealing with masculine sports, the largest group included ladies identifying with a masculine gender, while there were no typically feminine women. Women training in masculine sports had a significantly lower femininity index than women training in other sports and highly significantly lower than women not practising sport. This fact may result from the requirements that are set for women training in boxing, wrestling, and judo. The effect of sports activity depends here on masculine features such as strength, endurance, agility, "sports anger", persistence, and aggression [9,19].

Summing up, women taking up masculine sports activity identify mainly with a masculine and androgynic gender scheme. Moreover, women practising masculine sports have a lower femininity index than women training in other sports and much lower index than women not practising any sport. It turned out that women who don't practise sports are the most feminine in terms of psychological gender. Women training in swimming and gymnastics basically use an androgynic gender schema and they less identify with masculine features than women training wrestling, boxing, and judo.

References

1. Anshel M.H., A.Porter, J.J.Quek (1998) Coping with acute stress in sport as a function of gender: An exploratory study. *J.Sport Behav.*, 21:363-369.
2. Bem S.L. (1974) The measurement of psychological androgyny. *J.Consult.Clin.Psychol.*, 42:155-162.
3. Burke K.L. (1986) Comparison of psychological androgyny within a sample of female college athletes who participate in sports traditionally appropriate and traditionally inappropriate for competition by women. *Percept.Mot.Skills*, 63:779-782.
4. Cashmor E. (2002) Sport Psychology. The Key Concepts. Routledge, London.
5. Fallon M.A., L.M.Jome (2007) An exploration of gender – role expectation and conflict among women rugby players. *Psychol.Women Quart.*, 31: 311-321.
6. Gierowski J., A.Porańska (2007) Dependencies between psychological gender, empathy, and interpersonal relations in juvenile girls and boys. *Problems.Forensic.Sci*, 72:379-403.
7. Giuliano T.A., K.L.Turner, J.C.Lundguist, J.L.Knight (2007) Gender and the selection of public athletic role models. *J.Sport Behav.*, 30:161-198.
8. Hartman, D. (2003) What can we learn from sport if we take sport seriously as a racial force? Lessons from C.L.R.James's, Beyond a Bounduary. *Ethnic.Racial Stud.*, 26(3):451-483.
9. Koivula N. (2001) Perceived characteristics of sports categorized as gender-neutral, feminine or masculine. *J.Sport Behav.*, 24: 377-393.
10. Krane V., P.Y.L.Choi, S.M.Baird, C.M.Aimar, K.J.Kauer (2004) Living the paradox: Female athletes negotiate femininity and muscularity. *Sex Roles*, 50:315-329.
11. Lantz C.D., P.J.Schroeder (1999) Endorsement of masculine and feminine gender roles: Differences between participation in and identification with the athlete role. *J.Sport Behav.*, 22:545-557.
12. Mroczkowska H. (2007) Conformity with the pattern of maleness and cognitive – motivational determinants of aspirations for success in women. *Biol.Sport*, 2:275-284.
13. O' Reilly J, S.K.Cahn (2007) Women and Sports in the United States. Northeastern University Press, New England.
14. Ozkan T., T.Lajunen (2005) Masculinity, femininity, and the Bem Sex Role Inventory in Turkey. *Sex Roles*, 52:103-111
15. Pedersen D.M., D.M.Kono (1990) Perceived effects on femininity of the participation of women in sport. *Percept.Mot. Skills,* 71:783-792.
16. Pratto F. (1996) Sexual politics: The gender gap in the bedroom, the cupboard, and the cabinet. In: D.M.Buss, N.Malamuth (eds.) Sex, Power and Conflict: Evolutionary and Feminist Perspectives. Oxford University Press, New York: 179-230.
17. Salminen S. (1990) Sex role and participation in traditionally inappropriate sports. *Percept.Mot.Skills*, 71:1216-1218.
18. Soroka A, J.Bergier (2011) Sense of gender identity in women practicing football with consideration of the formation. *Pol.J.Sport Tourism*, 18:45-58.
19. Terelak J., A.Górecki (2010) Relationship between personality traits and sporting success of judo athletes (in Polish). *Kultura Fiz.*, 5-8:1-9.
20. Terelak J., M.Siołkowska (2008) Physiological gender and aggressiveness in women practicing team sports (in Polish). *Kultura Fiz.*, 7-8: 1-11.

External and internal sport motivations of young adults

Sándor Bollók [1], Johanna Takács [2], Zsuzsanna Kalmár [1], Beáta Dobay [3]

[1] Semmelweis University, Faculty of Physical Education and Sport Sciences, Budapest; [2] Semmelweis University, Institute of Behavioural Sciences, Budapest, Hungary; [3] Selye University, Department of Physical Education, Komarno, Slovakia

Summary

Study aim: To determine and evaluate the spectrum of sport motivation of young adults.
Material and methods: A group of 600 subjects, aged 17 – 19 years, participated in the study. An *ad hoc* questionnaire was applied to assess the 4 motivational factors: competition and success-oriented motivation, external accommodation, physical fitness and health + sportsman-like attitude, and hedonistic.
Results: Competition, contest, victory and beating own benchmark were the important factors for male students. The female students preferred external adequacy and others' opinion. They believed in the importance of healthy living, physical strength and sports give them better appearance. The motivational factors had more importance amongst active than inactive youths. Young active students believed that sport performance would guide them to success.
Conclusions: It is important to keep healthy lifestyle and sport motivation before teenage years since it is a guidance to preserve the health and adequate personality development.

Key words: Exercise motivation – Intrinsic/extrinsic motivation – Adolescents – Individual sports – Team sports

Introduction

One of the prime questions of psychology is what are the driving motives behind human behaviour, why are we able to mobilise huge energy for certain actions and unable to do so for other ones. In the world of sport, motivation is one of the most frequently used words determining the degree of body activation, organisation and efficiency of behaviour.

Successes in sports are influenced not only by cognitive and motor skills but also by the motivational background of an individual. Sport activity, like any other health behaviour, is linked to early childhood patterns when sport-related motivations are established. Adolescence is a critical period from the point of view of sport motivation, as the youths undergo significant biological and psychological changes; however, their system of values is still unsettled and as a result their sport activity level decreases [5,9].

Two basic types of motivations – the intrinsic and extrinsic orientation have been discerned [2]. Extrinsic motivation is affecting behaviour through influences independent of personality, e.g. verbal praise, rewarding with an object, acknowledgement; verbal scolding, punishment, forbidding participation do not thus serve the satisfaction of needs, rather they play an important role in the adjustment to the expectations of the environment.

Intrinsic motivations serve the satisfaction of needs, irrespective of the expectations of the environment; hence the purpose of behaviour is not an external factor, but the behaviour itself. In intrinsically motivated activities the satisfaction of needs is continuous, they originate from the self. Extrinsic factors are required from the viewpoint of sporting skills, through them the athlete is capable of adjusting to external expectations. These rules are understood as a part of his/her own internal world and it is through this internal system of relations they become able to adjust to expectations, rules, while allowing them to form an objective image of their abilities [12].

As a matter of fact, the intrinsic-extrinsic orientation is strongly related to several socio-demographical factors. In adulthood, intrinsic motivation is significantly stronger, especially health motivation, than it is in the childhood. There is a wider spectrum of motivations affecting the youth: extrinsic and intrinsic, social and psychological influences which equally affect their sport-related behaviour and decisions. The most frequent are social motivations, popularity, fun, better psychological shape, good looks, athletic build. Social environment has a decisive influence on individual's motivation.

Author's address Dr Sandor Bollok, Táborhegyi út 16.D/24, H-1037 Budapest, Hungary

The importance of the environment was highlighted by Ames and Archer [1], who also identified 2 objectives – the ego performance and the task/mastery. According to Nicholls [8], individuals, in order to become successful, shape their performance themselves; the task-oriented environment increases motivation and self-confidence in sports. Other studies also demonstrated that in cases of task-oriented athletes, positive emotions and higher self-consciousness, and an objective perception of own performance can be observed [4,6].

According to Vlachopoulos [14], athletes with high intrinsic motivation have better self-appreciation and are more successful in their activities compared with their intrinsically less motivated mates. On the whole, task-oriented, environment-motivates athletes, in addition to being able to afford higher performance levels, are not adversely affected by long preparation. On the other hand, ego-oriented individuals compare their abilities with those of others or, if they have to perform well, they become overwhelmed by worries and tension [7]. In addition to the environmental social factors, gender plays a decisive role in sports, in the area of motivation. In case of girls, intrinsic motivation is more prevalent; they more often enjoy sports than having fun or social get-together. In case of boys, testing their abilities, the chance to display strength, competition, achieving success, constitute the dominant motivational effect [13].

In this study, 4 sport motivational factors, as specified by Piko *et al.* [11], were investigated. The first factor – the competition- and success-oriented motivation, which is primarily linked to extrinsic motivation, i.e. motives related to sport competitions and victories, is considered the most significant one. The second factor includes intrinsic motivations, which are mostly linked to physical shape, health and body shape, i.e. physical fitness, health and athletic attitude. The extrinsic accommodation motivational factor which clearly assumes extrinsic influences, a compliance with requirements set by the school and the parents, is the third factor. The fourth factor consists of social motivational influences, such as entertainment, circle of friends, cheering. This is the hedonistic motivational factor.

The aim of this study was to determine and evaluate the spectrum of sport-related motivation of young adults with emphasis on what motivational factors characterise youth, and how the sport-related motivation is determined by social factors such as gender or preferences for individual or team sports.

Material and Methods

The study was an empirical survey. A group of 347 male and 253 female youths aged 17 – 19 years, randomly selected from all Hungarian schools, participated in the study. Their distribution by residence contained the capital (21.5%), other towns (38.8%), villages (39.5%) and farms (0.2%). A specially designed questionnaire was administered; it contained 5 dimensions: appearance, social consciousness and adaptation, healthy diet, sport and sport habits, addictions (tobacco, alcohol, drugs). The 69 items related to sport and sport habits were classified into 4 motivational factors:

1. Competition- and success-oriented motivation (15 items);
2. Physical fitness, health and sportsman-like attitude factor (18 items);
3. External accommodation motivational factor (22 items) and
4. Hedonistic motivational factor (15 items).

The SPSS 15.0 for Windows software was used in data analysis. Non-parametric methods: Mann-Whitney's U-test and Kruskal-Wallis' H-test were used, the level of $p \leq 0.05$ being considered significant.

Results

Those who reported being engaged in exercising regularly, i.e. at least 3 times a week for an hour, constituted 48.3% of the sample; 43% preferred individual sports and 57% - team games. The results of the survey are presented in Table 1 and in Figs. 1 – 3.

The important factors for male subjects were competition, contest and victory, their female peers preferring external adequacy and opinions of others – of the coach, fans and sport media. They place importance on future and carrier perspectives. Those engaged in sport activities declared that performance would guide them to success. They acknowledged the importance of contest, of achievement and of good results. The inactive youth mentioned coaching and declared finding happiness in the exercise itself.

Considering the external accommodation motivational factors, the sport-active youths emphasised the importance of their sport peers' and friends' opinion. They also believed that sport enhanced their relationships with adults and resulted in a more positive attitude.

Those who preferred team games were driven by victory over others; for them the external accommodation motivation factors play the major role. They placed importance on co-operation, future and career perspectives. They preferred opinions of others – their parents, coaches, sport peers, sport media, friends and their love partners. Those preferring individual sports considered the contest and competition important. They declared being happier in team work and followed team's interest than functioning alone (Table 1 and Fig. 1).

Table 1. Values of the External Accommodation Motivational Factor obtained for various categories of subjects

Factor	Gender		Activity		Sports preference	
Item	Men	Women	Inactive	Active	Individual	Team
Co-operation	292.0	312.2	294.1	307.3	280.3	315.8*
Team work	309.2	288.6	303.2	297.6	349.3	263.7*
Believe in coaching	298.6	303.1	318.5	281.3*	313.2	290.9
Team's interest	299.0	302.6	304.1	296.6	332.2	276.6*
Exercise itself	296.0	306.7	332.0	266.8*	298.8	301.8
Parents' opinion	291.7	312.5	296.9	304.4	276.4	318.7*
Coach's opinion	276.6	333.3*	293.1	308.4	273.3	321.0*
Sport peers' opinion	289.9	315.1	387.4	314.5*	266.0	326.5*
Fans' opinion	288.5	317.0*	296.2	305.1	270.0	323.5*
Sport media's opinion	284.2	322.9*	309.1	291.3	275.8	319.1*
Friends' opinion	291.6	312.7	284.9	317.2*	279.7	316.2*
Your love's opinion	289.9	315.1	291.0	310.7	276.5	318.6*
Jittering	287.6	318.1*	305.9	294.8	294.4	305.1
Career perspectives	280.1	328.4*	298.2	303.0	275.2	319.6*
Relationship with adults	305.4	293.8	287.8	314.1*	301.4	299.8
More positive attitude	308.3	289.8	289.4	312.4*	295.8	304.0

* Significantly ($p<0.05$) different from the respective other category

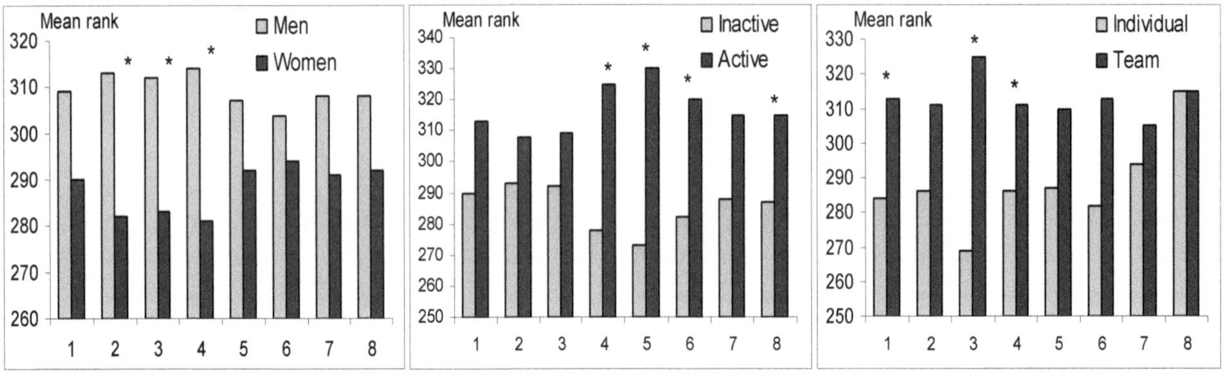

Fig. 1. Competition- and success-oriented motivational factors

Legend: 1 – Defeating others; 2 – Victory; 3 – Competition; 4 – Contest; 5 – Good result; 6 – Achievement; 7 – Sport-manifested achievement; 8 – I will be more successful; * Significantly ($p<0.05$) different from the respective other category

The important factor for male students was to beat own benchmark, while their female peers aimed at pleasing themselves. The latter also believed in the importance of healthy living and physical strength and, thus, to keep fit and healthy, sports giving them a better appearance (cf. Fig. 2).

Young active sportsman and women were inspired to improve their performance and to achieve independent good results. They believed that regular exercise and regular life would guide them to success in other areas of life. They felt sport as positively affecting their whole life and thinking (cf. Fig. 3). Young, active subjects perceived sport as bringing them pleasure, happiness and freedom.

Discussion

On the whole, the studied motivational factors proved of more importance amongst active than inactive youths. These factors (except physical fitness, and the health and sportsman-like attitude) were also significant in subjects preferring team sports. Interestingly, female subjects emphasised the external accommodation motivational factor.

As external motivation, competition, contest and victory proved important for male subjects while for the female ones the external accommodation motivation factor (such as acceptance and others' opinions) played a major role. Teenagers engaged in sports placed importance on achievements and good results. It was important

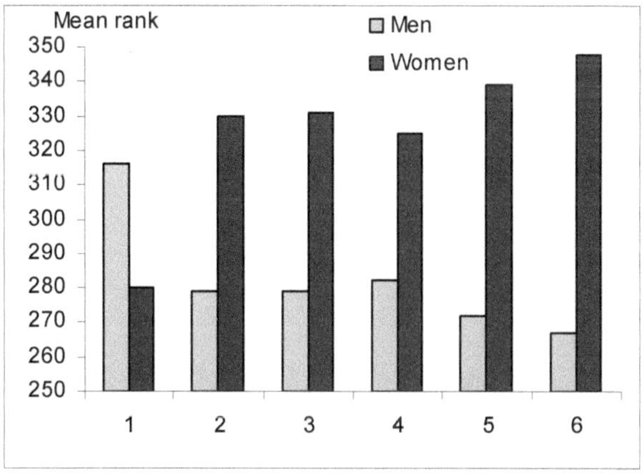

Fig. 2. Physical fitness, health and sportsman-like attitude as declared by young men (n = 347) and women (n = 253)

Legend: 1 – Beating own benchmark; 2 – Aim to please yourself; 3 – Do regular exercise; 4 – Be fit; 5 – Be healthy; 6 – Better appearance; In all cases, men differ significantly from women ($p<0.05$)

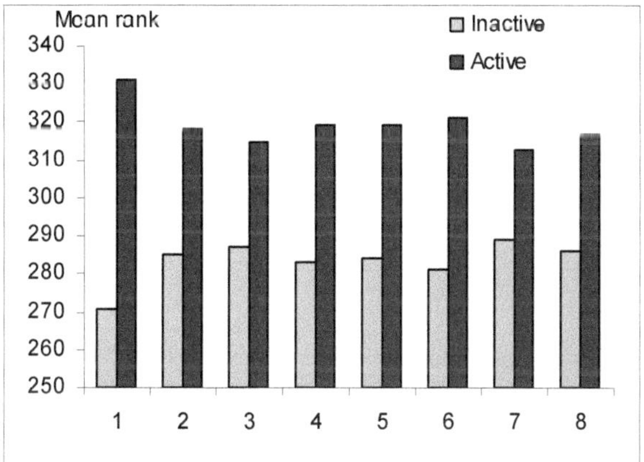

Fig. 3. Physical fitness, health and sportsman-like attitude as declared by active (n = 290) and inactive (n = 310) subjects

Legend: 1 – Beating own benchmark; 2 – Independent good results; 3 – Do regular exercise; 4 – Regularity; 5 – Success in other areas of life; 6 – Positively affects whole life; 7 – Long-term thinking; 8 – Positive thinking; In all cases, active subjects differ significantly from the inactive ones ($p<0.05$)

for them to have the approval of their peers and acquaintances. Those who were inactive believed that sport itself could offer them happiness. Those engaged in team sports were inspired to win over others, unlike those engaged in individual sports. The external motivational factor promoted those in team sports and helped them in co-operation, future plans, career; those preferring individual sports are gave more into following the team's interest.

The external and internal sport motivations varied between genders and age groups. The important milestone is the puberty age when sport can loose importance and gets replaced by fun with peers, especially for girls. They prefer the friends and fun in sports, while males enjoy physical ability, competition, victory and success [11].

In our study that included subjects aged 17 – 19 years similar results were noted. For male students it was important to beat their own benchmark, while female students were more interested in sport regarding health, fit body and nice appearance. Young active subjects believed that regular exercise will assist guiding them to success in other areas of life. Young active subjects loved sports for pleasure, happiness and freedom. Those who were active in team sports valued their team's companionship. Nowadays, the tendency to do regular exercise increases in young female adults. Naturally, in a consumer society, there are pressures from the media to many areas as body image and beauty [10] as the advertisements, TV and movie offer ideal body images [3]. Young adults are influenced by these role models and adjust their life styles to similar reference groups [10].

Real impressions of sports can give only those who live in it. Active young adults believe that sport will assist them in other areas of life and guide them to success (study, work, private life). They are characterised by social sensitivity and affected by opinions of their environment. Their sport and the time they send with sport characterise their motives to life. Those who are planning to make sport as their living are also differently approaching it than those who are using sport as recreation.

External correspondence are motivating mainly team sport players. They are more popular, have more audience and more noticed by media. For them teamwork and team dynamics are very important. In team sports motivation is based on shared goal, task, image and belonging to a group.

In conclusion, a right balance of internal and external motivations is decisive in choosing given sport. The other impact is the social group and cultural background of youths. All are rooted in the childhood model; what children receive and live by, will influence their later life. It is thus important to keep a healthy lifestyle and sport motivation before teenage years since it is a guidance to preserve the health and adequate personality development.

References

1. Ames C., J.Archer (1988) Achievement goals in the classroom: students' learninig stategies and motivation. *J.Psychol.* 80:260-267.

2. Deci E.L., R.M.Ryan (1985) Intrinsic Motivation and Self-determination in Human Behavior. Plenum, New York.

3. Featherstone M. (1991) The body in consumer culture. In: M.Featherstone, M.Hepworth, B.S.Turner (eds.) The Body. Social Process and Cultural Theory. Sage, London, pp. 170-197.

4. Huang C.R., H.Y.Kuo (1999) The sources of athletes' sport confidence. *Chinese Phys.Educ.* 13:60-66.

5. Luszczynska A., F.X.Gibbons, B.F.Pikó, M.Teközel (2004) Self-regulatory cognitions, social comparison, and perceived peers' behaviors as predictors of nutrition and physical activity: A comparison among adolescents in Hungary, Poland, Turkey and USA. *Psychol.Health* 19:577-593.

6. Mills J.S., K.R.Blankstein (2000) Perfectionism, intrinsic vs. extrinsic motivation, and motivated strategies for learning: A multidimensional analysis of university students. *Pers.Indiv. Diff.* 29:1191-1204.

7. Murcia J.A.M., E.C.Gimeno, D.G.Coll (2007) Young athletes' motivational profiles. *J.Sport Sci.Med.* 6:172-179.

8. Nicholls J.G. (1989) The Competitive Ethos and Democratic Education. Cambridge, MA: Harvard University Press.

9. Piko B. (2000) Health-related predictors of self-perceived health in a student population: the importance of physical activity. *J.Comm.Health* 25:125-137.

10. Piko B. (2002): The role of physical activity in university students' health . In: É.Martos (ed.): XXVII. FIMS World Congress of Sports Medicine. Monduzzi Editore, Bologna, Italy. pp. 149-152.

11. Piko B., N.Keresztes, Zs.Pluhar (2005) Sportmotivációs általános iskolások körében. (Sport motivation among primary school chidlren) V. Országos Sporttudományi Kongresszus, Válogatott Tanulmányok, Budapest, pp. 76-80.

12. Vallerand R.J., G.F.Losier (1999) An integrative analysis of intrinsic and extrinsic motivation in sport. *J.Appl.Sport Psychol.* 11:142-169.

13. Viira R., L.Raudsepp (2000) Achievement goal orientations, beliefs about sport success and sport emotions as related to moderate to vigorous physical activity of adolescents. *Psychol.Health.* 15:625-633.

14. Vlachopoulos S.P., C.I.Karageorghis, P.C.Terry (2000) Motivation profiles in sport: a self-determination theory perspective. *Res.Q.Exerc.Sport* 71:387-397.

Effect of consecutive aerobic and resistance exercise on cortisol, immunoglobulin A, and creatine kinase responses in male students

Hamid Arazi [1], Mohammad Azizi [2]

[1]Faculty of Physical Education and Sport Science, University of Guilan, Rasht, [2]Faculty of Physical Education and Sport Science, University of Razi- Kermanshah, Iran

Summary

Study aim: To investigate the effects of consecutive aerobic and resistance exercise on Cortisol, Immunoglobulin A (IgA), and Creatine kinase (CK) responses of male students.
Material and methods: Eight subjects (mean age 21.0 ± 1.5 years) completed two trail, aerobic ergometer exercises (60% VO2max; 45-min) and resistance (80% 1RM; 45-min) exercise concurrently; each subject was his own control. Blood samples were collected pre-exercise, post-exercise, and 3 hours after exercise. One-way ANOVA with repeated measure and LSD post-hoc tests were used to evaluate changes in Cortisol, IgA, and CK during baseline and exercise periods.
Results: During baseline, there were no differences between exercise day (ED) values and those obtained at rest day (RD) for Cortisol, IgA, and CK. After exercise, Cortisol concentration in ED was significantly higher than RD ($p<0.05$); however, changes in IgA and CK responses were not significant.
Conclusions: This type of consecutive exercise didn't increase susceptibility to upper respiratory tract infection and muscle damage. Therefore, it can be useful for the preparation phase of training for athletes.

Key words: Immunoglobulin – Mucosal immune – Stress hormone – Consecutive exercises

Introduction

The immune system is influenced by physiological and psychological stressors [12], including physical activity. The effects of exercise on the immune system are mediated through interactions between the nervous, endocrine, and immune systems [35].

Salivary immunoglobulin A (IgA) provides a valuable defense against potential pathogens by preventing colonization and replication on the mucosal surfaces of the upper respiratory tract [22]. Secretory IgA as an important component of saliva is produced in local plasma cells. The secreted IgA prevents antigens and microbes from adhering to and penetrating the epithelium (immune exclusion), interrupts replication of intracellular pathogens during transcytosis through epithelial cells (intracellular neutralization), and binds antigens in the lamina propria, thus facilitating their excretion through the epithelium back into the lumen (immune excretion) [11,19]. Reduced concentrations or reduction in the release of Salivary IgA may allow for increased pathogenesis via the mucosal surface [34]. It has been shown that lower concentrations of IgA or chronic IgA deficiencies are associated with an increased frequency of upper respiratory tract infection (URTI) episodes [10,11], recurrent URTI [15], or reduced protection against certain infections [2].

There are reports demonstrating that IgA concentrations are suppressed in response to high intensity exercise [10,39] remain either unaltered [26,42] or are elevated in response to moderate-low intensity exercise [20].

However, several studies have also shown a stable secretion rate of IgA following tennis drills [31], a soccer match [5], or cycling [6]. Jemmott and McClelland [16] concluded from a meta-analysis of nine studies that the level of IgA secretion might indicate vulnerability toward URTI. Mackinnon and Hooper [24] further suggested that the protective effect might depend not only on IgA concentration, but also on salivary flow rate.

Although the physiological mechanisms underlying the temporary suppression of various aspects of the immune function after high-intensity exercise are still unclear, it is likely that both neural and endocrine factors influence the immune response to exercise [8,35]. Cortisol is the end product of the neuroendocrine stress response in humans. Although high levels of Cortisol have been demonstrated to inhibit antibody production in vitro [1],

Author's address Prof. Hamid Arazi, Faculty of Physical Education and Sport Science, University of Guilan, Rasht, Iran P.O.Box: 41635-1438

studies have suggested that elevated glucocorticoids are necessary, but not sufficient, to suppress the antibody response [8]. However, while some studies have reported no acute changes in cortisol secretion in response to resistance exercise [7,29], others have reported changes [36].

Creatine kinase (CK) is found predominantly in muscle and is released into circulation during muscular lesions. Therefore, serum CK activity has been theoretically expected to be useful as a marker in exercise physiology and sports medicine for the detection of muscle injury and overwork [13]. However, previous studies on CK release have not clearly demonstrated its value as a marker for these states [27]. Numerous studies have evaluated changes in CK activity after exercise and found that it differs markedly according to exercise conditions. For example, in isometric muscle contraction exercise, peak serum CK activity is observed relatively early, 24–48 h after exercise [18], whereas it is seen 3–7 days after exercise in eccentric muscle contraction exercise [27], and a biphasic pattern is observed in weight training [40].

Totsuka et al. [25] reported that CK response depends on individual fitness level. They show that peak CK values during the bicycle exercise correlated with workload/cross-sectional area of the quadriceps femoris muscle, workload/volume of the quadriceps femoris muscle, and knee extensor strength/body mass.

However, according to inconsistency in previous results, there are no quantitative results concerning immune response to exercise. To our knowledge there is no study that evaluates the effect of single bout of consecutive aerobic and resistance exercise on immune response. Therefore, the purpose of this study was to determine the effect of a single bout of consecutive aerobic and resistance exercise on Cortisol, IgA, and CK responses in male students.

Material and Methods

Participants: Eight male physical education students took part in the study. They were not specifically endurance or resistance trained but were actively involved in various kinds of sports for 6-8 hours weekly on average. Characteristics of the subjects are reported in Table 1. Before the start of the study, subjects provided written informed consent. They were asked not to perform any strenuous exercise or consume medication for 2 days before each trial. Each subject was his own control. The protocol was approved by the Guilan University Ethics Committee.

Preliminary measurements: Maximal aerobic capacity ($\dot{V}O_2max$) was estimated using the Fox protocol (heart rate response to 5 min of cycle ergometry at 150 W (6300 − 19.26×(HR5min) = $\dot{V}O_2max$); [9]). Also, muscular strength was measured at the beginning of the study. Strength was assessed by one repetition maximum (1-RM) for bench press, leg press, leg extension, leg curl, lats pull-down, and biceps curl.

Table 1. Characteristics of subjects (mean ±SD)

Variable	Male students (n=8)
Age (years)	21.0± 1.51
Body height (cm)	178.0±5.0
Body mass (kg)	74.0± 8.8
Body fat (%)	12.3 ± 3.6
BMI (kg/m^2)	23.3 ± 1.0
$\dot{V}O_2$max (ml/kg/min)	46.2 ± 6.7

Following warm-up for the 6 resistance exercise testing, subjects selected a weight with which they felt they could complete three repetitions. At this weight, they only performed one repetition. Subjects then selected a weight they felt would be their 1-RM and attempted one repetition with this weight. Following successful attempts, weight was increased by 2-5 kg for subsequent 1-RM attempts. The 1-RM was usually reached in less than 6 sets, including the warm-up set. There was 3 min of rest between attempts, and two assistants changed the weight on the bar between attempts.

Procedures: The subjects completed trials in a counterbalanced order. For the afternoon exercise trial, subjects reported to the laboratory at 14:00 after fasting from 22:30 the previous day to 10:30 a.m. They then performed 45 min cycling at 60% $\dot{V}O_2$max and 45 min 6 free-weight resistance exercise in the following order: bench press, leg press, leg extension, leg curl, lats pull-down, and biceps curl. Exercises consisted of 3 sets of 8 repetitions (80% 1-RM), with a 2-min rest between sets and a 3-min rest between exercises. The laboratory temperature and relative humidity were 21.4 ± 0.4°C and 64 ± 3%, respectively. Blood and saliva samples were taken during baseline, immediately after exercise, and 3 hours after exercise. Samples were refrigerated until the end of the session and centrifuged, then refrozen at -20°C, and stored until all sessions for each subject were completed.

Salivary cortisol concentrations were measured in duplicate by using a commercially prepared ELISA kit (Diagnostics Biochem Canada, Inc.) with modified procedures suggested by the manufacturer. A lower limit of detection for saliva cortisol was 1.0 ng/dl. CK was assayed spectrophotometrically through the use of commercially available kits (PARS AZMUN CO.TEHRAN, IRAN). The CV for CK was < 4%. IgA was assayed by immunodiffusion (SRID) method by use of IgA kit (The Binding Site Ltd., Birmingham, UK), The CV for IgA was < 3%.

Statistical analysis: All results are presented as mean values and standard deviation of the mean. Normality of data distribution was assessed by the Kolmogorov-Smirnov test. Data were analyzed using a repeated measure ANOVA and LSD post-hoc test. Statistical significance was set at $\alpha = 0.05$.

Results

Results of the analysis showed that during baseline, there were no differences between exercise day (ED) and rest day (RD) for Cortisol, IgA, and CK. After exercise, Cortisol concentration in ED were significantly higher than RD ($p<0.05$); however, IgA and CK responses were not significant between ED and RD. Also, 3 hours after exercise, the Cortisol concentration in ED was significantly higher than in RD ($p<0.05$); but, IgA and CK concentration 3 hours after exercise was similar in ED and RD (Table 2). In addition, there were no correlations between IgA and Cortisol responses to exercise in both days.

Discussion

This study focused on IgA, CK, and cortisol response to exercise. Consecutive aerobic and resistance exercise protocol were designed to present physiological stress similar to the preparation phase of training in most sports.

Our results shows that mean salivary concentration of IgA were unaffected by consecutive aerobic and resistance exercise. These results are in line with previous studies [4,28,42]. Some studies have reported decreases in IgA concentration following high-intensity exercise [21,38]. Their exercise protocols were undertaken during a period of overtraining [24]. However, a significant elevation in IgA concentration has also been reported after high-intensity exercise [6]. This increase seemed to result from the reduction of saliva flow rate. Previous studies have suggested that there is an intensity-dependent effect of acute exercise on IgA, i.e. strenuous exercise is suppressive and moderate exercise has no effect [23]. Therefore, the inconsistency in responses of IgA secretion rate to exercise may be attributed to different types of sympathetic nervous system stimulation during exercise [14]. It seems that neither aerobic exercise nor resistance exercise at the same moderate exercise intensity evokes sufficient stimulation of the sympathetic nervous system or of the hypothalamic-pituitary-adrenal axis to modify IgA transcytosis.

We found that consecutive aerobic and resistance exercise was associated with increased salivary Cortisol concentrations immediately and 3 hours after exercise. Post-exercise Cortisol concentration changes seems to be affected by several mechanisms including stimulation of the sympathetic nervous system, stimulation of hypothalamic-pituitary-adrenal (HPA) secretion, increase of body temperature, changes in blood pH, hypoxia, lactate accumulation, and mental stress [30,37]. A study reported that Cortisol concentration increases due to continued exercises. These researchers reported that physical exercise could stimulate HPA, increase body temperature, increase Cortisol secretion, and the release of Cortisol from the carrier proteins [3]. Therefore, the high concentration of salivary Cortisol accompanied by increase of saliva viscosity is the indicator of sympathetic nervous system activation [3]. The findings of this study are in line with findings of Ben-Aryeh et al. [3] and Kaciuba-Uscilko *et al.* [17], who found that consecutive aerobic exercise and resistance exercise increase Cortisol concentration. Furthermore, the results of this study do not support the data given by O'Connor *et al.* [33] and Sari-Sarraf *et al.* [37]. The equivocal nature of these observations may be due to the difference in intensity, duration, and mode of exercise, the place of exercise, and the age of the subjects in each study.

We found a lack of correlation between IgA and Cortisol concentrations. Specifically, we observed that IgA concentration after consecutive aerobic and resistance exercise did not change, while Cortisol concentration changed. Our findings match those of Sari-Sarraf *et al.* [37], reporting that during heavy and moderate exercises Cortisol secretion had no relationship with the inhibition of salivary IgA.

Table 2. Mean values (±SD) of Cortisol, CK and IgA recorded pre-, post- and 3 hours post exercise during rest and exercise day in male physical education students

Variable	Rest day			Exercise day		
	Pre-exercise	Post-exercise	3h-post exercise	Pre-exercise	Post-exercise	3h-post exercise
Cortisol (nmol/L)	1.26 ±0.3	0.67± 0.1	0.76± 0.2	1.23 ± 0.4	1.43± 0.2*	1.50± 0.1*
Creatine kinase (U/L)	200.1 ±12.5	196.2± 8.7	195.1± 9.1	199.6 ± 7.9	203.7± 10.3	206.6± 11.4
IgA (mg/dl)	72.2 ±8.3	67.4± 6.1	67.2± 4.2	72.4 ± 5.4	72.8± 7.1	72.9± 6.4

Legend: IgA - Immunoglobulin A * Significantly ($p<0.05$) different from the rest day

When the subjects work at a fixed loading, CK is released from the muscle when the loading exceeds a certain limit of muscle ability [25]. Although numerous studies [18,32,40] have examined the effects of exercise on serum CK activity under various exercise conditions, to our knowledge no study has addressed CK release during consecutive aerobic and resistance exercise. In the present study, we found that consecutive aerobic and resistance exercise could not increase CK concentration. Previous studies reported that during exercise, muscle repeatedly contracts and uses energy substrates. When exercise intensity is within the normal range of metabolism, the muscle tissue is exercised without marked changes in membrane permeability. However, when exercise intensity exceeds this permissible range, the membrane permeability temporarily changes, resulting in CK release from the active muscle [25]. Volfinger *et al.* [41] indicated the possibility of a threshold value for CK release, with a "distance" threshold for CK release.

Totsuka et al. [25] reported that CK response depends on individual fitness level, levels that are usually different between athlete and non-athlete. Our subjects were physical education students and maybe the intensity of consecutive aerobic and resistance exercise did not exceed the ability of their muscles, thus the CK concentration in serum did not increase due to consecutive aerobic and resistance exercise.

In conclusion, we showed that 90-min consecutive aerobic and resistance exercise led to increased salivary Cortisol, but there were no significant changes in salivary IgA and serum CK concentration. Therefore, we suggest that this type of consecutive aerobic and resistance exercise don't show a wide range of deleterious effects on the immune system. Finally, it can only be stated that this kind of consecutive aerobic and resistance exercise was well tolerated; it has demonstrated that this sub-maximal exercise did not lead to muscle damage or altered salivary IgA levels.

References

1.Ambrose C.T. (1996) Symposium on in vitro studies of the immune responses: III Biochemical agents affecting the inductive phase of the secondary antibody response initiated in vitro. *Bacteriol.Rev.* 30:408-417.

2.Asahi Y, T.Yoshikawa, I.Watanabe, T.Iwasak, H.Hasegawa, Y.Sato, S.Shimada, M.Nanno, Y.Matsuoka, M.Ohwaki, Y.Iwakura, Y.Suzuki, C.Aizawa, T.Sata, T.Kurata, S.Tamura (2002) Protection against influenza virus infection in polymeric Ig receptor knockout mice immunized intranasally with adjuvant-combined vaccines. *J.Immunol.,* 168: 2930–2938.

3.Ben-Aryeh H, N.Roll, M.Lahav, R.Dlin, N.Hanne-Paparo, R.Szargel, C.Shein-Orr, D.Laufer (1989) Effect of exercise on salivary composition and cortisol in serum and saliva in man. *J.Dent.Res.*, 68:1495-1497.

4.Bishop N.C, A.K.Blannin, P.J.Robson, N.P.Walsh, M.Gleeson (1999) The effects of carbohydrate supplementation on immune responses to a soccerspecific exercise protocol. *J.Sports.Sci.,* 17: 787–796.

5.Bishop N.C, A.K.Blannin, N.P.Walsh, E.Armstrong, M.Rickman, M.Gleeson (2000) Carbohydrate and fluid intake affect the saliva flow rate and IgA response to cycling. *Med.Sci. Sports.Exerc.,* 32:2046-2051.

6.Blannin A.K, P.J.Robson, N.P.Walsh, A.M.Clark, L.Glennon, M.Gleeson (1998) The effect of exercising to exhaustion at different intensities on saliva immunoglobulin A, protein and electrolyte secretion. *Int.J.Sports.Med.*, 19:547–552.

7.Dohi K., A.M.Mastro, M.P.Miles, J.A.Bush, D.S.Grove, S.K.Leach, J.S.Volek, B.C.Nindl, J.O.Marx, L.A.Gotshalk, M.Putukian, W.J.Sebastianelli, W.J.Kraemer (2001) Lymphocyte proliferation in response to acute heavy resistance exercise in women: influence of muscle strength and total work. *Eur.J.Appl.Physiol.*, 85:367-373.

8.Fleshner M. (2000) Exercise and neuroendocrine regulation of antibody production: protective effect of physical activity on stress-induced suppression of the specific antibody response. *Int.J.Sports.Med.*, Suppl1:14-19.

9.Fox E.L. (1973) A simple, accurate technique for predicting maximal aerobic power. *J.Appl.Physiol.,* 35:914-916.

10. Gleeson M., W.A McDonald, D.B.Pyne, A.W.Cripps, J.L.Francis, P.A.Fricker, R.L.Clancy (1999) Salivary IgA levels and infection risk in elite swimmers. *Med.Sci.Sports.Exerc.*, 31(1):67–73.

11. Gleeson M., D.B.Pyne (1993) Special feature for the Olympics: effects of exercise on the immune system: exercise effects on mucosal immunity. *Immunol.Cell.Biol.*, 78:536–544.

12. Herbert T.B., S.Cohen (1993) Stress and immunity in humans: a meta-analytic review. *Psychosom.Med.*, 55:364–379.

13. Houmard J.A., D.L.Costill, J.B.Mitchell, S.H.Park, W.J.Fink, J.M.Burns (1990). Testosterone, cortisol, and creatine kinase levels in male distance runners during reduced training. *Int.J. Sports.Med.*, 11:41–45.

14. Hucklebridge F., A.Clow, P.Evans (1998) The relationship between salivary secretory immunoglobulin A and cortisol: neuroendocrine response to awakening and the diurnal cycle. *Int.J.Psychophysiol.*, 31:69–76.

15. Isaacs D., A.D.Webster, H.B.Valman (1984) Immunoglobulin levels and function in pre-school children with recurrent respiratory infections. *Clin.Exp.Immunol.*, 58:335–340.

16. Jemmott J.B., D.C.Mcclelland (1989) Secretory IgA as a measure of resistance to infections disease: Comment on Stone, Cox, Valdimarsdottir, and Neale. *Behavioral.Med.*, 15:63-71.

17. Kaciuba-Uscilko H., B.Kruk, M.Szczpaczewsk., B.Opaszowski, E.Stupnicka, B.Bicz, K.Nazar (1992) Metabolic, body temperature and hormonal responses to repeated periods of prolonged cycle-ergometer exercise in men. *J.Appl.Physiol.,* 64:26-31.

18. Kirwan J.P., P.M.Clarkson, J.E.Graves, P.L.Litchfield, W.C.Byrnes (1986). Levels of serum creatine kinase and myoglobin in women after two isometric exercise conditions. *Eur .J.Appl.Physiol.,* 55:330–333.

19. Lamm M.E. (1998) Current concepts in mucosal immunity. IV. How epithelial transport of IgA antibodies relates to host defense. *Am.J.Physiol.,* 274:G614–G617.

20. Ljungberg G., T.Ericson, B.Ekblom, D.Birkhed (1997) Saliva and marathon running. *Scand.J.Med.Sci.Sports,* 7:214–219.

21. Mackinnon L.T., T.W.Chick, A.Van As, T.B.Tomasi (1987) The effect of exercise on secretory and natural immunity. *Adv.Exp.Med.Biol.,* 216A:869–876.

22. Mackinnon L.T. (1992) Exercise and Immunology. Champaign IL: Human Kinetics.

23. Mackinnon L.T. (1996) Immunoglobulin, antibody and exercise. *Exerc.Immuno.Rev.*, 2:1–34.

24. Mackinnon L.T., S.Hooper (1994) Mucosal (secretory) immune system responses to exercise of varying intensity and during overtraining. *Int.J.Sports.Med.*, 15:S179-S183.

25. Totsuka M., S.Nakaji, K.Suzuki, K.Sugawara, K.Sato (2002) Break point of serum creatine kinase release after endurance exercise. *J.Appl.Physiol.*, 93:1280–1286.

26. McDowell S.L., K.Chaloa, T.J.Housh, G.D.Tharp, G.O.Johnson (1991) The effect of exercise intensity and duration on salivary immunoglobulin A. *Eur J.Appl.Physiol.*, 63:108–111.

27. Newham D.J., D.A.Jones, P.M.Clarkson (1987) Repeated highforce eccentric exercise: effects on muscle pain and damage. *J.Appl.Physiol.*, 63:1381–1386.

28. Nieman D.C., D.A.Henson, O.R.Fagoaga, A.C.Utter, D.M.Vinci, J.M.Davis, S.L.Nehlsen-Cannarella (2002) Change in salivary IgA following a competitive marathon race. *Int.J.Sports. Med.*, 23:69–75.

29. Nieman D.C., D.A.Henson, C.S.Sampson, J.L.Herring, J.M.Suttls, M.H.Conley (1995) The acute immune response to exhaustive resistance exercise. *Int.J.Sports.Med.*, 16:322-328.

30. Nieman D.C., D.A.Henson, C.L.Dumke, R.H.Lind, L.R.Shooter, S.J.Gross (2006). Relationship between salivary IgA secretion and upper respiratory tract infection following a 160-km race. *J.Sports.Med.Phys.Fitness.*, 46:158-162.

31. Nieman D.C., M.W.Kernodle, D.A.Henson, G.Sonnenfeld, J.M.Davis (2000) Acute immune responses to tennis drills in adolescent athletes. *Res.Quartly.Exerc.Sport,* 71:403-408.

32. Nosaka K., P.M.Clarkson (1992) Relationship between post-exercise plasma CK elevation and muscle mass involved in the exercise. *Int.J.Sports.Med.*, 13:471–475.

33. O'connor P.J., W.P.Morgan., J.S.Reglin (1991) Psychobiologic effect of 3D of increased training exercise intensities on salivary cortisol. *J.Strength.Cond.Res.*, 16:286-289.

34. Ostergaard P.A. (1977) IgA levels, bacterial carrier rate, and the development of bronchial asthma in children. *Acta.Pathol. Microbiol.Scand.*, 85:187–195.

35. Pedersen B.K., L.Hoffman-Goetz (2000) Exercise and the immune system: regulation, integration, and adaptation. *Physiol.Rev.*, 80:1055–1081.

36. Rahimi R., M.Ghaderi, B.Mirzaei, S.Ghaeni, H.Faraji, D.Sheikholeslami-Vatani, F.Rahmani-Nia (2010) Effects of very short rest periods on immunoglobulin A and cortisol responses to resistance exercise in men. *J.Hum.Sport.Exerc.*, 5:146-157.

37. Sari-Sarraf V., T.Reilly, D.A.Doran, G.Atkinson (2007) The effects of single and repeated bouts of soccer-specific exercise on salivary IgA. *Arch.Oral.Biol.*, 52:526-532.

38. Tharp G.D., M.W.Barnes (1990) Reduction of saliva immunoglobulin levels by swim training. *Eur.J.Appl.Physiol.*, 60:61–64.

39. Tharp G.D. (1991) Basketball exercise and secretory immunoglobulin A. *Eur.J.Appl.Physiol.*, 63: 312–314.

40. Tokuda S., A.Iiboshi, S.Otsuji (1985) Biphasic changes and characteristics in serum creatine kinase activity due to transient weight training. *Jpn.J.Phys.Fitness.Sports.Med.*, 34:218–224.

41. Volfinger L., V.Lassourd, J.M.Michaux, J.P.Braun, P.L.Toutain (1994) Kinetic evaluation of muscle damage during exercise by calculation of amount of creatine kinase released. *Am.J. Physiol.Regul.Integr.Comp.Physiol.*, 266:R434–R441.

42. Walsh N.P., A.K.Blannin, A.M.Clark, L.Cook, P.J.Robson, M.Gleeson (1999) The effects of high-intensity intermittent exercise on saliva IgA, total protein and alpha-amylase. *J.Sports. Sci.*, 17:129–134

Health awareness, motor performance and physical activity of female university students

Csaba Konczos[1], József Bognár[2], Zsolt Szakály[1], István Barthalos[1], István Simon[3], Zsolt Oláh[2]

[1] University of West-Hungary, Faculty of the Apáczai Csere János, Győr, [2] Semmelweis University – Faculty of Physical Education and Sport, Budapest, [3] University of West Hungary, Faculty of the Benedek Elek, Sopron, Hungary

Summary

Study aim: To assess body composition, health awareness and cardiorespiratory fitness in female university students differing in volume of obligatory physical activity classes.
Material and methods: 109 female students of the University of West Hungary volunteered to participate in the study. The subjects were divided into two groups according to frequency and volume of obligatory physical activity: students of recreation and health education programmes (RHE; $n = 27$) and of social pedagogy, tourism and catering, and teacher training programmes (STT; $n = 82$). Basic somatic characteristics were measured, body composition was assessed by bioelectrical impedance, cardiorespiratory fitness was evaluated using the Rockport Fitness Walking Test and health behaviour was assessed by questionnaire method. Student's t-test for independent samples, the U Mann Whitney test or chi-square test were used in data analysis.
Results: RHE students had higher values of percentage muscle mass ($p<0.05$) and of cardiorespiratory performance ($p<0.001$), they also declared significantly more frequently ($p<0.001$) practicing leisure physical activity as compared with the STT group. However, in both groups the symptoms of unhealthy behaviour were observed.
Conclusions: Although beneficial effects of augmented physical activity on body composition, cardiorespiratory performance and attitudes towards taking up leisure-time activity was noted, attention should be paid to symptoms of unhealthy behaviour observed in female students. This support the need for including obligatory physical education classes in university curriculum and the importance of education and promotion of healthy behaviour among the students.

Key words: Health behaviour – Body composition – Motor performance – Female students

Introduction

Hungary has experienced remarkable change in its political system, general socioeconomic conditions and its physical environment over the past 30 years. As a consequence of such change the social expectations of women have also significantly increased in this period and studies of women's health issues and health behaviour are of constant interest [18,26]. Inevitably any positive changes this period brought about were also accompanied by negative aspects, namely a remarkable general decrease in people's habitual physical activity and changes in nutritional habits. The negative characteristics of this transitional period in Hungary can be found to a considerable extent in students of higher education. According to some human biologists many factors of environmental influence are difficult to specify or have less overall importance. Among these environmental factors however, definite emphasis and importance can be attributed to nutrition and regular physical exercise [4,6].

There is evidence that a certain level of physical fitness is a vital part of being healthy, yet a physically active lifestyle has real value when combined with healthy daily habits as well. The behaviour patterns which have a negative influence on health usually include stress, diet, drug abuse, alcohol consumption, smoking, medication and lack of sleep. It is the role and indeed responsibility of the educational system to raise awareness of health issues and educate children about a healthy way of life from an early age. Nowadays most curricula contain some sort of theoretical and practical knowledge of healthy active living [27].

Probably the most determinative segment of a healthy lifestyle in a student's life is the one in which education is carried out within an organised framework. The behavioural pattern mediated by the teacher (especially in the field of physical education) is a key factor. The lack of a healthy behavioural pattern or negative models harmfully influence the attitude and regular activity level of children and young adults [3]. The desired behavioural

Author's address Csaba Konzos, Faculty of Apáczai Csere János, University of West Hungary, Liszt Ferenc Street 42, 9022 Győr, Hungary

patterns can be developed only as a result of a long process for which society (on the macro level), and different educational spheres (family, school, friends, sport clubs, etc.), at the micro level, have a great responsibility [29]. The motivated, mentally and physically well-trained educator will be able to develop and devolve a constructive lifestyle pattern that involves tasks of prevention as well. It is believed that behavioural patterns learned and formed in educational institutes remain a part of us our whole life. If proper bases are built during youth, then one can build on them throughout higher education studies as well.

It is during late adolescence and young adulthood when most negative behaviour patterns become a regular habit of the individual [14]. It is known that the more people smoke, the worse their physical performance become lesser to a significant degree [8].

Regular physical activity, besides its general favourable effects, can be used in rehabilitation and for the prevention and treatment of certain illnesses [15,16,21,24,29], and has also been shown to decrease the harmfulness of overweight conditions and obesity [5]. Physically-active obese and overweight people tend to have a lower rate of morbidity and mortality than normal weight but hypoactive people [23]. An inactive lifestyle and the accompanying moderate cardiorespiratory performance ability carry the same source of risk as obesity.

During the academic years of college and university, sedentary lifestyles tend to be typical, the direct outcome of which is a change in body composition and cardiorespiratory performance. Since the 1970s, common changes in living standards and lifestyles have resulted in the decreasing physical performance of children, adolescence, and young adults, while body fat as a percentage of body mass has increased [7,20]. Gáldi [14] stated that only 30% of those aged between 15 and 84 perform regular physical activity in Hungary, and there is a linear decrease in practicing sports with the age. According to this study, regular physical activity is performed by 49.9% of those aged between 20 and 29, and there is a correlation between the frequency of physical activities performed and the level of education.

With the help of a motor test and the measurement of selected body parameters, the fitness level of a given age group can be determined. Although the application of motor tests and fitness measurements is part of curriculum requirements, it is not widespread in the higher education system, despite the fact that there are many opportunities to train future educators and experts in fields of health and fitness. The aim of this study was to assess body composition, cardiorespiratory fitness and health awareness in female university students differing in volume of obligatory physical activity.

Material and Methods

The study sample (n = 109) was selected from full-time female students in teacher training, social pedagogy, tourism and catering, recreation and health promotion courses at the University of West Hungary, who were enrolled for the 2006-07 academic year. A stratified random sample was used in selecting the year and date of enrolment. The sample was divided into two groups according to frequency and volume of obligatory physical activity classes. The first group was composed of the recreation and health promotion students (RHE; n = 27) who depending on the semester, were participating in compulsory regular physical activity 2-4 times a week (60-80 minutes per session), the second one comprised of students of teacher training, social pedagogy, tourism and catering (STT; n = 82) who did physical exercise 30-40 minutes 0 - 2 times a week. All subjects gave their written consents to participate in the study; the research was approved by the local Committee of Ethics.

In all subjects body height and body mass were measured according to standard anthropometric procedures, from these BMI (body mass index) was calculated. As in Hungary no current reference values of BMI are available, classification of BMI used are according to WHO recommendations. WHO has established 11 different categories of BMI, however in this study subjects were classified to one of the 3 following categories: underweight (<18.49), normal (18.50-24.99) and overweight (>25). For the estimation of percentage body fat content and muscle mass the InBody 720 bioelectrical impedance scanner was used [31]. InBody 720 (Biospace Co, Korea) is a multi-frequency impedance plethysmograph body composition analyser which takes readings from the body using an eight-point tactile electrode method, measuring resistance at five specific frequencies (1 kHz, 50 kHz, 250 kHz, 500 kHz, and 1 MHz) and reactance at three specific frequencies (5 kHz, 50 kHz, and 250 kHz). In the measuring process the technical prescriptions of the International Biological Program were followed [30].

Health behaviour of subjects was assessed using the Győr-Moson-Sopron County ÁNTSZ Health Protection Department's "Habitude survey of the Adult Population" questionnaire [2]. It consisted of closed-ended questions and scales in the following fields: self-evaluation (self-confidence, shyness), future prospects (hope, hopelessness), nutritional habits (quality, frequency), harmful addictions (smoking, drug abuse, and alcohol consumption), and physical activity (regularity, quantity) [25]. Questions were directed to determine frequency of free time physical exercise lasting for at least 20 minutes per day (0 – 7 days/week), the level of satisfaction in relation to perceived health status (3-point scale), the frequency of perceived fatigue per week (4-point scale), and any harmful addictions, such as smoking or alcohol consumption (5-point scale).

The motor performance test was used for the measurement of cardiorespiratory performance in the sub-max zone with the Rockport Fitness Walking Test (1-Mile) to estimate relative $\dot{V}O_2max$ (ml/kg/min). It was decided to select the test most suitable for hypoactive persons' in order to best assess their motor performance as, from a methodological point of view this is the primary criteria of objective data recording. Based on this, it was supposed that the walk test would be acceptable for the students, and at the same time it would motivate them to perform better. The equation to predict maximum $\dot{V}O_2$ according to Fox's physiological basis for exercise and sport is for the Rockport Fitness Walking Test as follows:

$$\dot{V}O_2max = 132.853 - (0.0769 \times \text{body mass}) - (0.3877 \times \text{age}) + (6.315 \times \text{gender}) - (3.2649 \times \text{time}) - (0.1565 \times \text{heart rate}).$$

The students covered the one-mile distance in windless weather conditions with fast walking, the time of which was measured and recorded by a time-measuring appliance. The maximum heart rate was assessed with the Polar Accurex Pulse Rate Monitor and processed with Polar Precision Performance 3.0 Software (Version 4.00.020). The relative aerobic capacity of the tested persons was estimated with the programme available on the website (http://www.brianmac.dempn.co.uk/rockport-htm).

Statistics for Windows (version 7.1, StatSoft Inc., Tulsa, OK 74104, USA, 2006) was used for the data analysis. In case of body characteristics and cardiorespiratory variables differences between the means were assessed by using t-test for independent samples, the data pertaining to health awareness were analyzed with the use of U Mann Whitney test. The frequencies were assessed by using the chi-square function. The level of $\alpha = 0.05$ was considered significant.

Results

The anthropometric characteristics of studied subjects are presented in Table 1. No significant differences between both groups were found for age and most of the somatic variables, however variability of body mass among STT students was relatively higher as reflected by higher coefficients of variability (CV = 19.6% and 11.7% for SST and RHE respectively) and ranges (40-99 kg and 45-74 kg, respectively). Moreover, students from STT group tended ($p = 0.087$) to have higher values of percentage body fat as compared to RHE students.

According to WHO classification, respectively 4 (14.8%) and 8 (9.7%) students from RHE and STT were classified as underweight, 21 (77.0%) and 54 (65.8%) had normal values of BMI, while 2 (7.4%) and 20 (24.4%) individuals were overweight ($p<0.05$).

Table 1. Mean (±SD) values and ranges of anthropometric features recorded in female university students

Group Variable	RHE (n = 27)	STT (n = 82)
Age (years)	19.5 ± 1.3 18 ÷ 23	19.3 ± 1.0 18 ÷ 22
Body height (cm)	167.0 ± 4.9 156 ÷ 176	165.3 ± 6.6 152 ÷ 183
Body weight (kg)	62.6 ± 7.3 45 ÷ 74	62.4 ± 12.2 40 ÷ 99
Body Mass Index	22.4 ± 3.0 17 ÷ 27	23.0 ± 4.4 16 ÷ 34
Muscle mass (%)	41.2 ± 4.6 35.0 ÷ 46.6	39.1 ± 5.0* 25.6 ÷ 46.5
Body fat (%)	25.2 ± 5.4 16 ÷ 37	28.0 ± 7.8 ° 13 ÷ 50

Legend: RHE - recreation and health development programmes, STT - social pedagogy, tourism and catering, teacher training programmes; ° Tends to differ from RHE group ($p = 0.087$); * Significantly ($p<0.05$) different from RHE group.

Characteristics of the groups' health behaviour are presented in Table 2. The frequency of taking up regular leisure physical activity was significantly higher in the RHE than in SST group (3.0 ± 1.4 and 1.3 ± 1.1 days/week, respectively). It is of interest that among the RHE students were as much as 9 (33%) subjects whose regular physical activity did not meet the recommended minimum of activity of at least 3 times a week, while in STT group the respective percentage amounted to 89% (72 subjects). In case of other health behaviour i.e. perceived health, feeling of morning fatigue and harmful habits – smoking or alcohol consumption no significant between-group differences were noted, however in both groups the symptoms of unhealthy behaviour were observed. Namely, about 22% of RHE and SST students (6 and 19 subjects, respectively) declared everyday smoking and more than ¼ of them admitted alcohol consumption at least once per week (26 and 28%, respectively).

The results of the cardiorespiratory performance test (Rockport Fitness Walking Test) was presented in table 3. Students from RHE group covered the one-mile distance by about 1.5 minute faster ($p<0.001$) than the female students from the SST group. According to classification made with the use website programme the RHE students' time obtained in one-mile walk was "excellent", while STT students' was "good". Moreover, the RHE students had significantly ($p<0.001$) higher values of estimated $\dot{V}O_2max$ as compared to their mates from SST group

(45.4 ± 3.5 and 39.8 ± 5.0 ml/kg/min, respectively), while the maximum heart rates were in both groups comparable.

Table 2. Mean (±SD) values, medians and ranges of health-related variables recorded in female university students

Variable / Group	RHE (n = 27)	STT (n = 82)
Physical activity (days/week)	3.0 ± 1.4 (3) 0 ÷ 5	1.3 ± 1.1 (3)*** 0 ÷ 6
Perceived health (3-point scale)	2.2 ± 0.6 (2) 1 ÷ 3	2.4 ± 0.5 (3) 1 ÷ 3
Perceived fatigue (4-point scale)	2.5 ± 0.8 (2) 1 ÷ 4	2.7 ± 0.8 (3) 1 ÷ 4
Smoking (5-point scale)	2.6 ± 1.6 (2) 1 ÷ 5	2.5 ± 1.7 (3) 1 ÷ 5
Alcohol consumption (5-point scale)	2.7 ± 1.1 (3) 1 ÷ 5	2.8 ± 1.0 (3) 1 ÷ 5

Legend: RHE - recreation and health development programmes, STT - social pedagogy, tourism and catering, teacher training programmes; *** Significantly ($p<0.001$) different from RHE group

Table 3. Mean (±SD) values and ranges of motor performance variables recorded in female university students

Variable / Group	RHE (n = 27)	STT (n = 82)
Time (min)	14.3 ± 0.3 13.4 ÷ 15.3	15.7 ± 1.0 *** 3.6 ÷ 19.4
Heart rate (bpm)	147.0 ± 21.1 100.0 ÷ 182.0	151.1 ± 18.8 112.0 ÷ 198.0
$\dot{V}O_{2\,max}$ (ml/kg/min)	45.4 ± 3.5 39 ÷ 52	39.8 ± 5.0 *** 24 ÷ 47

Legend: RHE - recreation and health development programmes, STT - social pedagogy, tourism and catering, teacher training programmes, *** Significantly ($p<0.001$) different from RHE group

Discussion

Studied female university students seem to be of average height and body mass as the mean values and variances of both somatic traits are similar to other Hungarian samples [28]. Relative high variance of the body mass observed mainly among STT students refer to the body compositional differences derivate from nutritional status. Although no differences between the groups according to BMI were found, relatively higher variance was observed among SST students reflecting heterogeneity of the students' nutritional status. In most of the studied subjects (RHE - 77.0%, STT - 65.8%), the body mass index was within normal limits, however especially among SST students the prevalence of overweight was relatively high and amounted to about 25%. Cole et al. [10] consider prevalence of thin subjects to be of equal importance while evaluating the nutritional status, although in developed societies it is rather a consequence of fashion than negligence; the percentages of underweight subjects were in both groups alike (about 11%).

There are many methods for the estimation of muscle mass, however when evaluating the data it was difficult to find valid reference values. In this study the recommendation of Drinkwater and Ross was used [12]. Although there were significant differences between the groups, the mean percentage muscle mass in the physically active group (RHE) hardly reached the minimum level which is physiologically required. The development of muscle mass in STT students are under the required level which can be attributed to the lowered physical activity. Therefore their results are not surprising, taking into consideration both body composition and lifestyle characteristics.

Significant differences between the two groups, regarding healthy behaviour, have only been found in the frequency of taking up leisure-time physical activity; the number of days in week devoted to physical exercises being significantly higher in RHE students (3.0 vs. 1.3 days/week). Although no significant between-group differences were found, in perceived health and perceived fatigue during the week in both groups the symptoms of unhealthy behaviour were observed. Among Hungarian college students smoking and alcohol consumption are the most frequent examples of harmful behaviour. Smoking was reported in 67% of boy and in 61% of girls while regular alcohol consumption was observed in 49% of males and 27% of females [1]. Our results are well comparable with the results of the European Health and Behaviour Survey reported by Kopp and Skrabski [17]. In healthcare, and more specifically preventive health activity, RHE students nearly reached the required level only in the field of physical exercise. Full awareness of being healthy can only be reached if students decide to make lifestyle changes; hence a physically active lifestyle is only complete if combined with healthy habits.

In the assessment of cardiorespiratory performance by using Rockport Fitness Walking Test, beneficial effects of augmented physical activity were found regarding achieved times and relative aerobic capacity values. An evident consequence of lowered activity is that the mean values of the estimated relative oxygen uptake in the STT group only reached the lower, required limit [7]. Relative variance of maximum heart rates were comparable in both groups (CV = 14.6 and 12.4% in RHE and SST students respectively), however the differences in scatter were prominent, which illustrate properly the differences of the fitness level. The state of the cardiorespiratory system greatly depends on regular physical activity, thus the inevitable decrease in aerobic performance can be slowed down. Maffeis *et al.* [19] claim that decreased aerobic activity is fundamentally the consequence of a lifestyle which put less emphasis on exercise factor. The question becomes more complex when comparing the development of aerobic performance in young people with normal body mass and in those who are overweight. Similar consequences are seen in reports of Fletcher *et al.* [13] and Cole *et al.* [9,10]. According to Cureton *et al.* [11], a person's body composition or at least relative body fat level has to be taken into consideration while evaluating the cardiorespiratory performance of hypoactive test participants. Among the students from RHE, the optimal muscle mass and the body fat level (which is within the normal range) prove the beneficial effect of desired body composition. The result of an unfavourable proportion of muscle mass and fat affecting aerobic performance can be clearly linked to the significantly lower performance level in cardiorespiratory test among STT students.

The certain limitation of presented study was the fact the examination was not representative for the Hungarian young women as it covered only a specific segment of society. Although the findings do not allow broader generalisation, the presented results give an outlook on somatic and fitness characteristics as well as on behaviour patterns among female university students. Results of performed tests were discussed with the students in theory lessons during which they were given advice on health and fitness. They were encouraged to accept the fact that sport and exercise are a vital part of a healthy lifestyle. A discussion was held on the effects of preventative health care, mental hygiene, proper diet, physical activity and sport and students learnt how body composition and the condition of the cardiorespiratory system can be significantly improved. These facts also support the need for including obligatory physical education classes in university curriculum and the importance of education and promotion of healthy behaviour among the students.

References

1. Audrain-McGovern J., D.Rodriguez, H.B.Moss (2003) Smoking progression and physical activity. *Cancer Epidemiol. Biomarkers Prev.*, 12:1121-1129.

2. Bajtay A. (1999) Győr- Moson- Sopron megye egészségtérképe 1991-1996. [Győr- Moson- Sopron county health map in 1991-1996]. ÁNTSZ Győr-Moson- Sopron county Instytute (in Hungarian).

3. Barnekow-Bergvist M., G.Hedberg, U.Janiert, E.Jansson (1998) Prediction of physical fitness and physical activity level in adulthood by physical performance and physical activity in adolescence - an 18-year follow-up study. *Scand.J.Med.Sci. Sports.* 8:299-308.

4. Beunen G. (2003) Physical growth, maturation and performance. *Rev.Portug.Cienc.Desport.*, 3:11-12.

5. Blair S.N., S.Brodney (1999) Effects of physical inactivity and obesity on morbidity and mortality: current evidence and research issues. *Med.Sci.Sports Exeerc., Suppl.* 11:646-662.

6. Bodzsár É.B., C.Susanne (1998) Secular Growth Change in Europe. Eötvös University Press, Budapest

7. Bouchard C. (2000) Physical Activity and Obesity. Human Kinetics, Publishers, Champaign, Illinois

8. Chin O.T. (1986) A comparative study of the aerobic fitness of smokers and non- smokers. *Asian J.Phys.Educ.* 3-4:13-23.

9. Cole T.J., M.C.Bellizzi, K.M.Flegal, W.H.Dietz (2000) Establishing a standard definition for child overweight and obesity worldwide: international survey. *Brit.Med. J.*, 320:1-6.

10. Cole T.J., K.M.Flegal, D.Nicholls, A.A.Jackson (2007) Body mass index cut offs to define thinness in children and adolescents: international survey. *Brit.Med.J.*, 335:194-202.

11. Cureton K.J., T.A.Baumgartner, B.G.McManis (1991) Adjustment of 1-mile run/walk test scores for skinfold thickness in youth. *Pediatr.Exerc.Sci.*, 3: 152-167.

12. Drinkwater D.T., W.D.Ross (1980) Anthropometric fractionation of body mass. In: Ostyn M,. G.Beunen, J.Simons (Eds.): Kinanthropometry II. University Park Press, Baltimore. 178-189.

13. Fletcher G.F., N.Blair, J.Blumenthal (1992) Statement on exercise. Benefits and re-commendations for physical activity programs for all Americans. *Circulation*, 86: 340-344.

14. Gáldi G. (2002) Fizikai aktivitás Magyarországon az ezredfordulón. [Physical activity in Hungary at the turn of the century] *Magyar Sporttud.Szemle,* 3-4: 16-18.

15. Kikkinos P. F., B.Fernhall (1999) Physical activity and high density lipoprotein cholesterol levels. *Sports Med.* 28(5):307-14.

16. King G.A., E.C.Fitzhugh, D.R.Jr.Bassett, J.E.McLaughlin, S.J.Strath,A.M.Swartz, D.L.Thompson (2001) Relationship of Leisure-Time Physical Activity and Occupational Activity to Prevalence of Obesity. *Int.J.Obese,.* 25:606-612.

17. Kopp M., Á.Skrabski (1995) Practical Behaviour Science. Corvinus.

18. Kopp M., Á.Skrabski (2007) Női szerepek a mai magyar társadalomban. [Women's role in present day Hungarian society] http://www.vigilia.hu/2007/7/kopp.htm. Accessed on 04.06. 2011.

19. Maffeis C., F.Schena, M.Zaffanello, L.Zoccante, Y.Schulyz, L.Pinelli (1994) Maximal aerobic power during running and cycling in obese and non-obese children. *Acta Paediatr.,* 83:113-116.

20. Malina R.M., C.Bouchard (1991) Growth, Maturation, and Physical Activity. Human Kinetics Books, Champaign, Illinois

21. Morris J., A.Hardman (1997) Walking to health. *Sports Med.* 23:306-332.

22. Nagy N.K., J.Mészáros, A.Farkas (1996/97) Assessment of body composition of physically active male youth. *Anthropologiai Közl.*, 38: 93-100.

23. Nindl B.C., E.A.Harman, J.O.Marx, L.A.Gotshalk, P.N.Frykman, E.Lammi, C.Palmer, W.J.Kraemer (2000) Regional body composition changes in women after 6 months of periodized physical training. *J.Appl.Physiol.* 6:2251-2259.

24. Owen G. M. (2003) Body mass index and body fat. *Am.J. Clin.Nutr.,* 78(2):348-349.

25. Page R.M., E.P.Zarco, J.Suwanteerangkul, C.M.Lee, N.F.Miao, J.Taylor (2005) Perceptions of the prevalence of cigarette smoking by peers: A study of Taiwanese, Filipino, and Thai high school students. *Southeast.Asian.J.Trop.Med.Publ.Health,* 36(5):1-5.

26. Pongrácz Tné (2001) A család és a munka szerepe a nők életében. http://www.tarki.hu/adatbank-h/kutjel/pdf/a503.pdf Accessed on 04.09. 2011.

27. Salvara M. I., J.Bognár, N.E.Bíróné (2002) Elementary school physical education curriculum in Greece. *Int.J.Phys.Educ.,* 39(3):29-37.

28. Szakály Zs. (2002) Physique, body composition and motor performances in college students. *Hungarian Rev.Sport Sci.* Special Issue: 24-29.

29. Twisk J.W.R., H.C.G.Kemper, W.Mechelen (2000) Tracking of activity and fitness and the relationship with cardiovascular disease risk factors. *Med.Sci.Sports Exeerc.,* 8:1455-1461.

30. Weiner J.E.S., J.A.Lourie (eds). (1969) Human Biology. A Guide to Field Methods. IBP Handbook, No. 9. Oxford: Blackwell Scientific Publishers

31. www.e-inbody.com/Tech/paper.html. Accessed on 04.06. 2011.

Anaerobic endurance of young swimmers aged 12 years

Małgorzata Stachowicz [1], Katarzyna Milde [1], Marcin Janik [2]

[1] University of Physical Education, Warsaw; [2] Department of Physical Education, University of Rzeszów, Poland

Summary

Study aim: To assess the effects of swimming training on anaerobic endurance, swimming velocity and chest girth in children aged 12 years.
Material and methods: Two groups of children aged 12 years were studied. Group S (14 boys and 6 girls) training swimming at a sport-oriented school 3 days a week, 90 min per session, and Group R (6 boys and 6 girls) engaged in competitive swimming for 4 years. Children from Group S were subjected twice (in September and in February) to a swimming test consisting of 6 bouts of swimming the 12.5-m distance, spaced by 30-s intermissions. Mean and maximum swimming velocities in the entire test were recorded together with their ratio (Performance Index, PI). In children from Group R the swimming velocity at one 12.5-distance was recorded.
Results: Apart from somatic indices, significant increases over the 5-month training period were noted in mean swimming velocity in boys and girls ($p<0.001$) and in maximum velocity in boys ($p<0.01$). No significant changes were noted in the performance index or in heart rate.
Conclusions: Performance index as a measure of anaerobic endurance may serve as a useful tool in assessing the adaptive performance changes in young swimmers.

Key words: Swimming – Endurance – Training – Work capacity

Introduction

Swimming even not intense, practiced by children and youths, enhances the development of the respiratory system and increases lung volume [9]. Swimming exercise forces the control of inspiration and expiration, as well as maintaining relatively long periods of apnoea. The hydrostatic pressure facilitates expiration but exerts some resistance to inspiration; in effect, the strength of respiratory muscles and chest mobility increase. Swimming is an example of the so-called early sports in which high training loads, especially the endurance ones, ought to be applied in the period of growth in order to achieve high results [4,5,10,11,13,20]. Endurance training applied in the pre-adolescence period may increase the $\dot{V}O_2max$ in swimmers by as much as 20 – 30%. Thus, steady monitoring of the effects of anaerobic and aerobic stimuli provides valuable information on metabolic reserves and of their potential shaping [3]. However, an assessment of changes in the aerobic capacity of children, especially under a regular endurance training, is not easy [6], due to the growth-related changes in skeletal muscle mass [8].

This study attempted at assessing the anaerobic capacity in 12-year old children attending curricular swimming classes in a sport-oriented school. Of particular interest were the effects of swimming training on anaerobic endurance, swimming velocity and chest girth.

Material and Methods

A group of 14 boys and 6 girls aged 12 years, attending sport-oriented school of swimming profile, volunteered to participate in the study (Group S); they attended curricular swimming classes (90 min each) 3 days a week. Another group of 6 boys and 6 girls aged 12 years, engaged in competitive swimming for 4 years, served as reference (Group R); they trained 6 days a week and among them were Polish champions in that age category. The parents of children submitted their written consents; the study was approved by the local Committee of Ethics.

Children from Group S were examined twice – in September and February; they were subjected to a swimming test consisting of 6 bouts of swimming the 12.5-m distance, spaced by 30-s intermissions. Heart rates (HR) were

Author's address Małgorzata Stachowicz M.S., Department of Biomechanics, University of Physical Education, Marymoncka 34, 00-968 Warsaw, Poland

determined using SportTester devices (Polar Electro, Finland) immediately before and after every swimming bout. Swimming times were converted to velocities; from all 6 bouts, maximum (V_{max}) and mean (V_{av}) velocities were recorded and from these the so-called Performance Index (PI) was computed [15] using the formula $PI = V_{av} / V_{max}$. Children from Group R were examined only once to determine the swimming velocity at 12.5-m distance. This served as a reference for the data recorded in Group S.

Body height was measured with the use of a standard anthropometer (accuracy – 0.1 cm) and body mass – using medical scales (accuracy 0.1 kg) Chest girth was measured using anthropometric tape (mean value of measurements at maximum inspiration and expiration was recorded) in children from Group S.

The data of Group S were subjected to two-way ANOVA. Student's *t*-test for dependent (between examinations) or independent (between groups) data was applied. The level of $p \leq 0.05$ was considered significant.

Results

The results of somatic and swimming performance variables in Group S, measured before and after a 5-month training period, are presented in Table 1. Body height and mass, BMI and chest girth increased over that period as expected. Mean swimming velocities in the consecutive bouts of swimming the 12.5-m distance are presented in Fig. 1. Maximum velocity was attained in all subjects in the first bout and in boys was significantly ($p<0.01$) higher on second than on the first examinations. Mean velocity computed from all 6 bouts was slightly (by 2%) but significantly ($p<0.001$) higher in all subjects on second examination. Yet, the performance index reflecting the anaerobic endurance did not differ significantly either between examinations or between genders. The same was true for heart rates (HR) recorded immediately after 6 swimming bouts and for the differences between HR values post-bout and immediately before the following bout; only in boys that difference in the first test was significantly ($p<0.05$) lower than on second examination or in girls (Table 1 and Fig. 2).

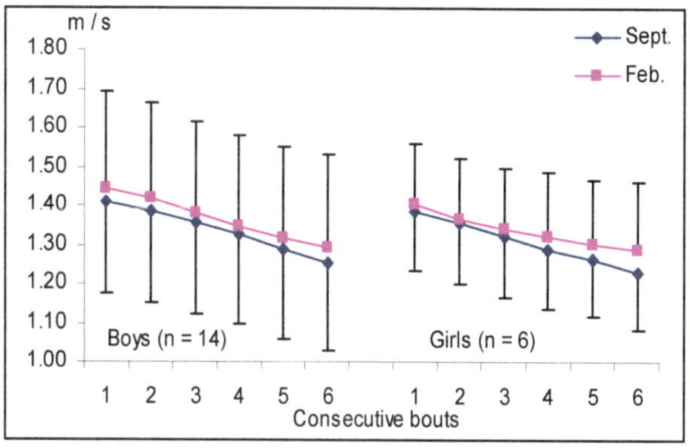

Fig. 1. Swimming velocities (means ±SD) recorded for 6 swimming bouts (12.5-m distance) spaced by 30-s intermissions before (Sept.) and after (Feb.) a 5-month training period

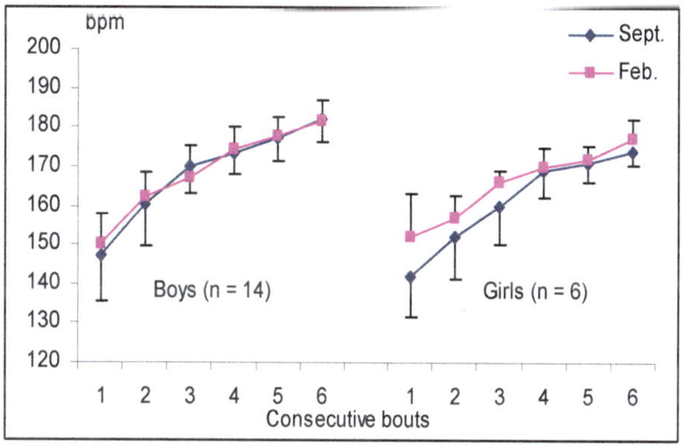

Fig. 2. Heart rates (means ±SD) recorded immediately after 6 swimming bouts (12.5-m distance) spaced by 30-s intermissions before (Sept.) and after (Feb.) a 5-month training period

Table 1. Mean values (±SD) of somatic and swimming performance variables in trained children aged 12 years (Group S) before (I) and after (II) a 5-month training period

Variable	Group / Period	Boys (n = 14) I	Boys (n = 14) II	Girls (n = 6) I	Girls (n = 6) II
Body height (cm)		153.8 ± 10.9	159.3 ± 11.9	156.1 ± 1.7	160.9 ± 1.8
Body mass (kg)		47.0 ± 12.6	52.5 ± 13.9	42.9 ± 5.7	49.4 ± 6.6
BMI		19.6 ± 3.7	20.5 ± 3.7	17.6 ± 2.2	19.1 ± 2.6
Mean chest girth (cm)		77.3 ± 8.3	81.8 ± 7.8	73.7 ± 3.9	81.4 ± 6.1
Maximum velocity (m/s)		1.41 ± 0.24	1.44 ± 0.25**	1.39 ± 0.15	1.41 ± 0.16
Mean velocity (m/s)		1.34 ± 0.23	1.37 ± 0.24***	1.31 ± 0.15	1.34 ± 0.16***
Performance index (PI)		0.947 ± 0.018	0.948 ± 0.017	0.943 ± 0.021	0.951 ± 0.017
Mean HR decrease (bpm)		25.6 ± 8.1	27.8 ± 9.2*	27.2 ± 6.2	28.3 ± 5.8
Post-exercise HR (bpm)		181.8 ± 6.0	181.8 ± 5.0	174.0 ± 3.8	177.0 ± 5.0

Significantly different from Period I (by ANOVA): * $p<0.05$; ** $p<0.01$; All somatic changes were significant ($p<0.001$)

When compared with competitive, elite swimmers of that age (Group R; Table 2), the non-competitive ones (Groups S) had comparable body height, body mass and BMI, although that latter tended to be lower in girls from Group R (p=0.07). On the other hand, mean swimming velocity attained by children from Group R was significantly higher than in Group S: 1.66 ± 0.04 vs. 1.44 ± 0.25 ($p<0.05$) in boys and 1.63 ± 0.04 vs. 1.41 ± 0.16 m/s ($p<0.01$) in girls, respectively. Yet, 3 boys from Group S were comparable with those from Group R with respect to swimming velocity they attained in the first bout, as their velocities ranged from 1.64 to 1.72 m/s and two of them attained very high PI values (0.948 and 0.972). The relationship between swimming velocity in the first bout on Examination II (Vmax) and the performance index (PI) in boys and girls from Group S is presented in Fig. 3.

Table 2. Mean values (±SD) of somatic variables and of swimming velocity in children aged 12 years engaged in competitive swimming (Group R)

Variable \ Group	Boys n = 6	Girls n = 6
Body height (cm)	159.9 ± 1.9	162.9 ± 4.7
Body mass (kg)	46.5 ± 2.6	42.7 ± 2.8
BMI	18.3 ± 0.6	16.9 ± 0.3
Max. velocity (m/s)	1.66 ± 0.04*	1.63 ± 0.04**

Significantly higher compared with Group S: * $p<0.05$; ** $p<0.01$

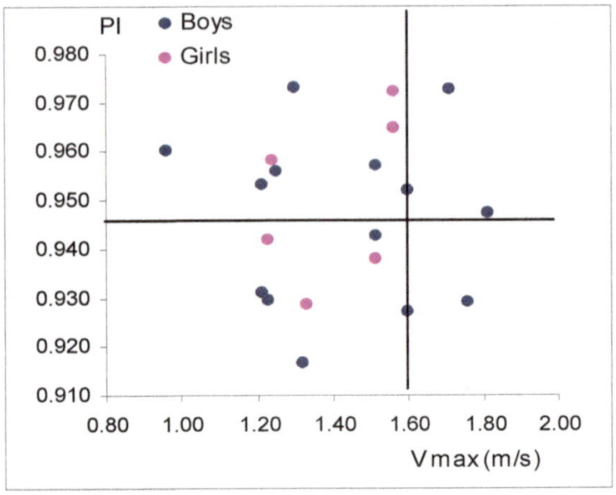

Fig. 3. Relationship between swimming velocity in the first bout on Examination II (V_{max}) and the performance index (PI) in boys (n = 14) and girls (n = 6) from Group S
Vertical line corresponds to lowest velocity recorded in Group R; Horizontal line corresponds to the mean PI value for boys and girls combined

When the results of mean chest girth were combined for boys and girls and analysed allometrically (log chest girth vs. log body mass), the post-training values proved to be by about 3% higher compared to the pre-training ones ($p<0.05$). This followed from the allometric regression computed for the pre-training values which was then applied to the post-training ones. Mean deviation of post-training values from that regression amounted to 0.011, i.e. over 2.5% (Fig. 4). On the other hand, no significant difference was found between the post- and pre-training states of the allometric relation between body mass and height.

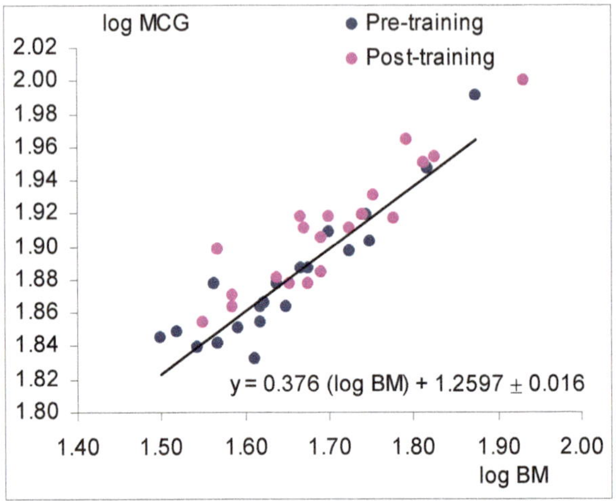

Fig. 4. Allometric relation between mean chest girth (MCG) and body mass (BM) in young male and female swimmers combined

Discussion

Sport training often includes repeated maximal bouts of exercise but their assessment with respect maintaining a high performance, i.e. anaerobic endurance [15,16,19], is usually neglected. The presented results suggest that measuring anaerobic endurance enables the assessment of adaptive performance changes in young swimmers. Inasmuch maximum swimming velocity, i.e. that attained in the first out of 6 repeated bouts of swimming the 12.5-m distance, significantly improved over the 5 months of training only in boys, the mean velocity determined from all 6 bouts significantly improved in both boys and girls. Moreover, girls tended to exhibit a higher stability of results than boys, as reflected by SD values and as reported by Åstrand [1].

Like reported by other authors [1,2,7,8,17], no training-induced somatic changes were noted except chest girth which slightly but significantly increased in relation to body mass. Similar changes were reported by others [9,13] in the early phase of swimming training.

The applied performance index (PI) enabled identifying those subjects (2 boys and 2 girls) who may portend well for the future as they attained both high swimming velocities and high performance in repeated swimming bouts. In practice, the intensity of exertion rating of sports takes place primarily on the basis of observation of heart rate, so the performance index as a measure of anaerobic endurance may serve as a useful tool in assessing the adaptive performance changes in young swimmers.

References

1. Åstrand P.O. (1985) Sexual dimorphism in exercise and sport. In: I.Ghesquiere, R.D.Martin, F.Newcombe (eds.) Human Sexual Dimorphism. Taylor & Francis, London, pp. 247-256.

2. Avlonitou E. (1994) Somatometric variables for preadolescent swimmers. *J.Sports Med.Phys.Fitness* 34:185-191.

3. Bernardi *et al.* (2000) Oxygen consumption and intensity of exercise in sports for disabled athletes. Proc. 5th Scientific Congress, Paraolympic Games, Sydney 2000, OR4C05.

4. Bompa T. (1994) Power Training for Sport: Plyometrics for Maximum Development. Mosaic Press, New York.

5. Colwin C. (2002) Breakthrough Swimming. Human Kinetics Publishers, Champaign IL.

6. Costill D.L., R.Thomas, R.A.Roberqs, D.Pascoe, C.Lambert, S.Barr, W.J.Fink (1991) Adaptations to swimming training: influence of training volume. *Med.Sci.Sports Exerc.* 23: 371-377.

7. Dybińska E. (2005) The learning and teaching efficiency of swimming as related to selected somatic predispositions. In: Scientific Fundaments of Human Movement and Sport Practice, Sports Kinetic, Rimini 2005, p. 121.

8. Dybińska E. (2006) Somatic conditions vs. swimming efficiency of 11-year-old boy and girl swimmers during the first year of the swimming training process. Ann.UMCS (Medicina, Sectio D)Lublin, 60(Suppl. 16/2):24-28.

9. Engstrom I. (1971) Preliminary report on the development of lung volumes in young girl swimmers. *A.Pediat.Scand.* 217: 73-276.

10. Maglischo E. (1993) Swimming Even Faster. Mayfield Publishing Co., Mountain View, CA.

11. Mujika I., T.Busson, A.Geyssant, J.C.Chatard (1996) Training content and its effects on performance in 100 and 200 m swimmers. In: J.P.Troup, A.P.Hollander, D.Strasse, S.W.Trappe, J.M.Cappaert, T.A.Trappe (eds.) Biomechanics and Medicine in Swimming VII. E.& F.N.Spon, London.

12. Narang I., E.Baraldi, M.Silverman, A.Bush (2006) Airway function measurements and the long-term follow-up of survivors of preterm birth with and without chronic lung disease. *Pediatr.Pulmonol.* 41:497-508.

13. Olbrecht J. (2000) The science of Winding. Planning, Periodizing and Optimizing Swim Training. Luton, England

14. Poprzęcki S., J.Cholewa, A.Zając (2005) Changes in anaerobic capacity of young swimmers in an annual training cycle. Ann. UMCS (Medicina, Sectio D)Lublin, 60(Suppl. 14/4):395-398.

15. Sienkiewicz-Dianzenza E., P.Tomaszewski, R.Stupnicki (2005) "Performance index" and its application to the assessment of multiple bouts of leg exercise. *Phys.Educ.Sport* 49:113-116.

16. Sienkiewicz-Dianzenza E., P.Tomaszewski, D.Iwańska, R.Stupnicki (2009) Anaerobic endurance of young untrained male and female subjects *Biomed.Hum.Kinetics* 1:16-19. DOI: 10.2478/v10101-009-0005-y.

17. Smoll F. (2002) Children sport development. In: Children and Youth in Sport. Kendall/Hunt Publishing Co., Dubuque IA.

18. Strzała M., A.Tyka (2009) Physical endurance, somatic indices and swimming technique parameters as determinants of front crawl swimming speed at short distances in young swimmers *Medicina Sportiva* 13:99-107.

19. Stupnicki R., E.Sienkiewicz-Dianzenza (2004) "Anaerobic endurance" and its assessment. *J.Hum.Kinetics* 12:109-115.

20. Sweetenham B., J.Atkinson (2003) Championship Swim Training. Human Kinetics, Champaign IL.

21. Wilmore J.H., D.L.Costill (1999) Training for Sport and Exercise. Human Kinetics Publishers, Champaign IL.

23

Conditions for preparations for the 2008 Beijing Paralympic Games in the opinion of the Polish national team

Joanna Sobiecka[1], Ryszard Plinta[2,3], Katarzyna Drobniewicz[4], Jadwiga Kłodecka-Różalska[5], Katarzyna Cichoń[6]

[1] Faculty of Motor Rehabilitation, University School of Physical Education, Krakow, [2] Department of Physical Education and Sport, Medical University of Silesia, Katowice, [3] Faculty of Physiotherapy, The Jerzy Kukuczka Academy of Physical Education, Katowice, [4] Non-Public Health Care Centre „Alma Spei", Cracow, [5] Department of Psychology, Institute of Sport, Warsaw, [6] Non-Public Health Care Centre for Autistic Persons „EFFATHA", Cracow, Poland

Summary

Study aim: To evaluate the process of preparing Polish athletes with disabilities for the 2008 Beijing Summer Paralympic Games.
Material and methods: The study included 31 women and 58 men representing 11 Paralympic disciplines, accounting for 97.8% of the Polish team taking part in the games. The average age was 32 years; the average amount of experience with sports training, 12 years. The method of diagnostic survey applied in the study was a questionnaire by J. Kłodecka-Różalska that was adapted to the needs of athletes with disabilities. The interpretation of the results was based on the arithmetic mean of individual evaluations. After checking the confidence interval, the factors were classified into one of three categories of conditions: satisfactory, sufficient, or unsatisfactory.
Results: Data analysis revealed different levels of care and conditions created for the Polish national team during their preparations for the Beijing Paralympic Games. The athletes were fully satisfied with the conditions of the central camps and consultation (food, accommodation, sports equipment) and social relations (atmosphere of cooperation between the athletes and cooperation between the athletes and national team coaches of various disciplines). Issues requiring more professional attention are the health of athletes nominated to participate in the Paralympic Games (medical care and individual orthopaedic equipment) and contact with the media, which shapes the image of sport of the disabled people.
Conclusions: In preparation for Paralympic Games, these athletes need to be provided with the constant and high-level assistance of a psychologist and a nutritionist. In the perspective of future athletic goals set for the representatives of our country, a high standard of sports facilities, individual sports equipment, transport to the central camps and consultation, as well as professional care in the field of wellness, physiotherapy and massage, should be taken into account for Paralympic Game preparations.

Key words: Preparation conditions – The Paralympic Games – Polish Paralympians

Introduction

Adapted physical activity tasks are carried out with people with disabilities as part of rehabilitation, special physical education, and sports. However, Paralympic sport has its own specific needs and it has become increasingly important not only to participate in the competition, but also to achieve results, including winning medals at the games.

Despite its distinctive nature, the requirements set out for the today's Paralympics basically do not differ from the training procedures followed for the Olympic Games [2]. According to Nunn [16], the training processes used to prepare for participation in the Paralympic Games should take place in conditions comparable to those of Olympic sports, which according to Sawicki [19] are designed not only to achieve success in sports, but above all else, to protect the athletes from injury and health risks.

In the culture of Polish athletes with disabilities there is a belief that to build their own sports career requires devotion [22]. But in the literature there is no information about the conditions under which the national team athletes trained for the Olympics from 1972 to 2002. The first studies were finally conducted among the athletes training for the 2004 Athens Paralympic Games [23]; those results are compared with the results obtained in our work, in the Discussion part of the paper.

Expectations and working hypotheses were associated with the observations conducted among the Olympic team

Author's address Joanna Sobiecka, Faculty of Motor Rehabilitation, University School of Physical Education, Al. Jana Pawła II 78, 31-571 Cracow, Poland

sportswomen in the period preceding their participation in the 2000 Sydney Olympic Games, the 2002 Salt Lake City Games, and the 2008 Beijing Games. Kłodecka-Różalska concluded that it is not only the modern facilities and optimal training programs that are necessary for the proper realisation of training and preparation for the event at the highest level. Instead, the following issues also require special attention and provision: medical care; specialist support of psychologists, physiologists, physiotherapists, dieticians; providing sportswomen with professional supervision of trainers who are highly qualified and experienced in working with women; care for the good emotional atmosphere and positive interpersonal relations; and the effective promotion of women's sport in the media and training organization that enable women athletes to reconcile their personal life, school, and professional preparation required to do sports [8,9].

Taking the above observations and recommendations into account, the present research assumes that to achieve sporting success on a scale of the Paralympians' dreams and fan expectations, it is not enough to secure the conditions met on an average or even good level. The process of preparation for big events must take place in circumstances that are satisfying and highly rated by the players in all areas that affect achievements in the Paralympic Games. The aim of this study was to evaluate the process of preparing Polish athletes with disabilities for the 2008 Beijing Summer Paralympic Games.

Material and Methods

The study involved 89 athletes, including 31 women and 58 men, i.e., 97.8% of all Polish athletes preparing for the 2008 Beijing Paralympic Games. The average age of respondents was 32 ± 9.7 years: 29 ± 10.3 years (15-51) for women and 32 ± 9.32 years (16-61) for men. The average duration of sports training experience was 12 ± 6.0 years: 10 ± 2.6 years (2-20) for women and 13 ± 7.0 years (1-47) for men. The youngest group of athletes were swimmers (mean = 21 years); the oldest, archers (mean = 51 years). People with damage to the musculoskeletal system accounted for 85.4% of the respondents, and those with damage to eyesight, 14.6%. The subjects had various education degrees, but most of them had completed general secondary school (about 34%) and higher education (about 22%). Some 14% of the Paralympians had finished technical or vocational secondary school, and 13% of them primary or lower secondary school. The surveyed athletes, who regularly trained up to 12 times a week, won nominations to the Paralympic Games in the following disciplines: horse riding – 1.1%, cycling – 3.4%; athletics – 32.5%, archery – 7.9%, swimming – 12.4%, lifting weights – 11.2%, shooting – 5.6%, wheelchair fencing – 7.9%, wheelchair tennis – 4.5%, table tennis – 11.1%, and rowing – 3.4 %. It is worth noting that repeat participants in the Paralympic Games were the majority of respondents (approximately 57%).

The study was mainly conducted during the camps that occurred about 30 days before leaving for the Paralympic Games. The study was preceded by detailed instruction. Visually impaired or amblyopic athletes could ask the researchers for assistance. The method of diagnostic survey was applied through the use of a questionnaire by J. Kłodecka-Różalska [6,7], which with the consent of its author was adapted to the needs of athletes with disabilities by J. Sobiecka and entitled "Survey for female and male athletes training for the Paralympic Games" (see Appendix A). It should be noted that the survey was verified in pilot studies, performed on a group of 91 athletes four years earlier, during preparations for the 2004 Athens Paralympic Games.

The questionnaire consisted of two parts. The first was comprised of 20 closed questions in which the respondents rated the preparation conditions on a scale of 1 to 5 (5 – very high, 4 – high, 3 – average, 2 – low, 1 – very low). The questionnaire also included open questions with which athletes could describe other needs that in their opinion should be secured in preparation for the Paralympic Games. The second part contained the subjects' socio-demographic and sports data.

The arithmetic mean was calculated from a sum of individual results for each of the evaluated factors by classifying the averaged opinions to three categories of conditions: satisfactory (5.0-4.1), sufficient (4.0-3.0) and unsatisfactory (2.9-1.0).

Furthermore, for each averaged opinion describing the preparation conditions, we examined the concordance of ratings of the respondents. The opinions were considered concordant in a statistically significant way if the width of the confidence interval for the mean was less than 1.0 ($\alpha = 0.05$).

Results

The first analysed data concerned sports infrastructure and individual equipment (Table 1). Both female and male athletes found having the opportunity to use high-quality sports equipment the most satisfactory, while sportswomen also evaluated individual sports equipment as the most satisfactory. For majority of the Paralympians, the most unsatisfactory factor was individual orthopaedic equipment used in their disciplines. Sports facilities received a generally positive assessment, being categorized as sufficient.

Among the factors considered were the conditions of the stay on central camps and consultation. The data in Table 2 shows that the respondents were mostly satisfied with provided food and accommodation. Duration of camps and transport were rated as sufficient. Women more often than men expressed a higher degree of satisfaction with these conditions.

Questions related to the conditions in which Polish national team athletes were preparing for the Paralympics also included the area of interpersonal relations. The data in Table 3 demonstrate the cooperation of the respondents with the national team coaches; atmosphere; and interaction between the athletes themselves. The responses relating to social dimension received a positive assessment; there were differences, however, between the polarized attitudes of women and men. None of the sportswomen evaluated the atmosphere of cooperation as destructive.

Table 1. Evaluation of the facilities, sports equipment, individual equipment, and sports orthopaedic equipment that the athletes used during their preparations for the Paralympic Games

Respondents	n	Rating categories*					Mean rating	Categories of conditions
		5	4	3	2	1		
Sports facilities								
Women	31	10	14	5	2	0	4,0	Sufficient
Men	58	13	31	11	2	1	3,9	Sufficient**
Total	89	23	45	16	4	1	4,0	Sufficient**
Sports equipment								
Women	31	13	9	8	1	0	4,1	Satisfactory**
Men	58	22	24	7	5	0	4,1	Satisfactory**
Total	89	35	33	15	6	0	4,1	Satisfactory**
Individual sports equipment								
Women	31	11	14	5	1	0	4,1	Satisfactory**
Men	58	16	23	11	8	0	3,8	Sufficient**
Total	89	27	37	16	9	0	3,9	Sufficient**
Sports orthopedic equipment								
Women	20	3	4	3	2	8	2,6	Unsatisfactory
Men	39	6	5	8	8	12	2,6	Unsatisfactory**
Total	59	9	9	11	10	20	2,6	Unsatisfactory**

* Ratings: 5 - very high, 4 - high, 3 - average, 2 - low, 1 – very low; ** Level of significance of mean rating: $p < 0.05$

Table 2. Evaluation of transport, accommodation, food, and planned duration of stay on the central sports camp and consultation that would allow for optimal preparation of athletes for the Paralympic Games

Respondents	n	Rating categories*					Mean rating	Categories of conditions
		5	4	3	2	1		
Transport								
Women	30	12	7	6	5	0	3,9	Sufficient
Men	55	13	26	10	6	0	3,6	Sufficient**
Total	85	25	33	16	11	0	3,7	Sufficient**
Accommodation								
Women	30	11	12	6	1	0	4,1	Satisfactory**
Men	55	18	26	10	1	0	4,1	Satisfactory**
Total	85	29	38	16	2	0	4,1	Satisfactory**
Food								
Women	30	18	10	2	0	0	4,5	Satisfactory**
Men	55	22	22	7	1	3	4,1	Satisfactory**
Total	85	40	32	9	1	3	4,2	Satisfactory**
Planned duration								
Women	30	9	10	7	3	1	3,8	Sufficient
Men	55	13	17	16	4	5	3,5	Sufficient**
Total	85	22	27	23	7	6	3,6	Sufficient**

For explanation of symbols see Table 1.

Table 3. Evaluation of cooperation between the national team coaches and Paralympic athletes, atmosphere, and interaction between the athletes themselves while preparing for the Paralympics

Respondents	n	Rating categories*					Mean rating	Categories of conditions
		5	4	3	2	1		
Cooperation with coaches								
Women	31	17	8	3	1	2	4,2	Satisfactory**
Men	58	30	10	10	4	4	4,0	Sufficient**
Total	89	47	18	13	5	6	4,1	Satisfactory**
Atmosphere and interaction between athletes								
Women	31	14	12	4	1	0	4,3	Satisfactory**
Men	58	20	30	5	1	2	4,1	Satisfactory**
Total	89	34	42	9	2	2	4,2	Satisfactory**

For explanation of symbols see Table 1.

Table 4. Evaluation of medical care and assistance of specialists the athletes received when preparing for the Paralympics

Respondents	n	Rating categories*					Mean rating	Categories of conditions
		5	4	3	2	1		
Medical care								
Women	31	7	1	6	11	6	2,7	Unsatisfactory
Men	58	5	9	7	8	29	2,2	Unsatisfactory**
Total	89	12	10	13	19	35	2,4	Unsatisfactory**
Wellness treatments after trainings and competitions								
Women	31	6	5	11	6	3	3,2	Sufficient
Men	58	10	15	12	8	13	3,0	Sufficient**
Total	89	16	20	23	14	16	3,1	Sufficient**
Assistance of physiotherapist								
Women	20	5	6	3	4	2	3,4	Sufficient
Men	30	8	6	5	4	7	3,1	Sufficient
Total	50	13	12	8	8	9	3,2	Sufficient**
Assistance of masseur								
Women	28	8	6	6	6	2	3,4	Sufficient
Men	38	14	7	4	7	6	3,4	Sufficient
Total	66	22	14	9	13	8	3,4	Sufficient**
Assistance of dietician								
Women	12	2	2	2	1	5	2,6	Unsatisfactory
Men	13	1	0	2	4	6	1,9	Unsatisfactory
Total	25	3	2	4	5	11	2,2	Unsatisfactory**
Assistance of psychologist								
Women	5	1	4	0	0	0	4,2	Satisfactory**
Men	5	2	0	0	2	1	3,0	Sufficient
Total	10	3	4	0	2	1	3,6	Sufficient

For explanation of symbols see Table 1.

The opinions of the respondents about medical care and assistance of specialists varied from very positive to strongly negative (Table 4). Every second man and fifth women expressed deep dissatisfaction with the medical care. As a result, it fell into a category "unsatisfactory". In the opinion of the Paralympians, wellness treatments after trainings and competitions only satisfied their needs at a sufficient level, and one in five respondents put them in the "very low" category. Only 56% of the athletes could count on the assistance of a physiotherapist: one in four persons rated this at the highest level, while one in five, strongly negative. This means that the guaranteed offer of assistance was far from the expectations of Polish Paralympians. Moreover, not all persons on the national team had the opportunity to work with a masseur. About 74% of the athletes received this assistance. Most of them expressed satisfaction with it; however, some women and men gave it low or very low ratings. In preparation for the games, the Polish athletes were not provided with the direct support of a dietician or a psychologist. Only a small portion of the respondents could use it (25 used a dietician; 10 used a psychologist). The sportswomen and sportsmen felt that the level of service of dietician was unsatisfactory. With regard to the assistance of psychologist: these conditions were satisfactory for women and sufficient for men.

The experience of the Paralympian team concerning their interaction with the media also proved unsatisfactory. Most of the ratings were low and very low for men, while average for women. Generally, the level of cooperation with the media was evaluated as unsatisfactory (Table 5).

The last of the studied issues was the relationship between obligations arising from practicing sports and the sphere of personal life, career, and education (Table 6). Most of the Paralympians managed to combine personal life with a sports career at a sufficient level. Juggling professional responsibilities and education with regular sports practice proved more difficult.

work and rest. The opinions expressed by the respondents – from very positive to strongly negative – confirmed the fact that not all areas of support and organization satisfied the Polish national team.

It should be noted that in preparation for the Paralympics, the adequate adaptation of facilities to the functional capabilities of persons with disabilities plays a crucial role. According to Depauw and Gavron [3], such facilities should provide the athletes with easy and unfettered access to every place in the infrastructure and its facilities. It is even more true in the eye of the norms used to design sports centres, which must address the needs of athletes with disabilities. Whether the facilities meet their requirements, according to Hanrahan [4], depends primarily on the national team coaches, because they are responsible for the organising training process, including planning and selecting optimal training facilities.

Table 5. Evaluation of contacts the athletes with the media during preparations for the Paralympic Games

Respondents	n	Rating categories*					Mean rating	Categories of conditions
		5	4	3	2	1		
Women	29	6	3	10	7	3	3,1	Sufficient
Men	47	2	5	9	17	14	2,1	Unsatisfactory**
Total	76	8	8	19	24	17	2,6	Unsatisfactory**

For explanation of symbols see Table 1.

Table 6. Evaluation of the possibility of reconciling personal life, professional, academic and school responsibilities with sport by the athletes preparing for the Paralympic Games

Respondents	n	Rating categories*					Mean rating	Categories of conditions
		5	4	3	2	1		
Combining personal life with sport								
Women	31	2	17	9	2	1	3,6	Sufficient**
Men	58	15	19	21	0	3	3,7	Sufficient**
Total	89	17	36	30	2	4	3,7	Sufficient**
Combining work with sport								
Women	20	1	9	5	2	3	3,2	Sufficient
Men	38	9	9	14	3	3	3,5	Sufficient**
Total	58	10	18	19	5	6	3,4	Sufficient**
Combining school and university with sport								
Women	21	3	6	9	2	1	3,4	Sufficient
Men	30	5	7	12	3	3	3,3	Sufficient**
Total	51	8	13	21	5	4	3,4	Sufficient**

For explanation of symbols see Table 1.

Discussion

Steadward and Sheri [25] pointed out that only the hard work of the athletes and their coaches, intensive training, and a well executed period before a competition have a significant impact on success in the Paralympic Games, but also the high standards of conditions created for both

The sports, individual, and orthopaedic equipment is also of great importance to the athletes preparing for the games. Pallis [17] and Vanlandewijck [27] are convinced that ensuring that this equipment is at the highest possible level will enable athletes with disabilities to not only achieve significantly better results during the competition, but it will also guarantee their safety. In addition, the appropriate adaptation of equipment with regard to the individual needs of each competitor will prevent or reduce the likelihood of injury and increase comfort during training and competition. The considered research results become very important when referring to the opinion expressed by Burkett and Mellifont [1]. In their view, an athlete's fitness and safety may be increased by simple but effective modifications in design techniques of basic sports equipment. Laing and Carr were of the same opinion [11], claiming that appropriate sports clothing is not only comfortable for athletes, but also minimises the risk of injury in case of a fall.

The opinions of the national team on the state of individual orthopaedic equipment that they used during the Paralympic competition are highly alarming. On the basis of the obtained results, it can be concluded that the athletes were not satisfied with it both during the Beijing and the Athens Olympic Games [23].

Before the Paralympic Games, sport training for the athletes nominated for national team are based on central camps and consultation, thus their satisfaction with the comfort of accommodation and the use of sports equipment is essential. The duration of stay at camps and sports consultation should be carefully thought out, with optimal possible access (transport). In the case of Polish Paralympians, this is particularly important due to the fact that the athletes who were nominated to participate in the Beijing Olympic Games combined their sports careers with family lives and parenting (about 26%), professional lives (about 65%), and/or school-academic responsibilities (about 57%).

It is believed that sports success is affected not only by properly realised training and athletic skills, but also – due to high levels of stress – by satisfying the area of human relations, including cooperation with coaches and a favourable atmosphere and interaction between the athletes themselves. The thesis of the impact of coach-athlete relationships on sports results has been confirmed by many researchers, including Smith and Smoll [20], Lavoie [12], and Martens [14].

A study conducted by Sobiecka et al. [24] showed that communication between coaches and participants of the Paralympic Games was at a very good level. It should be assumed then that the atmosphere and cooperation in this area proved to be satisfactory to the members of the Polish national team who were preparing for the Beijing Games.

According to Depauw and Gavron [3] and Makowski [13], in order to ensure the appropriate conditions for training, competition, and above all else, safety for the athletes with disabilities, it is necessary to appoint a medical team, which will include a doctor and other specialists in the following areas: wellness, physiotherapy, massage, physiology, and nutrition. They should fulfil their tasks not only during preparations for major competitions, but through systematic controlling and promoting the athletes' health and, if necessary, administering proper treatment and rehabilitation. From the point of view of mission, which has to be accomplished by a medical team while preparing the national team representatives to participate in the Paralympic Games, the results of the present study proved to be unsatisfactory. A low evaluation of the medical care provided to Polish athletes raises concerns. It is especially alarming in the face of Regulation of the Minister of Sport of 8 January 2007 regarding the scope of medical care for athletes of the national team – persons with disabilities and Paralympians – which was to provide athletes with disabilities with medical care, including all health-related prevention, treatment, and rehabilitation.

The key factors in the process of Olympic preparations include mental support. Kłodecka-Różalska [8,9] and Porter [18] argue that the success in significant events is not only an effect of physical fitness and mental preparation, but also the actual disposition of an athlete. Unfortunately, the data demonstrated that only one in ten Paralympians had the assistance of a psychologist ensured. Not everyone was satisfied with it.

There is a general belief that multilateral cooperation of the sports community of the disabled with representatives of the media has the greatest impact on promoting positive ideas about adapted physical activity, including Paralympic sports [3,15]. The results revealed the dissatisfaction of the Paralympians and negative opinions on contact with the mass media. This situation requires consideration and modern transformation, since the media, especially television, significantly affects social perceptions of the value of sport for the quality of life of people with disabilities.

According to Jones and Howe [5], special attention should be paid to the personal lives of athletes, as this factor is an essential element of the existence of every person, the disabled person's life in particular. Our findings in this field showed that preparations of a large group of athletes for the Paralympic Games were performed at the expense of their personal lives.

Key issues also remain including the ability to combine a professional career with other fields of activities as well as including people with disabilities into society [21,22]. Tasiemski and colleagues drew attention to the importance of a professional career for the functioning of disabled athletes [26]. According to them, in addition to the social benefits, a career provides financial independence for people with disabilities. The authors also pointed out that the athletes taking part in competition are hard workers. Systematic training and therefore sense of duty connected with it is reflected in their conscientiousness and efficient work organization. Similar views were demonstrated in a paper by Sobiecka [21]. She assumed that experiences acquired during a sports career proved to be useful in the exercise of professional responsibilities. In addition, many athletes appreciated their promotions and professional prestige, which were supported by regular sports activities. Education and professional preparation for athletes was of similar importance. The paper by Kraemer and Fleck [10] suggested that what is most important in schooling is not only individualized education, as well as support from teachers, lecturers, and family, but also the attitude of the closest sports circles, especially coaches of young athletes.

Based on the obtained results he following conclusions can be formulated:

1. Different levels of care and conditions for the Polish national team were provided during their preparations for the Beijing Paralympic Games.

2. Most of the athletes were fully satisfied with the conditions of central camps and consultation (food, accommodation, sports equipment) and social relations (atmosphere of cooperation between the athletes and cooperation between the athletes and national team coaches of various disciplines).

3. The issues that require more professional attention are the health of athletes nominated to participate in the Paralympic Games (medical care and individual orthopaedic equipment) and contact with the media, which shape the image of sport of the disabled people.

4. In preparation for the next Paralympic Games the athletes need to be provided with constant and high-level assistance of both a psychologist and a nutritionist.

5. In the perspective of future athletic goals set for the representatives of our country, a high standard of sports facilities, individual sports equipment, transport to the central camps, and consultation, as well as professional care in the field of wellness, physiotherapy and massage, should be taken into account in the Paralympic preparations.

References

1. Burkett B.J., R.B.Mellifont (2008) Sport science and coaching in Paralympic cycling. *Int.J.Sports Sci.Coach.* 3:95-103.

2. Coaching Association of Canada (2005) Stages coaches may go through when working for the first time with an athlete with a disability. In: Coaching Athletes with a Disability. Investors Group, Canada, pp. 4-6.

3. DePauw K.P., S.J.Gavron (2005) Disability Sport. Human Kinetics Publishers, Champaign IL.

4. Hanrahan S. (2005) Able athletes with disabilities: issues and group work. In: M.B. Andersen (eds.) Sport Psychology in Practice. Human Kinetics, Champaign IL, pp.223-247.

5. Jones C., P.D.Howe (2005) The conceptual boundaries of sport for the disabled: classification and athletic performance. *J.Philos.Sport* 32:133-146.

6. Kłodecka-Różalska J. (2001) Advantages-obstacles-psychological costs of women s sport activity. In: A.Papaioannou, M.Goudas, Y.Theodorakis (eds.) In The Dawn Of The New Millennium. Proc. 10th World Congr. Sport Psychology, ISSP, Skiatos, pp. 279-281.

7. Kłodecka-Różalska J. (2002) Opinion of Polish female athletes on preparation conditions for the Olympic Games in Sydney 2000 and Salt Lake City 2002. (in Polish) *Kob.Sport* 3:6-9.

8. Kłodecka-Różalska J. (2006) Mental training achievements and future applications of psychology in Polish sports. *Phys.Educ. Sport* 50 (4):99-107.

9. Kłodecka-Różalska J. (2007) "Face to face" with the whole world: how to mentally prepare the team for the Olympics. *Pol.J. Sports Med.* 23:184-188.

10. Kraemer W.J., S.J.Fleck (2004) Creating individualized programs. In: Strength Training for Young Athletes. Human Kinetics Publishers, Champaign, pp. 52-61.

11. Laing R.M., D.J.Carr (2005) Is protection part of the game? Protection against impact using clothing and personal equipment. In: R.Shiho (eds.) Textiles in Sport. Woodhead Publishing, pp. 232-261.

12. LaVoi N.M. (2007) Expanding the interpersonal dimension: closeness in the coach-athlete relationship. *Int.J.Sports Sci.*, 2(4):497-512.

13. Makowski A. (2008) High performance preparation for athletes of diverse abilities. *N.Am.J.Sports Phys.Ther.* 3 (2):66.

14. Martens R. (2004) Communicating with your athletes. In: Successful Coaching. Human Kinetics Publishers, Champaign, pp. 95-119.

15. Molinatti B. (2006) TV, sports, & history. *Sports 'n Spokes* 32: 61.

16. Nunn C. (2009) Coaching at the Paralympic level: if only the administrators understood. In: O.J.Schantz, K.Gilbert (eds.) The Paralympic Games: Empowerment Or Side Show? Meyer & Meyer Verlag, Aachen, pp. 102-114.

17. Pallis J.M. (2003) Materials in Paralympic sports. In: M.Jenkins (eds.) Materials in Sports Equipment. Woodhead Publishing, Cambridge, pp. 376-398.

18. Porter K. (2003) Mental training for specific needs. In: The Mental Athlete: Inner Training for Peak Performance in All Sports. Human Kinetics, Champaign, IL, pp.153-188.

19. Sawicki O. (2008) Reflections on the Beijing Summer Paralympic Games - A Canadian Paralympic Committee perspective. *Coach.Plan* 15: 37-39.

20. Smith R.E., F.L.Smoll (2007) Behavioral research and intervention in youth sports. In: D.Smith, M.Bar-Eli (eds.) Essential Readings in Sport and Exercise Psychology. Human Kinetics Publishers, Champaign, pp. 135-144.

21. Sobiecka J. (2000) The role of sport in comprehensive rehabilitation of Polish participants of Paralympic Games (in Polish). Studies and Monographs No. 9, AWF Cracow.

22. Sobiecka J. (2005) Winter sports practice and its influence on the frame of mind and lifestyle of disabled persons as exemplified by Polish Paralympic competitors. *Pol.J.Environ.Stud.* suppl. II, 13:512-516.

23. Sobiecka J. (2005) Some selected aspects concerning the preparation of the Polish national team members for the summer Paralympic Games held in Athens in 2004. *Med.Sport.* suppl. 9 (2):163-164.

24. Sobiecka J., R.Plinta, K.Cichoń, K.Drobniewicz (2011) The relations that occurred between the athletes and coaches of the national team during their preparations for the Paralympics games (according to the athletes). *J.Orthop.Trauma.Surg.Relat.Res.* 26:52-70.

25. Steadward R.D., L.F.Sheri (2003) History of disability sport. In: R.D.Steadward, G.D.Wheeler, E.J.Watkinson (eds.) Adapted Physical Activity. University of Alberta Press, Edmonton, pp. 471-498.

26. Tasiemski T., P.Kennedy, B.P.Gardner, R.A.Blaikley (2005) Athletic identity and sports participation in people with spinal cord injury. *Adapt.Phys.Activ.Q.* 21:364-378.

27. Vanlandewijck Y. (2006) Sport science in the Paralympic movement. *J.Rehabil.Res.Dev.* 43: 17-24.

Appendix A

Questionnaire for female and male athletes training for the Paralympic Games

(Based on "Survey for female athletes training for the Olympic Game",*
modified by Dr. J. Sobiecka for the needs of the athletes with disabilities)

Please rate the conditions under which you have been preparing for the Beijing Summer Paralympic Games **on a scale of 5 to 1 (5 – very high, 4 – high, 3 – average, 2 – low, 1 – very low).** If an issue does not concern you, underline the answer "**not applicable**". However, when the assistance of specialists has not been provided during your preparations or there was no interest from the media – please choose the answer "**none**".

1/ Sports facilities **5 4 3 2 1**

2/ Sports equipment **5 4 3 2 1**

3/ Individual sports equipment (clothing, shoes, bags, etc.) **5 4 3 2 1**

4/ Sports orthopaedic equipment **5 4 3 2 1 not applicable**

5/ Transport to the central sports camps and consultation **5 4 3 2 1**

6/ Standards of accommodation during the central sports camps and consultation **5 4 3 2 1**

7/ Food during the central sports camps and consultation **5 4 3 2 1**

8/ Planned duration of your stay on the camps and consultation, allowing the optimum preparation for the Paralympic Games **5 4 3 2 1**

9/ Cooperation with the Paralympic national team coaches **5 4 3 2 1**

10/ Atmosphere and interaction between the athletes themselves **5 4 3 2 1**

11/ Medical care **5 4 3 2 1 none**

12/ Wellness treatments after trainings and competitions **5 4 3 2 1 none**

13/ Assistance of a physiotherapist **5 4 3 2 1 none**

14/ Assistance of a masseur **5 4 3 2 1 none**

15/ Assistance of a dietician **5 4 3 2 1 none**

16/ Assistance of a psychologist **5 4 3 2 1 none**

17/ Contact with the media **5 4 3 2 1 none**

18/ Possibility of combining personal life with sports **5 4 3 2 1**

19/ Possibility of combining professional responsibilities with sports **5 4 3 2 1 not applicable**

20/ Possibility of combining school and academic responsibilities with sports **5 4 3 2 1 not applicable**

21/ Name other needs that should be met in your preparation for the Paralympic Games:

a/..

b/..

c/..

---

* *Kłodecka-Różalska J. (2002) Opinion of Polish female athletes on preparation conditions for the Olympic Games in Sydney 2000 and Salt Lake City 2002. (in Polish) Kob.Sport 3:6-9.*

Personal Data

Gender *(underline as appropriate):* female, male **Year of birth** ....

Weekly participation in training *(how many times per week)* ....

Experience with sports training *(in a number of years)* ....

Discipline *(underline as appropriate):* horse riding, cycling, athletics, archery, swimming, weightlifting, shooting, wheelchair fencing, wheelchair tennis, table tennis, rowing

Multiple participation in the Paralympic Games *(underline as appropriate):* 1 2 3 4 5

Start group - medical classification *(underline as appropriate):* visual impairment, amputations of at least one limb, paraplegia, other injuries of the musculoskeletal system, Cerebral Palsy

Education *(underline as appropriate):* higher education, general secondary education, vocational education (including post-secondary), basic vocational education, primary education (including lower secondary school *gimnazjum*)

Marital status (*underline as appropriate):* single, married, widowed, divorced, unmarried partners

Working life *(underline as appropriate):* working, unemployed, not working, pupil, student

Disability categories *(underline as appropriate):*
visual impairment – blind, amblyopic; injuries of the musculoskeletal system of the lower limbs – in a wheelchair, not using a wheelchair; injuries of the musculoskeletal system of the upper limbs; other (what?)........................

Disability levels *(underline as appropriate):* severe, moderate, light

Thank you very much for completing the survey. We wish you success in the Games and look forward to our further cooperation.

Increasing pupil physical activity: a comprehensive professional development effort

Pamela Hodges Kulinna

Mary Lou Fulton Teachers College, Faculty Affiliate Program of Kinesiology, Arizona State University

Summary

Study aim: To determine if pupil physical activity and Body Mass Index classifications maintained or improved after a one-year professional development program involving both classroom and physical education teachers. Guskey's model of teacher change guided this study.
Material and methods: Indigenous children from ten schools (N = 320) in grades 3-12 from one community participated in this year-long comprehensive school change effort. Classroom (n = 31) and physical education teachers (n = 7) participated in this study as intervention (n = 27) or comparison (n = 11) teachers. Intervention teachers participated in a year-long professional development program to increase physical activity and healthy behaviour knowledge of pupils.
Results: ANOVA results for pupil physical activity (measured using pedometry) indicated that both groups of pupils (intervention and comparison) became significantly more active over time. The intervention groups' behaviour was less stable ($\alpha = 0.71$) over time versus the comparison group ($\alpha = 0.86$), suggesting positive behaviour changes. No significant Body Mass Index changes were found.
Conclusions: Although the intervention resulted in physical activity increases for both intervention and comparison pupils at the schools, change takes time and these initial findings show progress in increasing physical activity behaviours at school in an understudied and disadvantaged population of indigenous USA youth.

Key words: Children – Health – Physical activity – Intervention

Introduction

The negative pattern of reduced physical activity and increased dietary consumption has led to the current childhood overweight crisis [20]. This national trend of youth's decreased physical activity and increased body mass have been seen in Poland [8], USA [9], Australia [11], England [7], Canada [17] and most other developed countries. The negative health effects related to inactivity (i.e., obesity, diabetes) have been more severe for minority populations, especially for indigenous youth [16]. When compared to an age and gender-matched reference population 5 to 10 years of age, indigenous children were heavier and had a higher percentage of body fat [16]. Diabetes in the indigenous tribe of Pima Indian children is growing at about 2% per year with nearly half of the adult population over the age of 35 having Type II diabetes [4].

One intervention strategy for working with schools on public health issues is to implement ongoing, embedded comprehensive professional development sessions with classroom teachers and physical education teachers focused on helping teachers change behaviours.

Guskey's Model of Teacher Change [6] is a theory about how teacher change happens in schools. It begins with staff development, which leads to changes in teachers classroom practices, which, in turn, leads to changes in pupil learning outcomes and finally to the creation of new teacher belief systems. This model is guided by three principles. First, teacher change takes time and is not easy. Second, it is necessary for teachers to see positive changes in pupil learning in order to buy into program effectiveness. Finally, support and follow-up are needed for teachers in the process of change.

The current paper grounded in Guskey's Model of Teacher Change focuses on pupil physical activity and body composition outcomes of this teacher change project (interviews are presented elsewhere [3]). The purpose of this study was to determine if pupil physical activity and Body Mass Index (BMI) classifications maintained or improved after a year long, professional development program involving both classroom and physical education instructors teaching healthy and active content (physical activity and nutrition). It was hypothesized that: (a) pupils would increase their physical activity levels at

Author's address Prof. Pamela Hodges Kulinna, Mary Lou Fulton Teachers College, Arizona State University, 7291 E. Sonoran Arroyo Mall, Santa Catalina Bldg., Mesa, AZ 85212

school and (b) pupils would maintain or decrease their BMI as a result of their teachers' lessons changes as an outcome from participation in ongoing healthy and active professional development experiences over one year.

Material and Methods

Guskey's model of teacher change and corresponding principles [6] were used to frame the current study. Based on Guskey's first principle, teachers were given time to implement changes in their teaching. For example, both classroom and physical education teachers participated in five workshops spread across the academic year (about 35 hours) to help them prepare to teach ten healthy behaviour lesson ideas (i.e., physical activity and nutrition content knowledge) and daily physical activity breaks, while Physical Education teachers were also trained to teach the Dynamic Physical Education curricular model. Wei et al. [22] reported that 30-100 hours of teacher training spread over six to 12 months resulted in significant positive effects on pupil outcomes. Based on Guskey's second principle, intervention teachers were able to observe and assess pupil changes taking place (i.e., pedometers were used to track physical activity). Finally, addressing Guskey's third principle, teachers were provided with extensive support. Mentor teacher support was provided to both classroom and physical education teacher participants on a monthly basis. Furthermore, administrative support was present at the school level.

Participants

Youth. Children and youth participants were 320 indigenous boys (n = 136) and girls (n = 184) at the primary (n = 200) and secondary (n = 120) levels, ranging from seven to twenty years of age (mean age 10.30 ± 3.06) from a single indigenous community in the USA. Participants in the intervention group (n=234) and comparison group (n = 86) were from ten schools: five were primary, three were middle, and two were high school, governed by Tribal Administrators, the Catholic Church, or the State Department of Education (two public schools). The project was approved by Tribe Administrators and the University IRB committee. Parents/guardians also provided consent and pupils assented to participate.

Teachers and recruitment. Thirty-one classroom teachers and seven physical education teachers (11 male and 27 female) from the ten schools who taught pupils in grades 3-12 participated in this project. Teachers were invited to participate in either the intervention (n = 27) or comparison (n = 11) group and only interested teachers participated. There were one to two intervention and comparison teacher participants at each school as per Tribal Administrators' requirements. Teachers in the intervention group had between one and 27 years of teaching experience (mean 9.40 ± 7.67) and teachers in the comparison group had between two and 27 years of teaching experience (mean 12.75 ± 11.02). Physical Education teachers met with classes two to five days/week depending on the school.

Overview and school district needs

Participation in this year-long teacher change initiative required intervention teachers to attend five after-school workshops (spread across the year) that were either focused on infusing physical activity and healthy behaviour knowledge into the curriculum or on the Dynamic Physical Education curriculum (a multi-activity K-12 Physical Education curricular model [5,14]). Teacher input was sought at workshops. Brainstorming time was also provided with other teachers who taught at similar grade levels. Teachers were given classroom sets of pedometers (all intervention teachers), physical activity equipment appropriate for the classroom, e.g., poly spots for the floor, soft balls, dice with words (classroom teachers), physical education class equipment, i.e., Dynamic Physical Education school equipment sets (see gophersport.com, physical education teachers), and a small stipend (participation incentive). For the comparison teachers, pre/post pupil data were collected and the teachers did not participate in any other aspects of the project.

Two experienced mentor teachers (external to the school district) who had taught indigenous pupils in Physical Education and in classroom settings were assigned to all intervention teachers. They visited the intervention teachers' classrooms/gymnasiums at an agreed upon date/time each month. Teachers also submitted monthly electronic reflections to their mentor teachers. Teachers in the intervention group were required to teach a minimum of ten lesson ideas (e.g., establishing a baseline for physical activity using pedometers) that integrated physical activity and healthy behaviour knowledge with academic content (please refer to Table 1). The lesson ideas were very general in order for teachers to modify the lessons as needed as well as to fit the content into their regular curriculum in logical places.

To complement and supplement the physical activity based lesson ideas that were being taught, classroom teachers also provided daily activity breaks for pupils (3-10 minutes). Primary classroom teachers were provided with the Activity and Healthy Schools® [15] classroom physical activity break cards (e.g., cards with physical activity break instructions see www.gophersport.com) that they used for lessons to teach physical activity breaks in the classroom). All teachers were also provided with over 40 classroom activity breaks that integrated content from various subjects (e.g., writing, math).

Table 1. Lesson objectives

State Standards Met	Title	Objective
Physical Education Standard 5 Technology Standard 3	Recording Pedometer Data	Pupils will demonstrate their understanding of pedometers by recording their daily accumulated step count and if required, their daily activity time.
Mathematics Standards 3 & 6	Establishing a Baseline	Pupils will learn how to establish a baseline by using teacher-designed data. When pupils can successfully establish a baseline with teacher designed data, they are now ready to work with their own data.
Self-Regulation Standard 1 Mathematics Standard 3	Goal Setting	Pupils will learn how to establish their own personal goals for increasing their activity level.
Language Arts Standard 1	Establish a Activity Word Wall	Pupils and teachers working together will establish a word wall of activity words they have learned while working with their new pedometers. This wall will be added to throughout the school year.
Mathematics Standard 1	Walking versus Jogging	Pupils will determine how walking and jogging differ in accumulating steps and activity time with their pedometer.
Physical Education Standard 3	Fitness Concepts	Pupils will understand why each of the five components of health related fitness are essential to improving the length and quality of their own life.
Mathematics Standards 2 & 8	Incorporating Math and Graphing Skills	Pupils will reinforce their math critical thinking skills and computation skills by using pedometer data to solve math problems.
Arts Standard 1 Language Arts Standard 2	Incorporating Writing Activities	Pupils will reinforce their writing skills by incorporating their pedometer information into their writing.
Science Standard 12 Life Skills Standard 4	The Scientific Process	Pupils will demonstrate their understanding of the scientific process by completing a walking and jogging activity.
Geography Standard 2 Mathematics Standard 4	Integrating Social Studies	Pupils will use their social study skills and pedometer step count to determine the distance and/or time it will take them to travel from point to point.

In addition to the ten lessons, physical education teachers were taught lessons and management techniques to adopt the Dynamic Physical Education curricular model [5,14]. The Physical Education teachers also provided support for the classroom teachers who were at the same school. Fidelity by Physical Education teachers to the Dynamic Physical Education curricular model was assessed by the mentor teachers during their monthly observations/meetings as well as by mentor teachers who read/corresponded with teachers regarding their reflections.

Instruments

The current study used pedometers to track pupils' physical activity patterns at school. Pedometers measure vertical oscillations of body movement from the hip, thus providing a total count of accumulated ambulatory movement of steps taken [19]. All pupil participants in the current project wore a Walk4Life 2505 pedometer shown to provide valid and reliable estimates of youth physical activity and steps [1].

Data collection procedures

Pedometer preparations. Guidelines [21] were followed in pedometer preparations and data collection procedures using sealed pedometers. Pupil participants in this project were informed that their physical activity was being measured. Prior to data collection, pupils practiced wearing pedometers in several physical education classes and/or in their classrooms (varied by school) to diminish potential novelty and reactivity effects. Refresher lessons were also provided the week prior to data collection.

Pedometer protocol. Pupils were instructed to wear pedometers at all times at school and not to tamper with them. Pupils who tampered (e.g., shook) with pedometers lost the privilege of participation (1-2 pupils per school). All pupils wore pedometers (Walk4Life 2505) for four consecutive school days in both September and May in order to give a representative sample of school based physical activity. Four days have been shown to be adequate time in order to accurately measure children's physical activity patterns [18]. At the end of each day, research team members recorded steps for each pupil, reset the pedometers to zero, and resealed them for the following day. The team members were present at the schools all day to ensure that pupils were accurately wearing pedometers.

BMI data. Demographic information (i.e., age) was collected from the parents or schools. BMI measurements, body mass (kg) and height (cm) were directly measured without shoes using a calibrated digital scale (Seca 882 Digital BMI Scale) and stadiometer (Seca 214 Portable Stadiometer). These measurements were taken during non-pedometer data collection days at each school pre and post intervention by members of the research team.

Data analyses

Data analyses began with *t*-tests investigating potential pre-test differences between the intervention and comparison groups for physical activity and BMI. Since groups were not significantly different at pre-test, Analysis of Variance (ANOVA) tests were performed to investigate pre/post group changes in physical activity and BMI by group (intervention versus comparison). ANOVA was also run to investigate possible gender and grade level differences in physical activity. Due to multiple ANOVA analyses, Bonferroni adjustments were made (k=4). Internal consistency reliability analyses were conducted to investigate the stability of physical activity behaviours; that is, high (e.g., >0.80) internal consistency reliability suggests little behaviour change. Finally, descriptive statistics were also run on the variables. The level of $p \leq 0.05$ was considered significant.

Results

ANOVA results investigating physical activity changes showed both groups (intervention and comparison) became significantly more active over time ($F_{1, 319} = 20.10$, $p < 0.001$), partial $\eta^2 = 0.06$). There was no significant group main effect ($F_{1, 319} = 3.10$, $p = 0.079$). Mean change scores were (622 steps/day) and (474 steps/day) for the intervention and comparison groups, respectively. For BMI, both groups had a slight increase in their BMI with no significant group main effect ($F_{1, 307} = 1.01$, $p = 0.36$). At post-test, BMI results showed 66.7% (girls) and 69.4% (boys) in the "at risk for overweight" and "overweight" categories using the Centres for Disease Control (USA) classifications [10]. Although BMI was lower for primary (25.16 ± 6.68) than secondary pupils (27.93 ± 7.97) it was not statistically significantly different. There were no gender differences in physical activity patterns ($F_{1, 319} = 1.73$, $p = 0.189$). There were, however, grade level differences in physical activity patterns ($F_{1, 319} = 5.56$, p<001; partial $\eta^2 = 0.14$). Grade level differences were due to large change scores or deltas for sixth (3884.4) and seventh grade pupils (2480.5).

Looking at an indicator of behavioural stability, the intervention groups' behaviour was less stable ($\alpha = 0.71$) over time versus the comparison group ($\alpha = 0.86$). This indicates that more change was occurring in the intervention group. In other words, the intervention group was comparatively less stable in behaviour over time, which is characterized by a less predictable shifting in rank order between time points. Interpreting the stability finding alongside an increased mean steps/day in the intervention group suggests that the observed instability was the result of a positive change in physical activity behaviour. This measure has also been used to show stability/lack of stability in physical activity patterns for adults [19].

Discussion

Results lend support to the generally favourable changes in pupils' physical activity patterns as a result of a year-long teacher change intervention in an indigenous community, with intervention pupils showing less stability in their physical activity patterns after the intervention. Utilizing the ratio of 100 steps is equivalent to one minute of physical activity [13], the indigenous pupils in the current sample averaged 53 (intervention) and 45 (comparison) minutes of physical activity per day at school. At post test, these pupils were coming close to accumulating the minimum recommendation of 60 minutes of daily physical activity for youth [20]. It is important to keep in mind, however, that pedometers do not measure the intensity of the physical activity performed; thus it is not known if the pupils met the intensity part of the recommendation for moderate-to-vigorous physical activity, which is a limitation of the current study.

In alignment with Guskey's second principle [6] teachers were able to see pupils' physical activity increasing, which might have persuaded them to integrate physical activities into their classrooms even more the following year. Supporting interview data are reported elsewhere [3] which are in alignment with Guskey's first principle that teachers who were able to buy into the program were able to see the program in "support of their work" rather than as additional work. Finally, in accordance with Guskey's third principle, the teachers in this project were provided support at all levels including: (a) teachers may have also had colleagues at their own school involved in the intervention, and (b) an external support team of mentor teachers and researchers were available to them.

In the current study, it was also hypothesized that pupils' BMI levels would be maintained or decrease for the intervention group. This investigation did not show a significant influence on pupils' body mass. It is important to address both increased physical activity patterns and improved eating behaviours in order to affect body mass. Nutrition content was taught along with physical activity knowledge by classroom teachers in the current study. The comprehensive Pathways Obesity Prevention Program project assessed both eating behaviours and physical activity behaviours. Researchers reported that pupils had a reduction in dietary fat intake but no significant reduction in percentage body fat [2]. In the present study, the relatively modest changes in physical activity were clearly not enough to influence pupils' entering body mass status. It is important to note, however, that both before and after the investigation over 65% of the pupils were classified as "overweight" or "at risk for being overweight". This was valuable baseline data for the community and other researchers.

As clearly stated by Guskey [6], p. 9, we should "recognize that change is a gradual and difficult process for teachers. Learning to be proficient at something new and finding meaning in a new way of doing things requires both time and effort…" This teacher change effort with pedometer lessons/activity breaks taught by all teachers and the Dynamic Physical Education curricular model taught by physical education teachers may take years to be fully understood as the first year of an investigation is almost always a challenging one for all involved partners with few large scale successes immediately apparent.

The results of this study are significant for several reasons. First, school based interventions are a logical and cost effective means of changing children's health behaviours, but educators know little about how to implement or assess such programs. The unique collaboration between physical education and classroom teachers in an indigenous community to build a healthy behaviour culture in their schools is a promising but little understood option that needs more investigation. Second, indigenous people around the world have significantly higher health risks than other ethnic background groups, which may make creating a healthy and active school culture more critical for indigenous communities. Finally, this investigation also provides insights into both a specific at-risk group as well as more generally the influence of context and its impact on change. Future work is needed with indigenous youth focusing on both in and out of school physical activity contexts in short and long term physical activity and nutrition interventions. For example, the Coordinated Approach to Child Health project (CATCH), had success in increasing physical activity in Physical Education programs, increasing physical activity during the school day and improving youth eating patterns with more than half of the teachers still consistently using the curriculum at a five year follow up study [12].

In conclusion, although the results of this study were modest gains in physical activity and no significant BMI changes, the study still provides important information. Any physical activity change is a positive one as physical activity behaviours are hard to change and the need for change in this community was great. Given the limited scope of the intervention, it is exciting to see that change did occur. It is also important to note that the data collected provided benchmark data on an understudied population.

References

1. Beets M.W., M.M.Patton, S.Edwards (2005) The accuracy of pedometer steps and time during walking in children. *Med.Sci.Sport Exerc.*, 37(3):513-520.
2. Caballero B., J.H.Himes, T.Lohman, S.M.Davis, J.Stevens, M.Evans, S.Going (2003) Body composition and overweight prevalence in 1704 schoolchildren from 7 American Indian communities. *Am.J.Clin.Nutr.*, 78: 303-312.
3. Cothran D.J., P. H.Kulinna A.Garn (2010) Classroom teachers and physical activity integration. *Teach.Teacher Ed.*, 26: 1381-1388.
4. Dabelea D., R.Hanson, P.Bennett, W.Roumain, W.Knowler, D.Pettitt (1998) Increasing prevalence of type II diabetes in American Indian children. *Diabetologia* 41: 904-910.
5. Darst P.W., R.P.Pangrazi (2009) Dynamic Physical Education for Secondary School Pupils. Pearson/Benjamin Cummings, San Francisco, California, USA.
6. Guskey T. (1986) Staff development and the process of teacher change. *Educ.Researcher*, 15(5): 5-12.
7. Hughes J.M., L.Li, S.Chinn, R.J.Rona (1997) Trends in growth in England and Scotland 1972-1994. *Arch.Dis.Child.*, 76: 182-189.
8. Jarosz M., E.Rychlik (2008) Overweight and obesity among adults in Poland, 1983-2005. *Adv.Med.Sci.*, 53(2): 158-166.
9. Keddie A.M. (2011) Associations between severe obesity and depression: Results from the National Health and Nutrition Examination Survey, 2005-2006. *Prev.Chronic Dis.*, 8(3): A57.
10. Levin S., R.Louwry, D.R.Brown, W.H.Dietz (2003) Physical activity and body mass index among US adolescents. *Arch. Pediatr.Adolesc.Med.*, 157: 816-820.
11. Marshall A.L., N.Owen, A.E.Bauman (2004) Mediated approaches for influencing physical activity: update of the evidence on mass media, print, telephone and website delivery of interventions. *J.Sci.Med.Sport*, 7(1): S74-80.

12. McKenzie T.L., D.Li, C.A.Derby, L.S.Webber, R.V.Luepker, P.Cribb (2003) Maintenance of effects of the CATCH physical education program: Results from the CATCH-ON study. *Health. Educ.Behav.*, 30: 447-462.

13. Miller R., W.Brown, C.Tudor-Locke (2006) But what about swimming and cycling? How to 'count' non-ambulatory activity when using pedometers to assess physical activity. *J.Phys. Act.Health*, 3: 257-266.

14. Pangrazi R.P., A.Beighle (2010) Dynamic physical education for elementary school children (16th ed.). San Francisco, California, Pearson Education.

15. Pangrazi R.P., A.Beighle, D.Pangrazi (2009) Promoting Physical Activity and Health in the Classroom. Pearson/Benjamin Cummings, San Francisco, California, USA.

16. Salbe A.D., C.Weyer, I.Harper, R.S.Lindsay, E.Ravussin, P.A.Tatranni (2002) Assessing risk factors for obesity between childhood and adolescence: II. Energy metabolism and physical activity. *Pediatr*ics, 110: 307-314.

17. Tremblay M., J.Wilms (2003) Is the Canadian childhood obesity epidemic related to physical inactivity? *Int.J.Obes.*, 27: 1100-1105.

18. Trost S.G., R.R.Pate, P.S.Freedson, J.F.Sallis, W.C.Taylor (2000) Using objective physical activity measures with youth: How many days of monitoring are needed? *Med.Sci.Sport Exerc.*, 32: 426-431.

19. Tudor-Locke C., B.Giles-Corti, M.Kuiman, G.McCormack (2008) Tracking of pedometer-determined physical activity in adults who relocate: results from RESIDE. *Int.J.Behav.Nutr.Phys. Act.*, 7: 5-39.

20. United States Department of Health and Human Services [USDHHS]. Physical Activity Guidelines for Americans (2008) Retrieved from http://www.health.gov/paguidelines/guidelines/summary.aspx.

21. Vincent S.D., R.P.Pangrazi (2002) Does reactivity exist in children when measuring activity levels with pedometers? *Pediatr.Exerc.Sci.*, 14: 56-63.

22. Wei R.C., L.Darling-Hammond, A.Andree, N.Richardson, S.Orphanos (2009) Professional Learning in the Learning Profession: A Status Report on Teacher Development in the United States And Abroad. National Staff Development Council, Dallas, Texas, USA.

Measurement of cognitive ability and thinking level of 10- and 13-year-old football players with football-specific tasks

István Kun, Laszlo Toth

Faculty of Physical Education and Sport Science, Semmelweis University, Budapest, Hungary

Summary

Study aim: To assess whether in a special area, such as football, formal thinking may appear as early as at the age of 10 years.
Material and methods: In total 50 children divided into three groups took part in the study: 10-year-old football players from the Premier League Team - level 1 (Group 1; n = 22), 10-year-old football players from the Football League Team - level 3 (Group 2; n = 13) and 13-year-old football players from the Premier League Team - level 1 (Group 3; n = 15). With the help of specific motor tests, the kinetic memory, level of thinking and technical level were assessed.
Results: The 10-year-old children representing lower levels of football proficiency (Group 2) were significantly ($p<0.05$) inferior to their mates from the Premier League in both the level of thinking as well as in kinetic memory. No significant differences were found between members of Group 1 and Group 3 in any of the studied variables.
Conclusions: The results support the thesis that 10-year-old children are able to use formal thinking in a particular area, such as football. To be aware of this would be of great importance to those experts who deal with selection and talent identification.

Key words: Football - Developmental psychology - Thinking level - Cognitive ability

Introduction

According to Bloomfield [3], sport experts and coaches from many relatively small countries think that talent identification is essential for their programme to develop the sport. In these countries, the question arises whether there are enough people to reach the elite levels seen in countries with large populations selecting by means of choosing.

Peltola [19] claims that competition itself is the best way to identify talent; it is during competition that one can register the best performances and talent fulfils itself in its own chosen branch of sport. Several authors mention that regular and systematic talent identification is part of sports from all over the world [1,11,14].

In our opinion, it is necessary in Hungary to have accurate and scientifically established football talent identification. The size of the country, the number of its people, and the number of footballers cannot allow sport leaders of football to ignore the fact that each and every child should take a place that is appropriate for his/her knowledge. It means that the most talented children should be trained by clubs having the best circumstances and by the best coaches, experts, and teachers.

Coaches and scientists have argued that perceptual-cognitive skills play a crucial role in sports performance, particularly at the highest levels. It is widely accepted that skilled performers are not endowed with superior visual skills per se, but rather enhanced cognitive knowledge bases that enable them to pick up and interpret perceptual information more effectively than their less skilled counterparts [13,26].

Based on the topics discussed above, it is clear that countries which play a leading role in football place great emphasis upon the standard of thinking when selecting the players. Helsen et al. [13] examined differences in tactical decision-making skills between experienced and intermediate-level adult football players. Participants watched open and closed (i.e., set plays) offensive football simulations and were asked to respond quickly and accurately. The experienced players were faster and more accurate in responding and employed fewer fixations of shorter duration when compared with their less skilled counterparts. Ward et al. [23] assessed the role of expectations (i.e., situational probabilities) in decision-making by requiring young football players to view filmed sequences taken from competitive matches, and then highlight the key players in a good position to receive the ball. The results revealed that elite football players demonstrated superior perceptual-cognitive skills compared to their sub-elite counterparts; these differences were evident

Author's address Dr Laszlo Toth, Faculty of Physical Education and Sport Sciences, Semmelweis University, Alkotás utca 44, 1123 Budapest, Hungary

as early as 9 years of age. Vaeyens et al [21] in their study examined the mechanisms underlying decision-making skill in football. They analysed differences in decision-making skill and visual search behaviour using simulations involving different microstates of the game and groups of adolescents matched by age and playing experience. It was shown that the visual search behaviour employed during decision-making varies as a function of playing experience, skill level, and the unique constraints of the task. The number of players involved and the relative proportion of offensive to defensive players all play a part in constraining the emergent search behaviour. They provided evidence that confirmed that an increase in the number of players and a greater relative proportion of offensive to defensive players changed the perceptual and cognitive demands of the task. The measures employed were able to successfully discriminate between football players and non-players, and more importantly, between elite and sub-elite players and their regional counterparts.

In the golden age of the Hungarian football this was typical of the Hungarians and our training system as well. This is why it is necessary and timely to establish a unified selecting system that focuses on standards of thinking as well as physical abilities.

By creating a series of training practice exercises, we intended to test the standard of thinking (which can be an essential element of selection) during the game. The level of technical knowledge hinders the possibilities for teamwork, the signs of which become visible at the very early age. Consequently, those children who can think at a higher level than others can learn the special motions, techniques, and tactics more easily and quickly [18,20]. The aim of this survey was thus to assess whether in a special field, like football, formal thinking may appear as early as at the age of 10. To answer that question the following hypotheses were tested: (1) the level of thinking differs between 10-year-old children representing different levels of football proficiency, (2) the level of thinking differs between 10-year-old and 13-year-old children representing different levels of football proficiency, (3) 10-year-old and 13-year-old children representing the same levels of football proficiency demonstrate the same levels of thinking, (4) children demonstrate the same technical level irrespectively of their age and level of football proficiency.

Material and Methods

In total 50 children divided into three groups took part in the study: 10-year-old football players from the Premier League Team - level 1 (Group 1; n = 22), 10-year-old football players from the Football League Team - level 3 (Group 2; n = 13) and 13-year-old football players from Premier League Team - level 1 (Group 3; n = 15). The survey was conducted on the pitches and laboratories of TF (Semmelweis University Faculty of Physical Education and Sport Sciences, Budapest, Hungary). With the help of motor tests, children's kinetic memory, level of thinking, and technical level were measured; the study was approved by the local Committee of Ethics.

Level of thinking (cogitation) - a task in which the presence of concrete or formal thinking is measured was recorded by a video camera. Nine direction-buoys were placed at an equal distance on a circle with a diameter of 10 meters. Eight children were standing by the buoys – one buoy was left free. One child had the ball; he had to pass it without stopping it to any of his team-mates other than the one standing next to him. Right after the pass he had to run to the buoy left free. Those who solved the task successfully could pass accurately with one contact and then leave towards the buoy in time [5]. With the help of the recording, the task was analysed according to the following criteria: passing accuracy; leaving for the good place; and leaving his position in time.

Technical level - a bench of 3 meters was leant against the wall: the top surface, where one usually sits, became the area to score onto. A line was painted 3 meters from the scoring area and in 60 seconds players had to pass the ball to that surface as many times as they could.

Kinetic memory: a buoy was placed one meter from the post of a handball goal. From a distance of 6 meters, they had to shoot the ball between the buoy and the post 5 times with eyes open and 5 times blindfolded [12].

Statistical analysis were conducted according Knapp's procedure [15]; to compare the results, a 5-level scale for the basic data was created. Then, these data were analysed with the use of the Kruskal-Wallis test, followed by the Tukey-b test. SPSS was used in data analyses; the level of $p<0.05$ was considered significant.

Results

The results of the study are presented in Table 1. No significant differences between groups were noted for the task measuring technical level ($Chi^2=1.7$; $p=0.432$) while these for the kinetic memory and the level of thinking the differences proved to be significant ($Chi^2=16.7$; $p<0.001$ and $Chi^2=17.6$; $p<0.001$, respectively).

The results of the post hoc analyses show the 10-year-old children representing lower levels of football proficiency (Group 2) were significantly ($p<0.05$) inferior to their mates from Premier League in both, level of thinking as well as in kinetic memory, while in any of the studied variables no significant differences were found between the younger (Group 1) and older (Group 3) football players from the Premier League (Table 1).

Table1. Mean (±SD) values of kinetic memory, level of thinking, and technical level recorded in young football players

Variable	Group 1 (n = 22)	Group 2 (n = 13)	Group 3 (n = 15)
Kinetic memory	3.18 ± 0.85	2.23 ± 0.44*	3.53 ± 0.83
Level of thinking	4.14 ± 1.04	2.77 ± 0.60*	4.20 ± 0.68
Technical level	4.27 ± 0.70	4.00 ± 0.82	4.07 ± 0.46

Legend: Group 1 - 10-year-old football players from the Premier League Team - level 1; Group 2 - 10-year-old football players from the Football League Team - level 3; Group 3 - 13-year-old football players from Premier League Team - level 1; * Significantly less than in other groups

Discussion

The special movements of football require special ways of thinking, the presence of which could and should be a filter when selecting players. According to Williams *et al.* [24], to determine which child has poor or good abilities concerning decision-making specific to football is possible as early as at the ages of 7-9 years. Ward *et al.* [23] suppose that the following processes take place in a player during a situation in the game: the player realizes the situation with the help of his perceptual abilities, he analyses it using his cognitive abilities, then executes his decision through his technical and kinetic abilities. Finally, using his visual abilities again, he collects information about the effect and the correctness of his action. In their opinion, the perception – decision-making – execution circle plays the most important part in recognizing the talented persons and selecting them. Apart from the laboratory studies and researches, they try to put their methods of measuring into practice and examine players through exercises that are designed to be performed during training sessions [9].

The child can only execute the task measuring the level of thinking perfectly if he creates a plan (at the very moment he notices and senses the ball heading towards him) about what to do next, to whom he shall pass the ball, and where he shall run after the pass. Making plans is one of the results of formal thinking [4,20]. The child can only execute the task perfectly if he recognizes the rule. Sensing where the ball comes from and where the empty area on the pitch is, is not enough; they have to know the rule. The rule is the following: they have to run and occupy the place of the person from whom the ball came, because there is the empty area on the pitch, since that is the place from where their fellow player had run away. If he does not know the rule he only notices where the empty buoy is and this is the direction he will head to after the pass (which means he can only react to concrete things) and he will notice only during running that his fellow player has already taken that place. In this moment he may try to change directions and search for an empty buoy and run towards it or continue to run to the original buoy in spite of the fact that his fellow player is standing there. One of the criterion of formal thinking is that children can imagine those things that have not happened yet. They order, classify, group the information they perceive, and thus they can understand the connections between them [6]. The young player who applies formal thinking – that is, in a particular situation analyse a particular moment of the game – can observe the connection that by the time he receives and then passes the ball – that is, when he has to run to the free buoy – the player who passed the ball him reaches that buoy that was free at the moment of the pass. Therefore, the player who received and passed the ball has to run to the buoy that has just become free [2]. Consequently, after sorting the perceived information the player can understand the connections and notices that the player who passes him the ball will run to the free buoy. Furthermore, he could also notice that the buoy – which the player who passed him the ball just left – will become free. In other words, the player can predict what will happen according to the perceived information [17].

Regarding the technical level, there is no difference among the three groups, which means that the execution of the task measuring the level of thinking does not depend on the technical standard of the players. The technical elements are the basis of football, which are taught everywhere independent of the quality and class of the team the children are learning to play football. In spite of this, there is a difference between the 10-year-olds from Group2 (aged 10 years) and Group1 (aged 10 years), which resulted in Group1 (aged 10 years) scoring more goals than Group2 (aged 10 years) during the matches. If there is no technical difference, still, there is some difference regarding the quality of the playing, what can be the root of this disparity? The results of the survey show that the truth can be found in the standard of thinking.

According to Knapp's [16] theory, kinetics can only be used from the third stage (the stage of refinement, the foundation of movement coordination). It seems to be clear that the received results show us the differences between the 10-year-old children and the 13-year-old children, and the existence and presence of this difference stems from the normal pace of children's natural development. The data also show that the task measuring the thinking actually measures the thinking during the game; that is to say, the execution of this task does not depend on the level of technical skills. The technical element is considered to be those movements that belong to the repertoire of a particular sport. Technique is the practical and efficient execution of these technical elements in a game situation. Knowing a technical element does not mean that a player can use it during the match; that is, a technical element does not turn into automatically technique. Sixty percent of traditional football technical elements are practiced. Besides this fact, the vast majority of the players would not be called "skilled players". In order to apply technical elements during a football match, game-related thinking is necessary. This game-related thinking transforms technical elements into technique [22]. Furthermore, the data can prove that children may start to use formal thinking during the game even at the age of 10 years. The presence of formal operational thinking at an early age can be an important factor when selecting players in football [8]. As a result, those children who use formal thinking have an advantage in learning movements, as opposed to the others who use only the concrete operations. These children learn the tactical-cognitive abilities faster; therefore, they can learn more about football than their fellow players [7,10] who only use formal thinking. The main difference between amateur and professional teams is whether or not simple technical elements are converted into technique during training sessions. Amateur players are only able to react to the actions during the game, and thus the speed of their play is slow. On the contrary, professional players continuously analyse the match situations and bear in mind those elements that have yet to occur. Therefore, their play is faster and continuous [25].

Based on the results it can be concluded that 10-year-old children can use formal thinking in a particular field, such as football. To be aware of these factors would be of great importance for those experts who deal with selection [27]. Certainly, game-related thinking is a complex process, and our research cannot fully measure its complexity. This complexity could be the reason to the observed high dispersion of the data. Other studies are in progress, and we endeavour to measure, examine, and understand in deeper levels this complex issue. In order to be sure that the exercise – which was presented previously – measures the existence of formal thinking, other measurements should be fulfilled. Additionally, more accurate data could be presented about the actual movements, passing, and decision-making of the players if the abovementioned exercise was recorded and analysed with a match analysis system. What is more, in order to prove the accuracy and authenticity of the measurement, it would be useful to assess the level of thinking, technical skills, and kinetic memory among the children who do not play football at all.

References

1. Baur J. (1986) Talent Identification and Development in Sport: An Interim Evaluation, Part 1. Unpublished translation – (Australian Institute of Sport, Belconnen), 1988, 1-26.
2. Bell-Walker J., A.M.Williams (2008) The effect of memory recall on perceptual-cognitive skill in elite soccer: Development of long term working memory. In: T.Reilly, F.Korkusuz, E.Ergen (eds): Science and Football. VI. Taylor and Francis, London. pp. 340–343.
3. Bloomfield J., T.R.Ackland, E.L.Bruce (1994) Applied Anatomy and Biomechanics in Sport. Blackwell Scientific Publ.
4. Cabrini M. (1999) The Psychology of Soccer. Reedswain INC. Spring City Pennsylvania.
5. Caruso A. (1996) Soccer Coaching Ages 5 to 12. Reedswan INC. Spring City Pennsylvania.
6. Chi M. (1978) Knowledge structures and memory development. In: R.Siegler (ed.) Children's Thinking: What develops? Hillsdale, NJ: Lawrencw Elbaum, pp. 73-96.
7. D'Ottavio S. (2003) La presentacione del giovanile calciatore. Societá Stampa Sportiva, Roma.
8. D'Ottavio S. (2004) Guida technica per le ccuole di calcio. F. I. G. C. - Settore giovanile e scolastico.
9. Fenoglio R. (2003) The Manchester United 4 v 4 pilot scheme for U9s. *FA Coaches Assoc.J.*, 6 (3):18-19.
10. Ford P.R., P.Ward, N.J.Hodges, A.M.Williams (2009) The role of deliberate practice and play in career progression in sport: The early engagement hypothesis. *High Abil.Stud.*, 20:65-75.
11. Hahn A. (1990) Identification and selection of talent in Australian rowing. *Excel*, 6 (3):5-11.
12. Hirtz P. (1985) Koordinative Fähigkeiten im Schulsport. Volk und Wissen Volkseigner Verlag. Berlin.
13. Helsen W.F., J.L. Starkes (1999) A multidimensional approach to skilled perception and performance in sport. *Appl. Cognit.Psychol.*, 13:1-27.
14. Hoare D. (1995) Talent Search. The National Talent Identification and Development Program, 13 (2):10-12.
15. Knapp B. (1963) Skill in sport. In: L.Killik (ed.) Basic Elements of Motor Learning. Sportpropaganda, MTS-OT, Budapest.
16. Knapp B. (1989) Basic Questions of Motor Learning. MTS-OT, 8:10-12.
17. Kun I., L.Toth (2010) The correlation of differential learning and the stage of cognitive development in football trough a game of three against one. *Int.Q.Sport Sci.*, 2:27-42.
18. Nunes T., A.D.Schliemann, D.W.Carraher (1993) Street Mathematics and School Mathematics. New York, Cambridge University Press.
19. Peltola E. (1992) Talent Identification. *New Stud.Athl.*, 7 (3):7-12.
20. Piaget J. (1999) Psychology of Children. In Hungarian. Osiris Budapest.
21. Vaeyens R., M.Lenoir, A.M.Williams, L.Mazyn, R.M.Philippaerts (2007) The effects of task constraints on visual search behavior and decision-making skill in youth soccer players. *J.Sport Exerc.Psychol.*, 29:147-169.
22. Ward P., A.M.Williams, (2003) Perceptual and cognitive skill development in soccer: The multidimensional nature of expert performance. *J.Sport Exerc.Psychol.*, 25:93-111.

23. Ward P., N.J.Hodges, A.M.Williams, J.L.Starkes, (2004) Deliberate practice and expert performance: Defining the path to excellence. In: A.M.Williams, N.J.Hodges (eds.) Skill Acquisition in Sport: Research, Theory and Practice. London: Routledge, pp. 231 – 258.

24. Williams A.M., K.Davids, L.Burwitz, J.Williams (1993) Cognitive knowledge and soccer performance. *Percept.Motor Skills*, 76:579-594.

25. Williams A.M., K.Davids (1998) Visual search strategy, selective attention, and expertise in soccer. *Res.Q.Exerc.Sport*, 69:111-128.

26. Williams A.M., A.Grant (1999) Training perceptual skill in sport. *Int.J.Sport Psychol.*, 30:194-220.

27. Williams A.M., T.Reilly (2000) Talent identification and development in soccer. *J.Sport Sci.*, 5:657-670.

Association between submaximal and maximal measures of aerobic power in female adolescents

Pantelis Theodoros Nikolaïdis

Laboratory of Human Performance and Rehabilitation, Department of Physical and Cultural Education, Hellenic Army Academy, Greece

Summary

Study aim: To examine the association between two submaximal (physical working capacity at a heart rate of 170 (PWC_{170}) on cycle ergometer test and YMCA Step Test) and maximal measures (maximal oxygen uptake (VO_2max)) of aerobic power, as well as to study the repeatability of the aforementioned submaximal measures in physically active female adolescents.
Material and methods: Ten female adolescents, aged 13.4 ± 0.7 years old, all members of a local track and field sport club, performed the PWC_{170} and YMCA Step Test twice. The tests were separated by an interval of one week. During the second laboratory visit, VO_{2max} was measured during a graded exercise test.
Results: Considering the repeatability of submaximal measures, intraclass correlation coefficient was 0.89 (95% CI 0.55-0.97) and 0.91 (95% CI 0.65-0.98) in absolute and relative to body mass values of PWC_{170}, while it was 0.69 (95% CI -0.27-0.92) with regard to heart rate at the end of step test and 0.78 (95% CI 0.11-0.95) at the end of the first minute of recovery after step test. PWC_{170} was associated significantly with VO_{2max} in absolute values ($r = 0.65$, $p = 0.04$), but not with VO_{2max} relative to body mass values ($r = 0.44$, $p = 0.20$). The corresponding relationships between relative PWC_{170} and VO_{2max} were $r = 0.39$ ($p = 0.27$) and $r = 0.60$ ($p = 0.06$). Heart rate at the end of the step test was non-significantly related to VO_{2max} in both absolute and relative values ($r = -0.53$, $p = 0.12$ and $r = -0.61$, $p = 0.06$), whereas respective values of heart rate at the end of the first minute after step test were $r = -0.72$ ($p = 0.02$) and $r = -0.69$ ($p = 0.03$).
Conclusion: These submaximal measures appeared to be valid and reliable, and they were recommended for further use in similar population with the assumption that a familiarization session was preceded.

Key words: Cardiorespiratory power– Maximal oxygen uptake– Test-retest

Introduction

While the lower spectrum of cardiorespiratory power (CRP) is associated with heart and pulmonary diseases (chronic obstructive pulmonary disease, coronary heart disease, chronic heart failure, and intermittent claudication) [27], its higher spectrum is linked not only to the absence of the aforementioned diseases, but also to well-being. Consequently, many national and international organizations that focus on health, e.g. the American College of Sports Medicine [10] and the World Health Organization [31], recommend exercise interventions targeting CRP. Because this health-related fitness parameter must be monitored periodically to evaluate its progress, appropriate tests should be applied.

Maximal oxygen uptake, i.e., the maximal quantity of oxygen received by human body through the respiratory system and transferred from lungs to tissues through the cardiovascular system where it is consumed, is regarded as the gold standard in the assessment of CRP. Nonetheless, the need for expensive equipment, a well-trained staff, and maximal effort that reaches exhaustion from participants raise the question for the usage of alternative assessment methods. It is thought that submaximal measures overcome certain limitations connected with maximal testing [24]; they are easier to administer, less expensive, and they demand much less effort from participants.

Physical working capacity at a heart rate (HR) of 170 beats per minute (PWC_{170}) is a submaximal test, which is performed on a cycle ergometer. The test evaluates the power corresponding to HR 170 beats per minute (bpm), i.e. the higher the PWC_{170}, the higher the CRP. The YMCA Step Test estimates the HR during the first minute of recovery after 3 minutes of stepping up and down, i.e. the lower the heart rate, the higher the CRP. In addition to the recording of the recovery HR, the HR at the end of the 3-minute step test can be used as an index

Author's address Dr Pantelis T. Nikolaïdis, 7 Thermopylon, Nikaia 18450, Athens, Greece

of CRP, too. To apply such measures in different populations, two parameters should be chiefly considered, validity and reliability. Validity is the degree to which a test measures what it purports to measure, while reliability is its characteristic to yield the same results on successive trials [30]. The validity of PWC_{170} was already examined in 12-year-old non-Caucasian females against VO_{2max} [18] and 15.6-year-old Caucasian female adolescents [4]. Additional relevant research conducted on schoolchildren did not discriminate between girls and boys and was excluded from further analysis [5].

Two null hypotheses were examined: first, that there was no agreement between test-retest of submaximal measures with interval of a week (reliability) and second, that there was no association between indices of submaximal measures and VO_{2max} (validity). Nevertheless, the aim of the study was not only to reject the null hypotheses and adopt their alternative, but to also achieve proper levels of affinity of the above parameters in order to ground validity and reliability in light of minimal values suggested by previous research [2,3,16]. Particularly, the acceptable level of intraclass correlation coefficient was proposed to be higher than 0.61 [2,3]. At least moderate ($0.30 < r < 0.50$) correlates with the criterion measures were suggested to lead to the validation of an instrument [16].

Material and Methods

Participants and procedures. Ten female adolescents, aged 13.4 ±0.7 years old, all members of a local track and field sport club, volunteered for this study. They visited our laboratory twice, with an interval of a week, they were informed of the protocols, and their parents provided oral informed consent. During their first visit, body composition, resting heart rate, blood pressure, and anthropometric data were obtained followed by a guided 15-minute warm-up (Table 1). Then, physical working capacity at a heart rate of 170 (PWC_{170}) and the step test were performed. During their second visit, the same procedures were repeated and, additionally, after a 15-minute break, a graded exercise test was performed.

Table 1. Mean values (±SD) of anthropometric variables in female adolescents studied (n = 10)

Variable	Pre	Post – Pre difference
Body height (cm)	161.0 ± 4.3	0.2 ± 0.6
Body mass (kg)	48.5 ± 6.6	0.3 ± 0.4
BMI (kg/m^2)	18.67 ± 2.12	0.06 ± 0.15
Body fat (%)	20.94 ± 3.50	-0.02 ± 1.16

Protocols and equipment. Height and body mass were measured using a stadiometer (SECA, Leicester, UK) and an electronic scale (HD-351, Tanita, Illinois, USA), respectively. Body fat percentage was calculated from the sum of 10 skinfold sites using a skinfold caliper (Harpenden, West Sussex, UK), based on the formula proposed by Parizkova [26]. Body circumference was measured using a measuring tape; humerus and femur biepicondylar breadth were assessed by caliper (Anthropometer 01291, Lafayette, USA).

PWC_{170} was performed according to Eurofit guidelines [11]. YMCA Step Test was performed in a 0.3 m height step for 3 minutes using a 24 ascent/min cadence [12]. A graded exercise test on a cycle ergometer (Ergomedics 828, Monark, Sweden), in which the initial workload was 1.5 W/kg, and was increased by 20 W every minute until exhaustion [13], was performed. Minute ventilation and oxygen uptake were recorded by a gas analyzer (Fitmate Pro, Cosmed, Italy). Anaerobic threshold was identified from ventilatory threshold, i.e. the relationship between minute ventilation and oxygen uptake. During test a cadence of 80 revolutions per minute was maintained through two means: visual contact with the monitor embodied in the cycle reporting cadence and the audio signal from a metronome set at 80 beats per minute. The duration of every flywheel revolution in cycle ergometer tests was measured with the help of electronic sensors; the power output of every revolution was computed by specialized software [25]. Blood samples were taken 5 minutes after termination of test, and lactate concentration was analyzed (Accutrend, Roche, Germany). Lactate concentration was employed as a criterion of VO_{2max} achievement (accepted values > 9 mmol/L). Predicted maximal heart rate was calculated by the formula $HR_{max,predicted} = 208 - 0.7 \times age$ [29] and it was employed as a criterion of VO_{2max} achievement, as well as an index of motivation level.

Statistical procedures and data analysis. All data were presented as mean ± standard deviation. Data sets were checked for normality using the Shapiro-Wilk normality test and visual inspection. Student pair *t* test was employed to compare values between trials. Pearson product moment correlation coefficient (r) was used to examine the association between VO_{2max}, PWC_{170}, and step test and therefore to ground the validity of submaximal measures. Intraclass correlation coefficient (ICC) was employed to examine the reliability of submaximal measures outcome and it was expressed in 95% lower and upper bounds of confidence intervals (CI). Student *t* test was employed to examine the differences between trials. Significance level was set at $\alpha = 0.05$. Statistical analyses were performed using SPSS v17.0.

Results

During the second visit to the laboratory, all submaximal indices improved, either significantly (PWC_{170} t_9 = 2.55, p = 0.03; PWC_{170} expressed in relative to body mass values, $rPWC_{170}$, t_9 = 2.62, p = 0.03) or non-significantly (HR at the end of step test t_9 = 0.41, p = 0.69; recovery HR after step test t_9 = 1.75, p = 0.11). With the exception of systolic arterial pressure (BP_s t=-2.71, p = 0.02), diastolic pressure and resting heart rate similar (BP_d t = 0.31, p = 0.76; HR_{rest} t = 0.73, p = 0.48). Considering the reliability of submaximal measures of CRP, ICC was 0.89 (95% CI 0.55-0.97) in PWC_{170} and 0.91 (95% CI 0.65-0.98) in $rPWC_{170}$, while it was 0.69 (95% CI -0.27-0.92) at the end of step test and .78 (95% CI 0.11-0.95) at the end of the first minute of recovery after step test (Table 2).

Table 2. Mean values (±SD) of cardiorespiratory parameters of participants (n = 10)

Variable	Pre	Post – Pre difference
BP_s (mmHg)	122.9 ± 9.1	-10.2 ± 11.9*
BP_d (mmHg)	60.8 ± 9.0	-0.8 ± 8.1
HR_{rest} (bpm)	79.8 ± 12.3	2.4 ± 10.4
Step $test_0$ (bpm)	158.9 ± 16.6	-1.9 ± 14.7
Step $test_1$ (bpm)	106.7 ± 22.1	-9.3 ± 16.8
PWC_{170} (W)	87.00 ± 23.97	13.06 ± 16.21*
$rPWC_{170}$ (W/kg)	1.81 ± 0.51	0.25 ± 0.30*
	Post	
VO_{2max} (mL/min/kg)	36.80 ± 5.09	
Ve (L/min)	59.43 ± 10.64	
HR_{max} (bpm)	195.0 ± 10.5	
HR_{thr} (bpm)	160.6 ± 10.9	
Lactate (mmol/L)	10.0 ± 3.1	
$HR_{max,pred}$ (bpm)	198.6 ± 0.5	
$HR_{max}/HR_{max,pred}$ (%)	98.2 ± 5.2	

Legend: BP_s – Systolic blood pressure; BP_d – Diastolic blood pressure; HR_{rest} – Heart rate in rest; Step $test_0$ – Heart rate at the end of step test; Step $test_1$ – Heart rate at the first minute of recovery after step test; PWC_{170} – Physical working capacity in heart rate 170 beats per minute; $rPWC_{170}$ – PWC_{170} relative to body mass; Ve – Pulmonary ventilation; HR_{max} – Maximal heart rate; HRthr – Heart rate at anaerobic threshold; $HR_{max,pred}$ – Maximal heart rate predicted from age; *p<0.05.

Heart rate at the end of graded exercise test reached over 98% of predicted value based on age, and lactate levels were in accepted levels. Therefore, end values of this test were considered maximal. PWC_{170} was associated significantly with VO_{2max} in absolute values (r = 0.65, p = 0.04), but not with VO_{2max} in relative to body mass values (r = 0.44, p = 0.20). The corresponding relationships between $rPWC_{170}$ and VO_{2max} were r =.39 (p = 0.27) and r = 0.60 (p = 0.06). Heart rate at the end of the step test was non-significantly related to VO_{2max} in both absolute and relative values (r = -0.53, p = 0.12 and r = -0.61, p = 0.06), whereas respective values of heart rate at the end of the first minute after step test were r = -0.72 (p = 0.02) and r = -0.69 (p = 0.03).

Discussion

It was examined whether the findings between trials, separated by one week, differed. Participants had better performance in all submaximal CRP indices during the second trial. This improvement was either statistically significant (PWC_{170} test) or non-significant (step test). Difficulty in pedalling at the required cadence and HR elevation from anxiety were mentioned previously as potential reasons for the discrepancy between maximal test and cycle ergometer measures based on HR [18]. However, adolescents were more accustomed to cycling and possessed a better sense of rhythm. Thus, it was proposed that the explanation for the lower HR responses to the same workloads during the second trial were attributed to both learning effect and lowered anxiety, and not to improvement of CRP. Consequently, these measures were acceptable to be applied in a sample of female adolescents to be tested once. However, if the purpose was to follow CRP longitudinally, a familiarization session was recommended.

The reliability of step test and physical working capacity at a heart rate of 170 bpm and their validity against VO_{2max} were also examined. ICC reached such levels in all submaximal indices, which grounded their reliability regarding desirable levels (> 0.61) [2,3]. Higher scores of ICC were observed in absolute and relative PWC_{170} than in step test, suggesting PWC_{170} to be more reliable than step test. Correlation between these measures and VO_{2max} ranged between 0.39 and 0.65, and were in agreement with suggested levels (at least 0.30 < r < 0.50 correlates with the criterion measures) [16]. Similar association between PWC_{170} and VO_{2max}, estimated by graded exercise test in treadmill, was observed in non-Caucasian female children (r = 0.54, n.s.; N = 8, aged 12 years, VO_{2peak} 38.5 ± 4.4 mL/min/kg, PWC_{170} 1.35 ± 0.42 W/kg) [18], and higher in Caucasian female adolescents (r = 0.84, p < 0.05; N = 18, aged 15.4 ± 0.7 years, VO_{2max} 42.6 ± 5.8 mL/min/kg, PWC_{170} 1.86 ± 0.39 W/kg) [4].

PWC_{170} and YMCA step test proved to be valid and reliable assessment methods of CRP in female adolescents, and they were recommended for further use. Recent findings, which revealed a decrease in CRP of girls during the last two decades, highlighted the need for monitoring using this physical fitness parameter [28]. CRP was inversely associated with BMI, it was lower in children and adolescents with higher BMI [1,8,9,14], and it was in close relationship with the parameters consisting the paediatric metabolic syndrome [7]. Increased risk for cardiovascular disease was found among adolescents with low CRP [15]. Children with chronic diseases had lower CRP than healthy controls [17]. Regarding the prevalence of inactivity [23] and obesity [21,22], particular levels of physical activity should be attained in order to have healthy CRP [19]. Therefore, the development of submaximal measures that are easy to be administered with low cost to large numbers of participants without demanding maximal effort, might contribute to better screening of CRP, especially in the context of its inverse association with many diseases. Since it has been shown that the level of exercise participation [20] and the response to exercise intervention is influenced partially (approximately 50%) by heredity [6], the effectiveness of an exercise intervention should be monitored periodically, where submaximal measures proved to be valid and reliable important assessment tool.

The number of participants in our study (n = 10) presents a limitation of our findings. This drawback has already been identified in previous relevant studies (n = 18, aged 15.4 years, [4]; n = 9, aged 12 years, [18]). It could be partially attributed to the inherent limitations of laboratory exercise testing, especially in child and adolescent populations.

In summary, the association with VO_2max and the repeatability of submaximal measures of cardiorespiratory power were examined. Both the PWC_{170} and YMCA step test proved to be valid and reliable in active female adolescents. Thus, their wide employment in cardiorespiratory power screening was encouraged. Because these CRP measures depended on heart rate, familiarization with testing procedures should be emphasized to minimize elevation of heart rate due to anxiety. However, these findings should be viewed with some caution until they are confirmed in larger samples.

References

1. Aires L., P.Silva, G.Silva, M.O.Santos, J.C.Ribeiro, J.Mota (2010) Intensity of physical activity, cardiorespiratory fitness and body mass index in youth. *J.Phys.Act.Health* 7:54-59

2. Badland H., G.Schofield (2006) Test-retest reliability of a survey to measure transport related physical activity in adults. *Res.Q.Exerc.Sport* 77:386-390.

3. Baranowski T., C.de Moor (2000) How many days was that? Intra-individual variability and physical activity assessment. *Res.Q.Exerc.Sport* 71:S74-S78.

4. Boreham C.A.G., V.J.Paliczka, A.K.Nichols (1990) A comparison of PWC170 and 20-MST tests of aerobic fitness in adolescent schoolchildren. *J.Sports Med.Phys.Fitness* 30(1):19-23.

5. Buono M.J., J.J.Roby, F.G.Micale, J.F.Sallis, W.E.Shepard (1991) Validity and reliability of predicting maximum oxygen uptake via field tests in children and adolescents. *Pediatr.Exerc. Sci.* 3:250-255.

6. Bouchard C., P.An, T.Rice, J.S.Skinner, J.H.Wilmore, J.Gagnon, L.Perusse, A.Leon, D.C.Rao (1999) Familial aggregation of VO_{2max} response to exercise training: results from the HERITAGE family study. *J.Appl.Physiol.* 87(3):1003-1008.

7. Brambilla P., A.Pietrobelli (2009) Behind and beyond the pediatric metabolic syndrome. *Italian J.Pediatrics* 35:41.

8. Dumith S.C., W.Ramires, M.A.Souza, D.S.Moraes, F.G.Petry, E.S.Oliveira, S.V.Ramires, P.C.Hallal (2010) Overweight/obesity and physical fitness among children and adolescents. *J.Phys.Act.Health* 7(5):641-648.

9. Dwyer T., C.G.Magnussen, M.D.Schmidt, O.C.Ukoumunne, A.L.Ponsonby, O.T.Raitakari, P.Z.Zimmet, S.N.Blair, R.Thomson, V.J.Cleland, A.Venn (2009) Decline in physical fitness form childhood to adulthood associated with increased obesity and insulin resistance in adults. *Diabetes Care* 32(4):683-687.

10. Ehrman J.K. (2010) ACSM resource manual guidelines for exercise test and prescription. Baltimore: Lippincott Williams & Wilkins, 6th ed.

11. Eurofit (1988) The Eurofit test of European physical fitness tests. Strasbourg: Council of Europe.

12. Golding L.A. (2000) YMCA fitness testing and assessment manual, 4th ed. Champaign: Human Kinetics.

13. Heller J. (2005) Laboratory manual for human and exercise physiology. Charles University in Prague:The Karolinum Press.

14. Huang Y.C., R.M.Malina (2010) Body mass index and individual physical fitness tests in Taiwanese youth aged 9-18 years. *Int.J.Pediatr.Obes.* 5(5):404-411.

15. Lobelo F., R.R.Pate, M.Dowda, A.D.Liese, S.R.Daniels (2010) Cardiorespiratory fitness and clustered cardiovascular disease risk in US adolescents. *J.Adolesc.Health* 47(4):352-359.

16. Kurtze N., V.Rangul, B.E.Hustvedt, W.D.Flanders (2007) Reliability and validity of self-reported physical activity in the Nord-Trondelag Health Study. *Eur J Epidemiol* 22:379-87.

17. Maggio A.B., M.F.Hofer, X.E.Martin, L.M.Marchand, M.Beghetti, N.J.Farpour-Lambert (2010) Reduced physical activity level and cardiorespiratory fitness in children with chronic diseases. *Eur.J.Pediatr.* 169(10):1187-1197.

18. Mahoney C. (1992) 20-MST and PWC170 in non-Caucasian children in the UK. *Br.J.Sports Med.* 26(1):45-47.

19. Martinez-Gomez D., J.R.Ruiz, F.B.Ortega, J.A.Casajus, O.L.Veiga, K.Widhalm, Y.Manios, L.Beghin, M.Gonzalez-Gross, A.Kafatos, V.Espana-Romero, D.Molnar, L.A.Moreno, A.Marcos, M.J.Castillo, M.Sjostrom (2010) Recommended levels and intensities of physical activity to avoid low cardiorespiratory fitness in European adolescents: the Helena study. *Am.J.Hum.Biol.* 22(6):750-756.

20. Nikolaidis P.T. (2011) Familial aggregation and maximal heritability of exercise participation: A cross-sectional study in schoolchildren and their nuclear families. *Sci.Sport* 26(3):157-165.

21. Nikolaidis, P.T. (2011) Overweight and obesity in male adolescent soccer players. *Minerva Pediatr.* 63(6) in print.

22. Nikolaidis, P.T. (2010) Obesity and sport in childhood - a case of a track and field club. *Acta Facultatis Educationis Physicae Universitatis Comenianae* 50(1):49-54.

23. Nikolaidis, P.T. (2009) Inactivity, nutritional and lifestyle habits: a cross-sectional study in Czech schoolchildren and their nuclear families. *Facta.Univ.Phys.Edu.Sport* 7(2):141-151.

24. Noonan V., E.Dean (2000) Submaximal exercise testing: clinical application and interpretation. *Phys.Ther.* 80:782-807.

25. Papadopoulos V., I.Kefala, P.Nikolaidis (2009) Mechatronic and software development of Wingate test. In: Papadopoulos C., Starosta W. (eds). Proceedings of 11th International Conference of Sport Kinetics, 25-27 September, Kallithea, Chalkidiki, Greece.

26. Parizkova J. (1978) Lean body mass and depot fat during autogenesis in humans. In: Parizkova J. Rogozkin V. (eds) Nutrition, Physical Fitness and Health: International Series on Sport Sciences, Baltimore, MA:University Park Press, pp. 22.

27. Pedersen B.K., B.Saltin (2006) Evidence for prescribing exercise as therapy in chronic disease. *Scand J.Med.Sci.Sports* 16(S1):3-63.

28. Saczuk J., A.Wasiluk (2010) Changes in the somatic and fitness variables in girls over two decades. *Biomed.Hum.Kinetics* 2:10-105.

29. Tanaka H., K.D.Monahan, R.Douglas, R.Seals (2001) Age-predicted maximal heart rate revisited. *J.Am.Coll.Cardiol.* 37: 153-156.

30. Thomas J.R., J.K.Nelson, S.J.Silverman (2011) Research methods in physical activity. Champaign: Human Kinetics, 6th ed.

31. World Health Organization (2010) Global recommendations on physical activity for health. Geneva: WHO Press.

Effects of isokinetic and isotonic training programmes on heart rate and blood pressure in high school students

Ahmet Ş. Őkmen [1], İbrahim Erdemir [2]

[1] School of Physical Education and Sports, Mugla University, Mugla; [2] School of Physical Education and Sports, Balikesir University, Balikesir, Turkey

Summary

Study aim: To compare the effects of 6-week isokinetic and isotonic training programmes on heart rate and blood pressure in high school students.
Material and methods: Twenty-nine healthy, untrained male student subjects aged 15 – 18 years participated in the study. They were assigned into 3 groups: control (C; n = 11), and subjected to isokinetic (IK; n = 8) or isotonic (IT; n = 10) training lasting 6 weeks, 3 days a week. Isokinetic exercises consisted of 3 sets of 20-s extensions/flexions (both knees) at 180°/s, spaced by 30-s intermissions, the isotonic ones - of 4 sets of extensions (both knees) at 50% of the predetermined one repetition maximum, spaced by 30-s intermissions. Heart rates (HR) and blood pressure were determined before and after the training period, both pre- and post-exercise.
Results: Mean resting HR and exercise-induced HR-increase significantly decreased post-training in IT group (by 19 and 24%, respectively; $p<0.001$). The exercise-induced HR increase significantly increased post-training in IK group (by 17%; $p<0.001$). Significant ($p<0.01$) training-induced decreases in the systolic pressure (SBP) were found in both training groups (IT and IK, by 7 and 6%, respectively).
Conclusions: The results may be of practical importance for athletes and health professionals who administer open-chain resistance exercises.

Key words: Isokinetic exercise – Isotonic exercise – Heart rate – Blood pressure – Knee joint

Introduction

Isotonic and isokinetic exercises are two modes of resistance training that can be used to improve muscle strength and performance. Isotonic exercise training is characterised by variable joint speed against a constant resistance. The amount of force generated also varies depending on the position of limb and its range of motion. Isotonic exercises are cost-effective and relatively simple to execute and have been used for many years to increase muscle strength in rehabilitation [7]. However, concentric isotonic exercises can only provide loads that can be overcome by weakest point in the range of motion and an accurate control of movement velocity can be difficult. In contrast, isokinetic exercise provides an accommodating resistance at constant velocity which, theoretically, allows for maximal force production at all points throughout the active range of motion and provides an angle-torque curve for each separate muscle action [2]. Isokinetic resistance training has also been used for strength testing and training in clinical settings [19]. Positive effects of weight training on changes in body composition, strength and power are known to occur [8,12]. However, traditional non-circuit weight training has not generally been regarded as important in producing increases in cardiovascular fitness. Most studies investigating cardiovascular fitness focused on aerobic power [8], few studies being devoted to the effects of non-circuit weight training on the heart rate [14]. Resting and recovery heart rates are elements of cardiovascular fitness and therefore will reflect positive changes in cardiovascular fitness as a result of training [20].

The heart rates at rest, exercise and recovery together with blood pressure are very important parameters in all types of sports activities and although more oxygen is consumed by large muscle groups, the rate response is essentially the same for e.g. knee or arm extensions [11]. Studies on the effects of resistance training on circulation

Author's address Dr Ahmet Şadan Őkmen, School of Physical Education and Sports, Mugla University, Turkey

parameters are, however, not numerous and this prompted us to undertake this study, aimed at demonstrating which training programme would be more effective in improving resting, exercise and recovery heart rates and blood pressure, as such information would be useful for specific patient populations and for athletes.

Material and Methods

Subjects: Twenty-nine healthy, untrained male student subjects aged 15 – 18 years volunteered to participate in the study. All subjects were non-smokers, used no drugs affecting the cardiovascular system and had no contraindications to exercise. All of them submitted their written consents to participate after having been informed about the study protocol and possible risks involved. The study was approved by the local committee of ethics.

Methodology: The subjects were randomly assigned into 3 groups. One of them served as a passive control (C; n = 11), the other ones were subjected to training – isokinetic (IK; n = 8) or isotonic (IT; n = 10). The trainings lasted 6 weeks, 3 sessions a week, lasting 15 min each and consisted of exercising knee flexors and extensors (IK group) or extensors only (IT group). One repetition of both kinds of exercises was applied at maximum resistance (1RM); isokinetic exercises consisted of 3 sets of 20-s extensions/flexions (both knees) at 180°/s, spaced by 30-s intermissions, using Cybex II dynamometer (Lumex Inc.USA). Isotonic exercises consisted of 4 sets of extensions (both knees) at 50% of 1RM, spaced by 30-s intermissions. No exercise was applied to the control group.

Before and after training period, heart rates were measured pre- and post-exercise, as well as 15, 30, 45 and 60 s post-exercise using a polar hearth rate monitor (Polar RS100, Finland). Blood pressure were recorded in sitting position pre-exercise when the right leg exercised using a sphygmomanometer and stethoscope.

Data analysis: One-way ANOVA was applied with the Duncan's multiple range post-hoc test in case of significant interaction. Student's *t*-test for paired data was applied to individual differences. The SPSS 15.0 software was used, the level of $p \leq 0.05$ being considered significant.

Results

The results are presented in Tables 1 – 3 and in Fig. 1. No significant between-group differences in physical characteristics were found except BMI (Table 1).

Table 1. Mean values (±SD) of age and basic somatic variables of young male subjects

Group / Variable	Isotonic n = 10	Isokinetic n = 8	Control n = 11
Age (years)	17.0 ± 0.9	17.7 ± 1.0	16.6 ± 0.7
Body height (cm)	172.2 ± 6.7	169.6 ± 7.5	173.2 ± 6.2
Body mass (kg)	59.7 ± 5.4	62.2 ± 12.0	60.3 ± 4.1
BMI	20.2 ± 2.0	22.6 ± 2.7*	20.1 ± 1.7

* Significantly (p<0.05) different from other groups

Mean pre-exercise heart rate was significantly lower post-training compared with the pre-training state in the IT group (by 19%; p<0.001) and the exercise-induced increase was in that group also significantly lower post-training (by 24%; p<0.001). In contrast, in the IK group no significant change in the pre-exercise HR was noted and the exercise-induced increase was in that group significantly higher post-training (by 17%; p<0.001) compared with the pre-training state (Table 2).

The post-exercise changes in the heart rate are presented in Fig. 1. All changes exhibit parallel courses, the between-group and training-induced changes corresponding to those presented in Table 2.

Table 2. Mean values (±SD) of heart rates (HR) and of individual, exercise-induced changes (Δ)

Variable	Group	Isotonic (IT) n = 10	Isokinetic (IK) n = 8	Control n = 11
Pre–training	Pre-exercise	90.6 ± 6.6	83.3 ± 17.1	84.0 ± 9.7
	Δ	31.8 ± 8.0*	24.0 ± 6.4*	28.4 ± 7.1*
Post–training	Pre-exercise	73.2 ± 6.8 °	78.0 ± 12.0	83.4 ± 7.8
	Δ	20.4 ± 8.6*	47.3 ± 15.5*^	28.0 ± 5.7*
Post-pre training	Pre-exercise	-17.4 ± 6.6*^	-5.3 ± 18.0	-0.5 ± 3.2
	Post-exercise	-28.8 ± 12.9*^	18.0 ± 8.5*^	-0.9 ± 4.9^

* Significant (p<0.001) exercise- or training-induced change; Significantly (p<0.01) different from: ° Control group; ^ Other groups

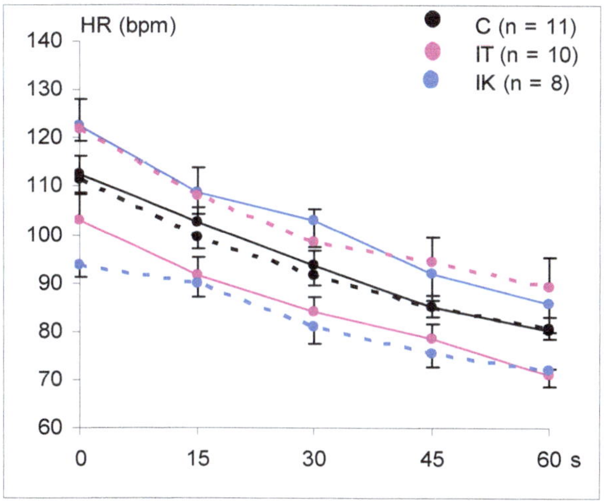

Fig. 1. Mean values (±SE) of post-exercise changes in heart rate (HR) pre-training (solid lines) and post-training (dotted lines)

Legend: C – Control group; IT – Isotonic training group; IK – Isokinetic training group

No significant between-group differences in blood pressure were noted pre-training. Significant ($p<0.01$) training-induced decreases in the systolic pressure (SBP) were found in both training groups (IT and IK, by 7 and 6%, respectively). No significant change was noted in the control group. Further, no significant training-induced changes were noted in the systolic-diastolic differences in either group (Table 3).

Table 3. Mean values (±SD) of systolic (SBP) blood pressure and of systolic/diastolic differences (SBP - DBP)

Variable	Group	Isotonic (IT) n = 10	Isokinetic (IK) n = 8	Control n = 11
Pre–training	SBP	118.6 ± 10.7	121.8 ± 5.8	115.8 ± 4.3
	SBP - DBP	44.6 ± 9.8	48.0 ± 7.7	45.6 ± 5.6
Post–training	SBP	110.4 ± 8.6	114.8 ± 8.1	116.0 ± 4.4
	SBP - DBP	42.4 ± 11.8	51.3 ± 11.7	44.7 ± 5.7
Post-pre difference	SBP	-8.2 ± 7.0*	-7.0 ± 4.9*	0.2 ± 2.4 ^
	SBP - DBP	-2.2 ± 10.8	3.3 ± 9.4	-0.9 ± 3.0

* Significant ($p<0.01$) training-induced change; ^ Significantly ($p<0.01$) different from other groups

Discussion

Heart rate increases in the IK-group may have resulted from the muscle contraction velocity affecting the cardio-respiratory responses during repetitive isokinetic exercises [10,13] since isokinetic concentric contractions elicit greater HR changes than isokinetic eccentric contractions in knee extension exercises [22]. However, Okamoto *et al.* [21] reported lower heart rates for isokinetic training than in this study and suggested that high-intensity eccentric contractions exert only a small stress to the cardiovascular system, thus being applicable to resistance training.

Reductions in the resting heart rate in the IT-group may be the result of an increase in the parasympathetic /diminished sympathetic input ratio [1]; this is likely accompanied by an increased stroke volume [14]. However, other authors [3,4,9,13,17,24] reported significant increases or no changes in HR and blood pressure in subjects practicing free weight, universal gym, nautilus training or conventional resistance training. Furthermore, some researchers [5,6,16,23] found significant decreases in resting HR in subjects practicing weight lifting, circuit weight training or nautilus training.

Isokinetic training induced a decrease in the resting blood pressure but had no significant effect on resting HR while isotonic training affected the resting heart rate. However, other authors [6,15,18,22] found significant increases in HR and blood pressure in subjects exercising on isokinetic ergometers (Cybex II, Kinetic Communicator Model 500-H, Cybex 6000 or Cybex Norm). No comparable data, however, were found in the available literature to evaluate the observed effects on resting HR.

The presented results may be of practical importance for athletes and health professionals who administer open-chain resistance training exercises, as well as to researchers who use isotonic and/or isokinetic training modes of resistance exercise to examine muscle functions. In addition, future studies should examine different types of resistance speed and of exercises to compare with IK training and IT training muscle action.

References

1. Blomqvist C.G, B.Saltin (1983) Cardiovascular adaptations to physical training. *Ann.Rev.Physiol.* 45:169-189.

2. Brown L.E. (2000) Isokinetics in Human Performance. Human Kinetics, Champaign IL.

3. Collins M.A, K.J.Cureton, D.W.Hill, C.A.Ray (1991) Relationship of heart rate to oxygen uptake during weight lifting exercise. *Med.Sci.Sports Exerc.* 23:636-640.

4. Connie C.C, J.E.Graves, M.L.Pollock, M.I.Phillips, C.Sumners, J.M.Hagberg (1991) Effect of exercise training on blood pressure in 70 to 79 years old men and women. *Med.Sci.Sports Exerc.* 23:505-511.

5. Dawson P.K, B.F.Hurley (1993) Effect of training on resting blood pressure in men at risk for coronary heart disease: Strength vs. aerobic exercise training. *Res.Q.* (Suppl.):A-27.

6. Degache F., F.Roche, P.Bernard, P.Calmels (2009) Cardiovascular responses during isokinetic knee extension testing in chronic heart failure patients. *Isokinet.Exerc.Sci.* 17:63-67.

7. Delorme T.L., A.L.Watkins (1948) Techniques of progressive resistance exercise. *Arch.Phys.Med.Rehabil,* 29:263-273.

8. Gettman L.R., M.L.Pollock (1981) A critical review of its physiological benefits. *Physician Sports Med* .9:45-60.

9. Haennel R.G, H.A.Quinney, C.T.Kappagoda (1991) Effects of hydraulic circuit training following coronary artery by pass surgery. *Med.Sci.Sports Exerc.* 23:158-165.

10. Hayashi N, S.Koba, Y.Yoshida (2003) The effect of muscle contraction velocity on cardiorespiratory responses to repetitive isokinetic exercise in humans. *Japan J.Physiol.* 53 (5): 327-333.

11. Hempell, L, and Wells, C.L (1985) Cardiorespiratory cost of the nautilus express circuit. *Phys.Sport Med.* 13:82-97.

12. Hickson R.C, M.A.Rosenkoetter, M.M.Brown (1980) Strength training effects on aerobic power and short-term endurance. *Med.Sci.Sports Exerc.* 12:336-339.

13. Iellamo F, J.M.Legramante, G.Raimondi, F.Castrucci, C.Damiani, C.Foti, G.Peruzzi, I.Caruso (1997) Effects of isokinetic, isotonic and isometric submaximal exercise on heart rate and blood pressure. *Eur.J.Appl.Physiol.Occup.Med.*75:89-96.

14. Kanakis C., R.C.Hickson (1980) Left ventricular responses to a programme of lower limb strength training. *Chest* 78: 618-621.

15. Karlsson J., K.Piehl, H.G.Knuttgen (1981) Performance and muscle metabolite changes in exercise with repeated maximal dynamic contractions. *Introd.J.Sports_Med.* 2:110-113.

16. Katz J, R.Bradley, A.Wilson (1992) The effect of a six week, low intensity Nautilus circuit training programme on resting blood pressure in females. *J.Sports Med.Phys.Fitn.* 32: 299-302.

17. Lamotte M., G.Strulens, G.Niset ,Ph.Van de Borne (2005) Influence of different resistive training modalities on blood pressure and heart rate responses of healthy subjects. *Isokinet. Exerc.Sci.* 13:273-277.

18. Lamotte M., A.Chevalier, A.Jamon, E.Brassine, Ph.Van de Borne (2009) Hemodynamic response of an isokinetic testing and training session. *Isokinet.Exerc.Sci.* 17:135-143.

19. Morrisey M.C., E.A.Harman, M.J.Johnson (1995) Resistance training modes: specificity and effectiveness. *Med.Sci. Sports Exerc.* 27:648-660.

20. Nelson J.K (1969) Fitness testing as an education process. In: J.Broedhoff (ed.) Physical Education Sports and the Sciences. Microform Publications, University of Oregon, Eugene OR, pp.66-73.

21. Okamoto T, M.Masuhara, K.Ikuta (2006) Cardiovascular responses induced during high-intensity eccentric and concentric isokinetic muscle contraction in healthy young adults. *Clin. Physiol.Funct.Imaging* 26:39-44.

22. Overend T.J, T.H.Versteegh, E.Thompson, T.B.Birmingham, A.A.Vandervoort (2000) Cardiovascular stress associated with concentric and eccentric isokinetic exercise in young and older adults. *J.Gerontol.A:.Biol.Sci.Med.Sci.* 55:B177-182.

23. Reynolds T.H, G.A.S.Forzo, P.A.Frye (1993) Cardiovascular responses of females to resistive exercise following training. *Res.Q.* S.A-44.

24. Staab J.S, M.A.Sharp, B.C.Nindl, K.R.Rarick, B.A.Spiering, D.L.Hatfield, L.M.Yamamoto, P.N.Frykman, E.A.Harman, D.J.Gutekenst, J.S.Volek, C.M.Maresh, W.J.Kraemer (2006) Comparison of three training programmes for improving aerobic performance in women. *Med.Sci.Sports Exerc.* 38(Suppl.) No. 2587.

Generational differences in the motivational factors that drive Cypriots to participate in sporting activities

Efstathios Christodoulides

Department of Social Sciences, Faculty of Physical Education and Sport Science, Semmelweis University, Budapest, Hungary

Summary

Study aim: To examine the factors that motivate Cypriots to participate in sport, particularly examining the differences between the last 3 generations regarding their motivations for sport involvement at the present and at the ages of 12-18 years.
Material and methods: The study was completed by survey method among 3 generational groups in Cyprus comprised of secondary school students, their parents, and their grandparents (N=1067). Data were collected via questionnaires that contained 3 open-ended, 16 multiple-choice, and 12 semantic differential scale questions. The response rate was 100% for the students, 77.4% for the parents, and 65.5% for the grandparents. The data were analyzed by the SPSS program for Microsoft Windows; factor analysis and one-way analysis of variance were used.
Results: The examined motivations were clustered into two factors: Joy Factor and Health Factor. Significant differences were found among the 3 generations in their sporting activities at present and the ages of 12-18 years. The students' participation motivations for sport are closely related to fun and enjoyment. Their parents have similar motives at present, but in their childhood they considered health enhancement as the most important reason for sport involvement. The oldest generation regarded the improvement of their health as a stimulating factor for sport in their childhood and youth; they did not change this during their whole life cycle.
Conclusions: Generational differences in the motivation for participation in sport are probably universal, but their elements are dissimilar depending on the value system in general and in sport in societies. The historical and cultural circumstances in Cyprus allow for the generalization of the conclusions only at the national level.

Key words: Sport participation - Motivation - Generational group - Value transmission

Introduction

Since the members of societies are continuously replaced by new members, generational changes occur over time in all areas of social life, including sport. Likewise, in other fields of society only some of the social norms, values, traditions and behavioral patterns are transmitted more or less unaltered from generation to generation; others are abandoned and/or replaced by new ones, also in sport. Everyday experiences suggest that since modern sport emerged at the end of the past century younger generations have been more and more interested in sport than their seniors. Notwithstanding generational differences in sport sciences have been rarely investigated in connection with sport. The few research works were related to sport administration [19], coaching [12], motivations of sport fans [11] and sporting values [5], and they only examined generational changes between two generations. According to our knowledge the sole sport sociological study dealing with the development and transmission of sporting traditions through 3 generations was carried out at the turn of the 1960s and 1970s in a housing estate in Warsaw [14]. The major conclusions of the latter emphasized the social nature of sport and the decisive impact of the social-political and economic systems the members of the 3 generations were living in on the mechanism of the transmission

Both society and within it sport as a social institution have undergone tremendous changes over the last centuries. In contrast with half a century ago, the modern lifestyle offers a vast assortment of conveniences such as the Internet, high-definition televisions, video games, and generally appliances that can easily keep anybody busy in a comfortable position on a couch. The technological advantages that the modern society offers its members are admirable, but they also have negative consequences. As the sedentary lifestyle gained ground, obesity became an overall problem. The lack of regular physical activity has become a significant risk factor; it endangers people's health in all age groups. Over the last decades individuals

Author's address Efstathios Christodoulides, Faculty of Physical Education and Sport Sciences, Semmelweis University, Alkotás utca 44, 1123 Budapest, Hungary

in most societies typically spend over five hours a day in front of the television. The media has gained tremendous power during the last decades and their touch on social life is influential on all aspects, including sports [8]. On the one hand it created consumers and not participants in sport, and its use highly contributed to a dramatic decline in physical activity [9]. On the other hand, the development of media and especially televised sport events and the mediated new sporting movements raised interest in, and up-staged the importance of, exercise. For instance, the so-called fitness boom can be thanked partly to the popularity of the fitness movement in the media.

During the same period, the concept of sport has also been modified. Elite sport diverged from leisure sports and recreational sporting activity. New sports, e.g. aerobic, risk sports and adventure sports, new types of movements, e.g. sport for all and fitness [20], and new target groups, e.g. disabled, elderly and immigrants, emerged. Sport was attributed to non-traditional values: post-modern values, excitement, and autonomy [17]. The social functions of sport broadened, and the set of motivations for sport participation became more complex [13]. Nowadays, many people do sport and exercise for different reasons or for different purposes than did their predecessors. The person's changing needs and expectations of people are also visible in the diverse and new motives of sport participants. Research has been undertaken to determine the individual participant's motivation for sport and exercise in different historical periods; however, neither the research focusing on 2 generations nor the study comparing sporting values with 3 generations examined motivations driving people in different generational groups to be involved in sport. Studies with a similar topic could not been found in the relevant literature.

Parallel with the slowly increasing importance of sport in the Cypriot society in the last decades, several research projects have been carried out regarding various social issues in national sport, but generational differences in sport related motivations have not been studied here, either. Taking into consideration that sport is a mirror of society and that in Cyprus sweeping social, political, cultural, and economic changes occurred successively within just few decades, it can be rightly assumed that these changes might also be reflected in the population's sporting values, habits, behaviors, and participation motivations for sport in a special way.

Research findings suggest that sport habits can generally be renewed or borrowed and adapted from the past [18]. Cypriot sport seems to have been changed partly according to traditions and to the national appreciation of sport, and partly to the changes in international sport and sport policies [1]. The opportunities for being involved in sports have enlarged; accessibility to sport by people of different age, gender, and socioeconomic backgrounds has improved recently on the inland. New needs in connection with sport were born and the ways satisfying the altered needs for sport also have been modified [4]. The Cyprus Sport Organization, which is the body responsible for developing sport at a national level, makes serious efforts to prepare right and adequate programs for sport for all and to make adequate suggestions to improve the physical education programs at school, but the efficiency of its activity is hindered by the lack of scientifically based information on the particular sporting values, norms, habits, motives, and behavioral patterns of the population's different age groups. In order to provide the decision makers in Cypriot sport with information on the basis of which they can plan their policy and with which they can realize their projects in a more effective way, a special topic out of the above-mentioned issues was chosen for investigation. Namely, we examined the factors motivating Cypriots to participate in sporting activities. We discovered the major differences between the last 3 generational groups regarding their motivations for being involved in sport at the present time and at the age of 12-18 years, respectively. The purpose of this paper is to give a brief report on this research and present the main results concerning the differences in motivations for sport of 3 successive generations.

Material and Methods

The research was carried out by survey method. The students attending Cypriot secondary schools in the academic year 2007-2008, their parents, and grandparents were regarded as the total population of the research. At first, the student sample was gradually selected by stratified sampling according to regions (mainland, coastal, and mountain areas of Cyprus), the type of the secondary schools (gymnasiums and lyceums), the gender, and the grade of the students. The students in the individual schools were randomly selected. Then a snowball selection followed for the parents' and grandparents' sample, via the students.

The sample consisted of 3 stratification schemes or sub-samples, more specifically 741 students, 229 parents, and 97 grandparents. Due to the gradual, stratified and random sampling methods that were used, all 3 sub-samples are heterogeneous with regards their education and other socioeconomic characteristics. The student sample is representative of the total student population regarding the region, the type of the secondary school, the gender, and the grade of the students. The parent and the grandparent sub-samples followed the student sample, but they were not representative according to gender. The mean age (±SD) of the students, parents, and grandparents were 15±3 years, 45±8 years, and 75±5 years, respectively.

The data were collected by questionnaires, which consisted of 3 open-ended, 16 multiple-choice, and 12 semantic differential scale questions. The latter were related to the motivational factors: the scoring scales provided respondents with 5 options to tick, with the middle point being the neutral answer. The following indices of motivation were constructed: to have fun, to relax, to meet people, to develop one's personality, to improve health, to improve physical achievement. The reliability was measured by the Cronbach's alpha coefficient (0.89). The answers given to the open-ended questions were categorized according to their frequency.

The students completed the questionnaires in the presence of the author during school time, and the parents and grandparents were subsequently given the questionnaires at home. The response rate was 100% for the students, 77.4% for the parents, and 65.5% for the grandparents.

The survey method was complemented by in-depth interviews (N=15), which were structured according to the age of the respondents, and the answers were categorized according to the type of the motivations (enjoyment or health prevention). The parents and grandparents were asked both about the attitudes and motivations that they have at the present time and those that they used to have at the age of 12-18 years, while students were asked only about the attitudes and motivations that they have at present.

The data were analyzed using the SPSS program for Microsoft Windows. In order to assess the motivation level for sport participation of the 3 generational groups at the present time and at the age of 12-18 years, a multivariant analysis (factor analysis) and one way analysis of variance (ANOVA) were used where appropriate. Due to the high number of variables, a data reduction method (factor analysis) was used in order to cluster the variables according to their characteristics. The assumptions for using ANOVA were verified; normality by Kolmogorov-Sminronov test and homogeneity of variance by Brown-Forsythe test. The Bonferroni post hoc tests were used to further indicate statistically significant differences between the 3 generational groups; the level of $\alpha=0.05$ was considered significant.

Results

The data processing started with factor analysis to assess motivation for participation in sporting activity at the present time and at the age of 12-18 years. The Kaiser-Meyer-Olkin (KMO) index was 0.719 and 0.811, respectively, which is a satisfactory value allowing to continue with the Factor analysis. In both cases the motivations that have been examined were clustered into 2 factors: *Joy Factor* and *Health Factor,* the respective factor loadings were presented in Tables 1 and 2. Although the total variance explained by the two factors was relatively low in both analyses (52.3% and 50.0% for activities at present and the age of 12-18 years, respectively), only the 2 of them were included in the model since the eigenvalues were under 1 for other components. Moreover, the goal of the research emphasized parsimony, that is, to explain variance with as few factors as possible. In this case, the criterion for determining the value of as low as 50% can be regarded satisfactory and hence, the model with the 2 factors could be sufficient to be representative of the variables related to motivational issues.

Table 1. Factor loading of the 2 factors against the motivation degree for participation in sporting activity at the present time

Items	Factors		Communality (h^2)
	I	II	
Joy Factor (a = 0.801)			
To have fun	0.784	0.171	0.64
To relax from day to day life	0.702	0.297	0.58
To meet other people	0.633	0.205	0.44
To develop my personality	0.582	0.129	0.35
Health Factor (a = 0.771)			
To improve health	0.145	0.989	0.99
To improve physical performance	0.493	0.560	0.55
Eigenvalue	3.28	1.06	
Percentage of variance explained	30.3	22.0	

Table 2. Factor loading of the 2 factors against the motivation degree for participation in sporting activity at the age of 12-18 years

Items	Factors		Communality (h^2)
	I	II	
Joy factor (a =0.784)			
To have fun	0.703	0.192	0.53
To relax from day to day life	0.670	0.350	0.57
To meet other people	0.645	0.208	0.45
To develop my personality	0.565	0.199	0.35
Health factor (a=0.808)			
To improve health	0.162	0.986	0.99
To improve physical performance	0.486	0.606	0.60
Eigenvalue	3.37	0.98	
Percentage of variance explained	28.2	23.8	

The results of ANOVA are indicative of significant differences between the 3 generational groups concerning the *Joy Factor* ($F_{(2, 1064)}$= 101.0, $p<0.001$) as well as the *Health Factor* ($F_{(2, 1064)}$= 4.77, $p<0.01$) at the present time. The post hoc analyses revealed that students attained significantly ($p<0.001$) higher values of the *Joy Factor* as compared to both parents and grandparents; the differences being 0.42 and 0.52, respectively (Table 3). Regarding the *Health Factor*, the highest values (0.60) were observed in the grandparents – significantly ($p<0.001$) higher than in students (0.20) or parents (0.25).

Table 3. Results of ANOVA analyses (mean values ±SD in z scores): Differences between the 3 generational groups regarding *Joy* and *Health* factors at the present time

Factor	Students (n = 741)	Parents (n = 229)	Grandparents (n = 97)
Joy	0.75 ± 0.19	0.33 ± 0.21***	0.23 ± 0.21***##
Health	0.20 ± 0.23	0.25 ± 0.25***	0.60 ± 0.23***###

*** Significantly ($p<0.001$) different from students; Significantly different from parents: ## $p<0.01$; ### $p<0.001$

Likewise, the present time, the *Joy Factor* ($F_{(2, 1064)}$ = 17.363, $p<0.001$) and *Health Factor* ($F_{(2, 1064)}$= 126.950, $p<0.001$) at the age of 12-18 years proved to be significantly differentiated in the 3 generational groups. The post hoc analyses indicated that in the *Joy Factor* significant ($p<0,001$) differences exist between students (0.52) and two other groups, but not between parents (0.41) and grandparents (0.38). Regarding the *Health Factor* the value for grandparents (0.78) was significantly ($p<0.001$) higher than observed in the parents or students; the value observed in the latter group was the lowest (0.26) amongst the 3 generational groups.

Table 4. Results of ANOVA analyses (mean values ±SD in z scores): Differences between the 3 generational groups regarding *Joy* and *Health* factors at the age of 12-18 years

Factor	Students (n = 741)	Parents (n = 229)	Grandparents (n = 97)
Joy	0.52 ± 0.19	0.41 ± 0.23***	0.38 ± 0.22***
Health	0.26 ± 0.23	0.46 ± 0.26***	0.78 ± 0.23***###

*** Significantly ($p<0.001$) different from students; ### Significantly ($p<0.001$) different from parents

Discussion

Generational differences were seldom approached from scientific perspectives in Cyprus. They are lacking not only from sport-related literature but from the other areas of social sciences as well. As an exception, Zopiatis *et al.* [21] investigated occupational differences and similarities between two generations that are currently active in hospitality workplaces. The findings of this research helped some elements of the existing generational gaps in contemporary Cypriot society to be understood, but it could not be used as reference material for the results presented in this article. The only research found on 3 generations in international sport literature was published 4 decades ago. It analyzed the sporting habits of people living in a housing estate [14], so it can hardly serve as previous research for comparison. The perceived motivational differences can be discussed in a historical and cultural context and participation motivations with different age groups are taken into consideration.

The grandparents' generation spent their childhood during the British colonial area. At that time, participation in modern sport was not a serious alternative for spending their leisure; they were more involved in traditional games and sports. Schools were not socializing agents for sport; most children had no early sport socialization in the current sense of the term. Besides, the prevailing traditional value system was puritan; enjoyment, fun and relaxation played much less importance in it as they did some decades later. All these reasons explain why the sporting motivations of the grandparents' generations were different from the next generation, when they were 12-18 years old. They considered health enhancement as a stimulating factor in their childhood and youth, and they did not change their mind during their whole life cycle.

The circumstances for sport socialization changed when Cypriot sport developed and became institutionalized after the inland became independent from colonial rulers in 1960. The parents' generation was growing up about that time. The children of this period received relatively more impulse for sport involvement, but this trend was interrupted when the Turkish forces invaded the inland and the country was separated in half. This historical event also had a decisive impact on the sporting values, attitudes, and motivations of Cypriot youth. Moreover, the value system in the Cypriot society was still traditional in the childhood of today's parents; their parents (today's grandparents) transmitted their puritan values and behavioral patterns in connection with sport. Consequently, in spite of the changing role of modern sport in society, today's parents' sporting motivations when they were aged 12-18 years did not differ significantly from their own parents' motivations, that is, they regarded health enhancement as the most important reason to practice sport. Comparing the findings with their parents' motivations, the only modification in their motives was that a few of them also found the improvement of their physical performance important. Paradoxically, the prospect to have fun, to meet other people, and to relax stimulate today's parents more to be involved in sport in their adulthood than it did in their childhood, as both sport and the Cypriot society have changed since then.

The members of the youngest generation, which consists of secondary school students, were brought up under entirely different social circumstances since as a result of globalization traditional social norms and values have been radically changing in Cyprus recently. Life-organizing values have also been modified, and motivations for gratification and filling one's life with joy came to the forefront in various field of social life, including sport. The majority of today's secondary school students who are interested in sport are not willing to work hard for achieving higher performance; rather, they regard it as a source of pleasure.

At the beginning, in the 1970s, research on participation motivations for sport focused on youth participation [6] and the work focused on constructs connected to the youngsters' physical ability; the social aspects of motivations were not studied in detail [2]. The findings of these investigations show that among the multiple reasons for young peoples' sport involvement to develop skill and fitness, to answer challenges, and to have fun can be found the most frequently. Later, from the latter half of the 1980s, when researchers' interest also turned to the participation motivations of adults, it was discovered that their most often cited motives were different from the youngsters' motives. Generally speaking, fun and enjoyment energize different types of sport involvement less frequently with adults than with young people.

Keeping in mind that the above-mentioned research examined the different generations' participation motivations for sport separately and under different social, cultural and economic circumstances, little similarity and considerable differences can be observed. Similarity is reflected by the fact that today among the young people's reasons for participating in sport fun and enjoyment play an outstanding role regardless of their nationality and they have a new concept on the meaning of sport [16]. There is a move towards adventure sports as a form of escaping or transcending the routines of life. Modern sport cannot be identified with competitive sport alone, but with a wide range of new sports called "sports modi," such as fitness, adventure, and health sports. Alternative and extreme sports are becoming formal sports, although such classification is not absolute [3]. Youngsters in particular are looking for unconventional activities, such as snowboarding and in-line skating, in their quest to become or remain active without the interference of undue authority. The peer motivational climate is of great importance in sport participation [13]. Like worldwide, young participants in Cyprus are looking for alternative sports activities with central values such as: freedom, experience of excellent movements, and creating an own youth culture.

However, the similarities stop here. Two major differences are worth mentioning. First, even a few decades ago the most significant motivators of Cypriot youth for sport were not related to pleasure but to health prevention, and contrary to international trend, when they became adults they placed greater importance on fun and enjoyment through sport than they did in their youth. The second main difference is related to the elderly's motivation for exercising. The health factor is generally a significant participation motivation for sport involvement with this age group [7,10]. However, with the Cypriot old generation the emphasis was put mostly on physical health; in other studies mental and social health were also referred as the older people's frequently cited motive. The Cypriot elderly seem not to be really aware of or interested in the beneficial impact of sport on their mental well-being. This statement is also supported by the contradictory results of a recent Eurobarometer on Sport and Physical Activity [15], which on the one hand show Cyprus as a health-conscious country regarding individuals' motivations for physical activity. On the other hand, in another chapter of the same study it is revealed that almost the half of the Cypriot population aged 15 years and over never plays sport or do it less than monthly, and Cyprus is one of the countries in the European Union where the sport participation of the 55+ age group decreases the fastest.

The particular characteristics of the historical and cultural circumstances in Cyprus allow the generalization of the conclusions only on a national level. The fact that there also are generational differences in motivations related to sporting behavior is probably universal but the elements of these differences can be dissimilar. In principle, some findings of this research could be relevant in those southern European states where traditional values and behavioral patterns have survived over a long period of time and the close family ties playing an outstanding role in early sport socialization loosened only recently as a consequence of globalization. In practice, not significant similarities can be observed because of the radical differences in their history and in the history if their sport. Unlike Cyprus the cited countries were not colonized, they were instead colonizers (e.g. Spain and Portugal). Besides, modern sport emerged much earlier in those counties. For instance Greece, the value system of which is the most similar to the Cypriot one, played a leading role in promoting the rise and the spread of the Olympic movement. Finally, all the considered counties are considerably larger than Cyprus, where daily life is usually more personal than in countries with large populations and the knowledge of other people's backgrounds and personalities might have a special impact on sport socialization throughout the life cycle. Notwithstanding, the question how the smallness of Cyprus and in connection with this the strong interpersonal networks as well as the closeness of the interpersonal relations do influence the participation motivations for sport is still open. This issue and the actual impact of the Cypriot people's social and economic background on their motivations for participating in sport need further studies.

References

1. Alexopoulos A. (2005) Recent sport-political decisions of the Council of Europe and Cypriot sport: A preliminary study. In: S.G.Foldesi, A.Gal (eds.) New Social Conditions in Sport 1990-2005. Hungarian Society for Sport Sciences, Budapest, pp. 50-70.

2. Allen B.J. (2003) Social motivation in youth sport. *J.Sport Exerc.Psychol.,* 25:551-567.

3. Baar P. (2001) Organized sport programs for children: do they meet the interests of the children effectively. In: J.Steenbergen, P.De Knop, A.Elling (eds) Values and Norms in Sport, Critical Reflections on the Position and Meanings of Sport in Society. Meyer and Meyer Sport, Aachen, pp. 323-336.

4. Christodoulides E. (2012) Impact of socializing factors on three Cypriot generations (in Hungarian). *Magy. Sporttud.Szle.,* 13:11-17.

5. Foldesi S.G. (1982) Sport in the hierarchy of values. (in Polish) *Kult.Fiz.* 4-6:27-30.

6. Frederick M.C., M.R.Richard (1993) Differences in motivation for sport and exercise and their relations with participation and mental health. *J.Sport Behav.,* 16(3): 124-146.

7. Gill K., V.Overdorf (1974) Incentives for exercise in younger and older women. *J.Sport Behav.*, 17(2):87-97.

8. Gal A. (2005) Sociological aspects of mediated women's sports. In: S.G.Foldesi, A.Gal (eds.) New Social Conditions in Sport 1990-2005. Hungarian Society for Sport Sciences, Budapest, pp. 94-115.

9.Hardman E.A., J.D.Stensel (2003) Physical Activity and Health: The Evidence Explained. Routledge, London.

10. Ibrahim, R.A. (2012) Motives of physical activity in elderly. *World J.Sport Sci.,* 6: 62-66.

11. Izzo G.M., C.Munteanu, B.E.Langford, C.Ceobanu, I.Dumitru, F.Nichifor (2011) Sport fans'motivations: an investigation of Romanian soccer spectators. *J.Int.Bus. Cult.Stud.*, 5. www.aabri.com/jibcs.html

12.McCrindle M. (2008) Engaging with the new generations. *Sports Coach*, 30(1):1-3.

13. Murcia M.A.J., L.M.Román, M.C.Galindo, N.Alonso, G.D.Cutre (2008) Peers' influence on exercise enjoyment: A self-determination theory approach. *J.Sports Sci. Med.* 7: 23-31.

14. Pudelkiewicz E. (1974) A need of sociological research on the problem of sport in housing estate in a family of three generations. In: I.Baly, F.Takács (eds) Sportszociológia. Közgazdasági és Jogi Könyvkiadó, Budapest, pp. 279-289.

15. Special Eurobarometer on Sport and Physical Activity. (2010) European Commission, Bruxelles.

16. Steenbergen J. (2001) The double character of sport. In: J.Steenbergen, P.De Knop, A.Elling. Values and Norms in Sport, Critical Reflections on the Position and Meanings of Sport in Society. Meyer and Meyer Sport, Aachen, pp. 33-56.

17. Stewart B., A.Smith (2000) Australian sport in a post-modern age. *Int.J.Hist.Sport* 17:2-3.

18. Struna L.N. (2000) Social history and sport. In: J.Coakley, E.Dunning (eds.) Handbook of Sport Studies. Sage Publications, London, pp. 187-203.

19. Williamson D.J., S.H.Song (2011) Understanding generational differences in sport administration: creating a cohesive work environment. Sport Entertainment & Venues Tomorrow. Conference abstracts, 32-34. www.hrsm.sc.edu/SEVT/PDFs/2011 SEVT PDFs/2011 SEVT Ab.

20. Volkwein A.E.K. (2000) Fitness as cultural phenomenon. In: J.Tolleneer, R.Renson (eds.) Old Borders, New Borders, No Borders: Sport and Physical Education in a Period of Change. Meyer and Meyer Sport, Aachen, pp. 83-94.

21. Zopiatis A., M.K.Kapardis, A.P.Varnavas, I.Pavlou (2010) Are X-ers from Mars and Y-ers from venus? Generations under the Microscope. The EuroCHRIE, Amsterdam 2010 Conference Proceedings. http://www.eurochrie2010.nl/publications/118.pdf

29

Anthropometric characteristics and somatotype of Greek male and female flatwater kayak athletes

Vassilios Diafas, Eleni Dimakopoulou, Vassiliki Diamanti, Danae Zelioti, Socratis Kaloupsis

Department of Physical Education and Sport Science, National and Kapodistrian University of Athens, Greece

Summary

Study aim: To investigate some anthropometric characteristics of male and female kayakers of four competitive categories.
Material and methods: Anthropometric characteristics of 83 kayak athletes were measured during the 2009 Greek Cup. Kayakers were divided into four groups according to their competitive category: Women (n = 13; mean age 22.7 ± 3.1 years), Junior Female (n = 15; mean age 16.2 ± 1.1 years), Men (n = 27; mean age 23.7 ± 4.6 years) and Junior Male (n = 28; mean age 16.3 ± 1.2 years).
Results: In both groups, the BMI, lean body mass, and relaxed and flexed arm girth were significantly different with respect to age group; body mass was significantly different, but only in male groups. No differences were found between groups on body fat.
Conclusions: The data provided in this study could be used as a guideline for talent identification from the general population and may help coaches establish a specific kayak anthropometric profile in order to distinguish an elite kayak athlete.

Key words: Anthropometry – Body fat – Somatotype – Flatwater kayak

Introduction

Flatwater kayaking is a very demanding outdoor activity, where physical structure, technique, fitness, and other factors (psychology, race strategy) are essential factors for winning a race [4]. Body dimensions are related to performance, and are thus very important [20]. Ackland *et al.* [1] suggested that the morphology of elite paddlers has altered over the past 25 years. Athletes tended to be heavier but leaner. When compared to untrained men, kayakers had greater sitting height, greater biacromial and chest breadths, less body fat, and smaller bicristal and bitrochanteric breadths [6]. Recent studies reported that kayakers are usually taller than average, they have large body mass, strong muscles, and solid skeletons [19]. Thus, it is recognized that optimal performance depends on the upper body build of the kayaker [1,12]. Although the anthropometric characteristics of kayakers have been extensively described [21], there is limited research comparing different flatwater competitive categories. Thus, the aim of this study was to examine selected anthropometric characteristics of male and female kayakers aged 15-29 (divided in four competitive groups). Furthermore, in order to provide a full description of the physique, Heath-Carter somatotype was calculated and compared between groups. These data of Greek kayakers can be used for the process of talent identification and may help coaches establish a specific kayak anthropometric profile in order to distinguish an elite kayak athlete. It should be emphasised that no other scientific data is been published regarding anthropometric characteristics of Greek kayakers.

Material and Methods

Participants: At the 2009 Greek Cup (Schinias Venue, Athens), anthropometric measurements were performed on 83 Greek male and female flatwater kayak athletes. This event provides the opportunity for national coaches to select the best athletes for the national development camps. The athletes were divided in four groups according to their competitive category: Women (n = 13; mean age 22.7 ± 3.1 years, 5-7 years of experience), Junior Female (n = 15; mean age 16.2 ± 1.1 years, 3-4 years of experience), Men (n = 27; mean age 23.7 ± 4.6 years, 5-7 years of experience) and Junior Male (n = 28; mean age 16.3 ± 1.2 years, 3-4 years of experience). All the subjects were highly trained and experienced kayakers who compete on the national and international levels. At the time of the investigation, the athletes were in their competitive training phase. A full description of the testing procedure was presented to the participants and each athlete read

Author's address Dr Diamanti Vassiliki, 185 Sofokleous str., 176 73 Kallithea, Athens, Greece

and signed a written and informed consent prior to participation. The Athens University Ethics Committee approved this study.

Anthropometric measurement: Each subject was tested in the morning. A full anthropometric profile of the participant was taken. Participants were registered by one of the authors, and then directed to the start of the procedure. The following anthropometric variables were measured: body mass, body height, torso length, arm and leg length, humerus and femur width, bi-iliac breadth, relaxed and flexed arm girth and shoulder breadth. Also, measurements of six skinfolds (triceps, biceps, subscapular, supraspinal, front thigh, and medial calf) were performed. All variables were measured on the right side of the body, and according to the methods of Claessens et al. [9]. The variables were measured by an experienced anthropometrist, who took the same measurements for all the surveyed athletes, and was assisted by a recorder. Ratings for the three somatotypes were calculated according to Heath-Carter somatotype method [5]. Using the skinfold data the percent body fat, fat mass, and lean body mass were calculated according to Durnin and Rahaman [10].

Equipment. Harpenden skin-fold calliper (to the nearest 0.01 mm) was used to obtain skinfolds, a bone calliper (Holtain, U.K.) to measure width dimensions. The athlete's height (cm) was measured by a wall stadiometer (Holtain, UK) to the nearest 0.1 cm, athlete's weight measured to the nearest 0.1 kg on an electronic scale (Tanita TBF 401 A, Japan). Limb lengths (cm) were obtained using a girth tape.

Statistical analysis: All statistical analyses were performed using the SPSS 15. Descriptive statistics (mean, standard deviation) were calculated for all variables for each competitive group of kayakers. Comparison between Women and Junior Female and between Men and Junior Male were performed using the independent t-test (two-tailed). The level of statistical significance was set at $p<0.05$.

Results

Descriptive statistics for absolute parameters of the four groups are presented in Table 1. The junior male kayakers had lower body mass than their men counterparts and the t-test results pointed to a statistically significant difference ($p<0.01$). Also, the female junior kayakers had lower body mass compared to women athletes, however the difference was not statistically significant. Men had higher values of lean body mass than the junior male ($p<0.01$).

Table 1. Mean values (±SD) of anthropometric variables in four groups of kayakers

Variable	Women (n=13)	Junior Female (n=15)	Men (n=27)	Junior Male (n=28)
Age (years)	22.7±3.1	16.2±1.1	23.7±4.6	16.3±1.2
Body mass (Kg)	65.9±10.1	59.0±9.0	78.8±7.3***	73.1±7.5
BMI (Kg/m^2)	23.8 ± 2.3***	21.04 ± 2.2	25.1 ± 1.8***	23.6 ± 2.3
Body Fat (%)	26.4±4.4	25.9±3.1	23.7±3.9	22.7±4.0
Lean body mass (Kg)	48.3±5.8**	43.5±5.4	59.6±5.8**	56.0±5.4
Height (cm)	165.8±7.2	167.1±6.1	176.9±4.5	175.6±4.4
Total Arm length (cm)	71.7±4.3	70.6±3.8	76.0±3.4	75.9±3.6
Total Leg Length (cm)	89.7±4.8	89.6±4.8	98.1±5.6	97.0±4.6
Torso Length (cm)	55.5±4.7	54.3±4.9	62.7±8.2	61.5±8.2
Biceps skinfold (mm)	10.3±4.1	11.3±2.8	8.8±3.8	7.5±2.7
Triceps skinfold (mm)	16.1±4.3	15.9±3.8	12.8±4.9	11.7±3.6
Subscapular skinfold (mm)	15.5±5.4	14.5±3.7	14.4±4.9	13.1±4.5
Suprailiac skinfold (mm)	20.7±9.1	16.5±6.5	15.0±5.4	14.0±4.6
Thigh skinfold (mm)	22.6±6.7	24.0±5.7	16.5±4.9	14.8±4.2
Calf skinfold (mm)	14.4±5.1	16.6±4.3	11.8±4.2	13.6±4.6
Relaxed Arm girth (cm)	27.6±2.8***	25.6±2.6	30.3±2.2***	28.3±2.3
Flexed Arm girth (cm)	30.2±3.8***	27.0±2.5	34.1±2.8***	31.2±3.5
Bio-iliac Breadth (cm)	27.4±2.2	28.6±2.3	28.6±1.8	28.0±2.3
Shoulder Breadth (cm)	38.9±3.1	38.6±2.1	42.0±8.1	41.3±7.5
Humerus width (cm)	6.2±0.7	6.0±0.4	6.6±0.6	6.5±0.8
Femur width (cm)	7.3±1.2	7.5±0.9	8.8±1.4	9.3±1.7

Significantly different from respective value in junior category* $p<0.05$; ** $p<0.01$; ***$p<0.001$

Moreover, women had bigger values of lean body mass compared to junior female ($p<0.05$). No differences were found between groups on body fat percentage. The women and men kayakers did not different statistically with junior female and junior male in height, arm, and leg length, respectively. Women had higher BMI than junior female ($p<0.01$); men also had higher BMI than junior male athletes ($p<0.01$).

Men kayakers had bigger relaxed and flexed arm girth than the junior male ($p<0.001$) and ($p<0.01$), respectively. Women differed significantly in flexed arm girth compared to junior female ($p<0.006$). Moreover, all groups had significant differences between relaxed and flexed arm girth ($p<0.001$).

Mean endomorphy, mesomorphy, and ectomorphy ratings for each group are shown in Fig. 1. Endomorphy ratings were the same between women and female junior. Mesomorphy ratings were higher in women ($p<0.01$) compared to junior female. The women and junior female had statistically significant differences in ectomorphy ratings ($p<0.001$). Men and junior did not differ significantly in endomorphy and mesomorphy ratings. Ectomorphy ratings were higher in junior athletes ($p<0.005$). The mean somatotype of women kayakers demonstrates that these athletes are described as mesomorph-endomorph, while the female junior kayakers are best described as balanced endomorph. Male paddlers were endomorphic mesomorph and junior males were showed to be balanced mesomorph.

Discussion

The individual data were compared with the reference group [8]. Male and female paddlers were taller and heavier than the reference group. Regular training, according to Malina [14], does not affect statural growth, but rowers are already taller than reference group during childhood, and this position remains during adolescence.

One finding of this study was that women and men kayakers had similar body height, arm and leg length, but higher lean body mass compared with the junior female and junior male kayakers. The height of the men is similar to those reported by Ridge *et al.* [18], but the body mass of our athletes is higher. Also, the height and body mass is similar with the values reported by Anca and Muniroglou [3]. However, our men kayakers are less tall and somewhat lighter than those in the study of Ackland *et al.* [1].

Regarding the breadth of shoulder, humerus, and femur of women and men, our results have small differences with those of Ridge *et al.* [18] and Ackland *et al.* [1]. In addition, flexed arm girth is almost similar with those of Ridge *et al.* [18] for both categories. Ackland *et al.* [1] reported higher values of flexed arm girth for both sexes (32.1 women, 37.6 men) compared to ours (30.2 women, 34.1 men). Moreover, body fat percentage of our kayakers is higher in all categories compared to the body fat percentage reported in other studies [3,11,20,21].

The somatotype of men is very similar to this reported by Anca and Muniroglou [3]. Men kayakers are best described as endomorphic-mesomorph. Compared to other studies [1,18] the value of mesomorphy is higher than endomorphy and ectomorphy. The somatotype of women in our study was found to be mesomorph-endomorph. Our result is not in line with other studies, in which women were found to be mesomorphic [16]. Comparison of the somatotype ratings across women and junior females showed that mesomorphy ratings were increased in women.

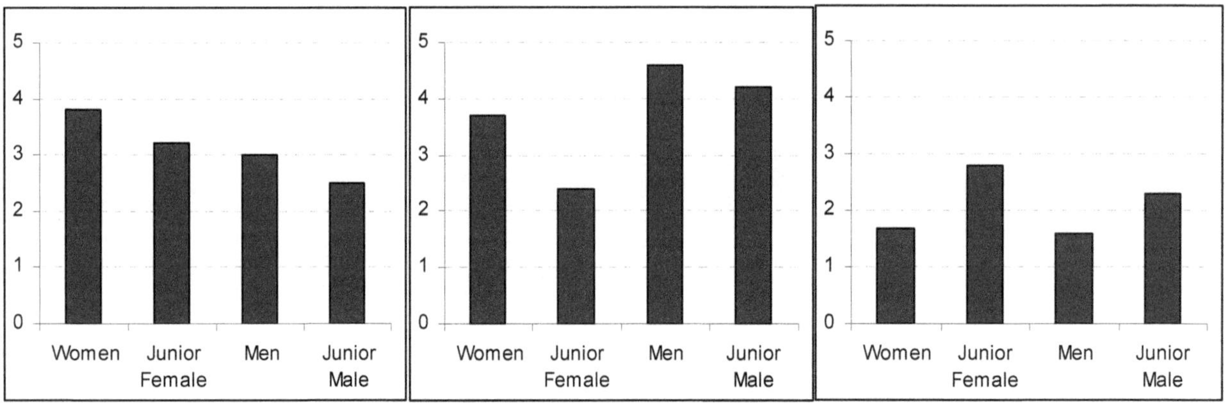

Fig.1. Mean endomorphy (left), mesomorphy (middle), ectomorphy (right) ratings in four groups of kayakers

Comparison of men kayakers with a Greek reference group [7,8] by means of percentiles (P) revealed that regarding height, weight, and BMI they belong to P50, P60, P60, respectively. Junior male belong to P30 of height, P47 in weight and P40 in BMI. Furthermore, women kayakers belong to P60 in height, P75 in weight, and P23 in BMI. Junior female kayakers belong to P70 in height, P58 in weight, and P37.5 in BMI.

On the other hand, mesomorphy was similar between men and junior male (cf. Fig. 1) [15].

There is no available data, as far as we know, for the ages of female and male junior kayakers. Most of the published studies present the anthropometric characteristics of high level kayak athletes. Thus, the present study tries to highlight the physical structure of male kayakers and male kayakers aged 15-17. Comparing junior male kayakers with rowers of the same age revealed that rowers are taller, with lower body fat and slightly higher lean body mass. Their body mass was very similar [13].

A recent study by Alacid *et al.* [2] describes the anthropometric characteristics of male and female elite sprint paddlers aged 13-14 and is useful for talent identification. Furthermore, the results of this study have shown that there are not large differences between male and female flatwater kayakers, and a reference population of non-athletes. For coaches and others who seek talent, there may be a large pool of potential kayakers to choose from the general population.

In conclusion, the present investigation has shown that male and female kayakers aged 16-17 had similar height, arm, and leg length, but lower lean body mass compared with men and women kayakers. Anthropometric characteristics and somatotype of our athletes were found to be almost similar when compared to kayakers at the international level. Anthropometric data is useful because some anthropometric variables are correlated with performance [12,21]. Additionally, coaches could use anthropometric variables to control the training process and to select the appropriate paddle and boat set up [17]. A comprehensive anthropometric description may help coaches to understand and to better select their athletes, as in Greece especially there is a paucity of this data in the investigation of kayaker profiles.

References

1. Ackland T.R., K.B.Ong, D.A.Kerr, B.Ridge (2003) Morphological characteristics of Olympicsprint canoe and kayak paddlers. *J.Sci.Med.Sport* 6:285-294.
2. Alacid F., M.Marfell-Jones, P.A.Lopez-Minarro, I.Martinez, J.M.Muyor (2011). Morphological Characteristics of Young Elite Paddlers. *J.Hum.Kinet.* 27:97-112.
3. Anca F., S.Muniroglu (2008) Anthropometric-somatotype and strength profiles and on-water performance in Turkish elite kayakers. *Int.J.Appl.Sports Sci,* 20 (1):22 34.
4. Bishop D. (2000) Physiological predictors of flat-water kayak performance in women. *Eur.J.Appl.Physiol.,* 82: 91-97.
5. Carter J.E.L. (1980) The Heath- Carter Somatotype Method. 3rd Ed. San Diego State, University Syllabus Service, San Diego.
6. Cermak J. I.Kuta, J.Parizkova (1975) Some predispositions for top performance in speed canoeing and their changes during the whole year training program. *J.Sports Med.Phys.Fit.* 15 (3): 243-251.
7. Chiotis D., G.Tsiftis, M.Chatzisymeon, M.Maniati, X.Krikos, A.Dakou-Voutetaki (2002) Growth charts for the Greek population: boys aged 0-18 years. A′ Pediatric Clinic. Medical School, University of Athens, Greece
8. Chiotis D., G.Tsiftis, M.Chatzisymeon, M.Maniati, X.Krikos, A.Dakou-Voutetaki (2002) Growth charts for the Greek population: girls aged 0-18 years. A′ Pediatric Clinic. Medical School, University of Athens, Greece
9. Claessens A.L., G.Beunen, R.M.Malina (2000) Anthropometry, physique, body composition and maturity. In: Armstrong N., van Mechelen W. (eds): Paediatric Exercise Science and Medicine. Oxford: Oxford University Press, 11-22.
10. Durnin J.V.G. A., M.M.Rahaman (1967) The assessment of the amount of fat in the human body from measurements of skinfolds thickness. *Br.J.Nutr.* 21:681-689.
11. Fleck S.J. (1983) Body composition of elite American athletes. *Amer.J.Sports Med.,* 11 (6):398-403.
12. Fry R.W., A.R.Morton (1991) Physiological and kinanthropometric attributes of elite flatwater kayakers. *Med.Sci.Sports Exerc.,* 23(11): 1297-1301.
13. Kaloupsis S., G..C.Bogdanis, E.Dimakopoulou, M.Maridaki (2008) Anthropometric characteristics and Somatotype of young Greek rowers. *Biol.Sport,* 25(1): 57-68.
14. Malina R.M.(1994) Physical activity and training: effects on stature and the adolescent growth spurt. *Med.Sci.Sport Exerc.,* 26:759-66.
15. Malina R.M., C.Bouchard (1991) Growth, Maturation and Physical Activity. Human Kinetics, Champaign, IL, pp.65-86
16. Michael J.S., K.B.Rooney, R.Smith (2008) The metabolic demands of Kayaking: A review. *J. Sports Sci. Med.,* 7, 1-7.
17. Ong K.B., T.R.Ackland, P.A.Hume, B.Ridge, E.Broad, D.A.Kerr (2005) Equipment set-up among Olympic Sprint and Slalom Kayak paddlers. *Sports Biomech.,* 4(1): 47-58.
18. Ridge B.R., E.Broad, D.A.Kerr, T.R.Ackland (2007) Morphological characteristics of Olympic slalom canoe and kayak paddlers. *Eur.J.Sport Sci.,* 7(2): 107-113.
19. Rynkiewicz M., T.Rynkiewicz (2010) Bioelectrical impedance analysis of body composition and muscle mass in advanced kayakers. *Hum.Mov.,* 11(1): 11-16.
20. Tesch P.A. (1983). Physiological characteristics of elite kayak paddlers. *Can.J.Appl.Sport Sci.,* 8(2). 87-91
21. Van Someren K.A., G.S.Palmer (2003). Predictor of 200m sprint kayaking performance. *Appl.Physiol.Nutr.Metab* 28 (4): 505-517

Correlations of handgrip strength with selected hand-anthropometric variables in university softball players

Shyamal Koley, Santhosh B. Kumaar

Department of Sports Medicine and Physiotherapy, Guru Nanak Dev University, Amritsar, Punjab, India

Summary

Study aim: To assess the handgrip strength in Indian university softball players as dependent on selected hand-anthropometric variables.
Material and methods: Indian university softball players (121 males and 122 females) and untrained controls (98 males and 102 females) aged 18 – 25 years participated in the study. The following variables were recorded: body height and mass, BMI, right hand width and length, lengths of the right 2nd, 3rd and 4th digits and right handgrip strength.
Results: One-way ANOVA showed significant differences ($p<0.05 – 0.001$) in all the characteristics studied, except body height, right hand length and right 2nd digit length among these four sets of data. The right handgrip strength was significantly correlated ($p<0.01 – 0.001$) with all the variables studied. Both in male and female softball players, the partition of R^2 into the contributions of individual independent variables revealed that body height (18%), hand width (11%), body mass (8%) and hand length (5%) significantly contributed to the total variance (44%) of handgrip strength.
Conclusions: The data might be useful in selecting players and in talent identification for softball.

Key words: Hand – Anthropometry – Handgrip strength

Introduction

Softball is a direct descendant of baseball. It requires speed, strength and endurance [27], handgrip playing a crucial role. The main basic aspects of the game, i.e. swing velocity and pitch speed, are greatly influenced by the grip strength of the player [9]. Softball players require a significant amount of upper body muscle balance due to the specificity of the forearm activity. Many athletes and coaches believe that the forearm plays a significant role both in hitting and throwing the ball [4].

Handgrip strength is the result of forceful flexion of all finger joints with the maximum voluntary force that the subject is able to exert under normal biokinetic conditions [3,23] using several hand and forearm muscles. The estimation of handgrip strength is of immense importance in sports like wrestling, tennis, handball, basketball, volleyball, baseball and softball, where sufficient degree of grip strength is necessary to be successful. For example, without adequate grip and forearm strength, tennis players may run the risk of developing lateral epicondylitis, commonly known as tennis elbow. Often overlooked or taken for granted, the grip strength plays a key role in injury prevention and overall strength development [5,8,31]. In many cases, strengthening the grip has been a prescription for rehabilitation from injuries such as golfers and tennis elbow [5]. These ailments are often caused by improper strength ratios between the elbow and the forearm muscles. If the elbow flexors, like biceps and brachialis, are too strong for the forearm flexors, uneven tension accumulates in the soft tissue and results in elbow pain [22].

Grip strength determines the handedness of an individual. It is often used as an indicator of the overall physical strength [7], muscle performance of the hand and forearm [20], and as a functional index of nutritional status [10-12,21,28,29] and physical performance [25]. Handgrip strength is a physiological variable that is affected by a number of factors including age, gender and body size. Strong correlations between grip strength and various somatic traits (body mass and height, hand length, etc.) were reported earlier [11,14,15,24].

Some reports related to morphological/anthropometric characteristics and handgrip strength of softball players are available [4,9,28,30]. But, from the best of our knowledge, the information related to the correlations of hand anthropometry and grip strength in softball players largely remains unreported so far. In the present study, an attempt has been made to estimate the handgrip strength of inter-university softball players, including its association with various hand anthropometric characteristics

Author's address Dr. Shyamal Koley, Department of Sports Medicine and Physiotherapy, Guru Nanak Dev University, Amritsar 143005, Punjab, India

Material and Methods

Subjects: This cross-sectional study was based on 243 randomly selected Indian inter-university softball players (121 males and 122 females) aged 17 – 25 years from Punjabi University, Patiala, Punjab University, Chandigarh, Guru Nanak Dev University, Amritsar, Kurukshetra University, Kurukshetra, Himachal Pradesh University, Himachal Pradesh and Delhi University, Delhi. The competition was organised at the Guru Nanak Dev University, Amritsar, Punjab, India. An adequate number of controls (98 males and 102 females, aged 17 - 25 years, with no competitive sport background were randomly selected from the same places. All subjects submitted their written consents to participate. The data were collected under natural environmental conditions in morning hours (8:00 – 12:00). The study was approved by the local ethics committee.

Anthropometric measurements: The following data were recorded: body height (cm), body mass (kg), BMI, right hand width (cm), lengths (cm) of the right hand and of the 2nd, 3rd and 4th digits, and right handgrip strength (kg) by using standard techniques [1,19]. All measurements were done in triplicates, the median values being taken for analysis. Body height was recorded during inspiration using a stadiometer (Holtain Ltd., Crymych, Dyfed, UK) to the nearest 0.1 cm, body mass was measured by digital medical scales (Model DS-410, Seiko, Tokyo, Japan) to the nearest 0.1 kg. Hand measurements were made using Vernier slide caliper (Starrett, 123 Series, U.S.A.).

Maximum handgrip strength was measured (in triplicates, at 30-s intervals) using a standard adjustable digital dynamometer (Takei Scientific Instruments Co., LTD, Japan) in standing position with shoulder adducted and neutrally rotated, elbow in full extension. The dynamometer was held freely without support, not touching the subject's trunk. The position of the hand remained constant throughout the measurement. Anthropometric equipment and handgrip dynamometer were calibrated before each assessment and the measurements were conducted after 3 min of a warm-up.

Data analysis: All measurements were converted to logarithms and analysed allometrically: hand length vs. body height and other measurements vs. hand length. One-way ANOVA followed by Bonferroni's *post-hoc* test was used. All variables proved to be normally distributed by Shapiro-Wilk's test. Pearson's coefficients of correlations between the right handgrip strength with other variables and contributions of the independent variables to the total variability of the dependent variable were computed [26]. The SPSS software V. 17.0 was used, the level of $p \leq 0.05$ being considered significant.

Results

Mean values (±SD) of hand anthropometric characteristics and grip strength of Indian inter-university softball players and controls are shown in Table 1. Significant differences ($p<0.05$ – 0.001) were noted between male softball players and their control counterparts (not shown in the table) in right hand width and length, right 3rd and 4th digit length, whereas highly significant differences ($p<0.001$) were found between female softball players and controls in all the variables studied except body height, right hand length, and right 2nd digit length. Highly significant gender differences ($p<0.001$) were found in softball players in all the variables studied. One-way ANOVA showed significant differences ($p<0.05$ – 0.001) in all the characteristics studied, except body height, right hand length and right 2nd digit length among these four sets of data.

Table 1. Mean values (±SD) of selected hand-anthropometric variables in Indian university softball players

Variable / Group	MS n = 121	MC n = 98	FS n = 122	FC n = 102
Age (years)	20.7 ± 1.5	21.4 ± 2.7	20.1 ± 1.6	23.2 ± 1.5
Body height (cm)	172.4 ± 7.0	172.3 ± 6.4	159.6 ± 5.3	159.2 ± 5.4
Body mass (kg)	63.9 ± 10.0	65.8 ± 10.3	51.4 ± 6.4	53.97 ± 7.3
BMI	21.4 ± 2.9	22.1 ± 3.0	20.2 ± 2.2	21.3 ± 2.8
RHW (cm)	8.41 ± 0.41	8.12 ± 0.43	7.51 ± 0.43	7.36 ± 0.35
RHL (cm)	18.9 ± 0.8	18.6 ± 0.8	17.2 ± 0.9	17.2 ± 0.7
R2ndDL (cm)	7.31 ± 0.39	7.24 ± 0.42	6.68 ± 0.47	6.59 ± 0.31
R3rdDL (cm)	8.16 ± 0.45	7.93 ± 0.48	7.43 ± 0.48	7.29 ± 0.35
R4thDL (cm)	7.58 ± 0.40	7.31 ± 0.43	6.87 ± 0.50	6.72 ± 0.35
HGR (kg)	41.4 ± 6.2	40.3 ± 6.2	26.6 ± 4.5	23.78 ± 4.2

Legend: M – Male; F – Female; S – Softball players; C – Control subjects; RHW – Right hand width (cm); RHL – Right hand length (cm); R2ndDL – Right 2nd digit length (cm); R3rdDL – Right 3rd digit length (cm); R4thDL – Right 4th digit length (cm); HGR – Right handgrip strength (kg)

Simple correlation coefficients, multiple correlations (R^2) and percentage contributions of independent variables (body height and mass, BMI and all hand-anthropometric variables) to the total variance of the right handgrip strength are shown in Tables 2 - 5. The R^2 values in male and female softball players were identical (R = 0.445) but higher than their control counterparts (R^2 = 0.272 and 0.350, respectively). The right handgrip strength was significantly correlated ($p<0.01 - 0.001$) with all the variables studied. All the hand-anthropometric variables were significantly correlated ($p<0.001$) with each other.

Table 2. Simple correlation coefficients, multiple correlations (R^2) and percentage contributions of independent variables to the total variance of the right handgrip strength in Indian inter-university male softball players

Variable	BM	BMI	RHW	RHL	R2ndDL	R3rdDL	R4thDL	HGR	%
BH	0.507***	-0.037	0.491***	0.645***	0.573***	0.543***	0.545***	0.422***	18***
BM		0.841***	0.466***	0.470***	0.354***	0.329***	0.334***	0.457***	8***
BMI			0.233*	0.139	0.054	0.043	0.045	0.260*	1
RHW				0.604***	0.570***	0.575***	0.636**	0.559***	11***
RHL					0.752***	0.794***	0.782***	0.576***	5***
R2ndDL						0.842***	0.777***	0.364***	0
R3rdDL							0.855***	0.438***	1
R4thDL								0.469***	0
								R^2 = 0.445***	

* p<0.05; ** p<0.01; *** p<0.001

Table 3. Simple correlation coefficients, multiple correlations (R^2) and percentage contributions of independent variables to the total variance of the right handgrip strength in control males

Variable	BM	BMI	RHW	RHL	R2ndDL	R3rdDL	R4thDL	HGR	%
BH	0.493***	0.020	0.417***	686***	0.457***	0.503***	0.518***	0.364***	13***
BM		0.878***	0.445***	0.522***	0.457***	0.420***	0.518***	0.383***	6***
BMI			0.290***	0.224*	255***	0.209*0.	0.125	0.246*	0
RHW				0.526**	0.526**	0.572**	0.480**	0.447**	7***
RHL					0.694***	0.714***	0.754**	0.335***	0
R2ndDL						0.770***	0.731***	0.357***	1
R3rdDL							0.775***	0.343***	0
R4thDL								0.312***	9
								R^2 = 0.272***	

* p<0.05; ** p<0.01; *** p<0.001

Table 4. Simple correlation coefficients, multiple correlations (R^2) and percentage contributions of independent variables to the total variance of the right handgrip strength in Indian inter-university female softball players

Variable	BM	BMI	RHW	RHL	R2ndDL	R3rdDL	R4thDL	HGR	%
BH	0.507***	-0.037	0.491***	0.645***	0.573***	0.543***	0.545***	0.422***	18***
BM		0.841***	0.466***	0.470***	0.354***	0.329***	0.334***	0.457***	8***
BMI			0.233*	0.139	0.054	0.043	0.045	0.260*	1
RHW				0.604***	0.570***	0.575***	0.636***	0.559***	11***
RHL					0.752***	0.794***	0.782***	0.576***	5***
R2ndDL						0.842***	0.777***	0.384***	1
R3rdDL							0.855***	0.438***	0
R4thDL								0.469***	0
								R^2 = 0.445***	

* p<0.05; ** p<0.01; *** p<0.001

Table 5. Simple correlation coefficients, multiple correlations (R^2) and percentage contributions of independent variables to the total variance of the right handgrip strength in control females

Variable	BM	BMI	RHW	RHL	R2ndDL	R3rdDL	R4thDL	HGR	%
BH	0.368***	-0.145	0.379***	0.625***	0.456***	0.487***	0.490***	0.273***	7***
BM		0.865***	0.406***	0.267***	0.282*	0.206*	0.245*	0.240*	3*
BMI			0.225*	-0.059	-0.046	0.054	-0.004	0.101	1
RHW				0.518***	0.441***	0.465***	0.516***	0.434***	11***
RHL					0.720***	0.812***	0.780***	0.500***	8***
R2ndDL						0.859***	0.893***	0.381***	0
R3rdDL							0.889***	0.433***	0
R4thDL								0.344**	5***
								$R^2 = 0.350$***	

* p<0.05; ** p<0.01; *** p<0.001

When allometric analysis was applied, the following results were obtained: male players had slightly (by about 3 – 4 mm; p<0.01) longer hand in relation to body height compared with control subjects; no difference was found in the female subjects. The players differed from controls in having slightly greater hand width, and lengths of the 3rd and 4th fingers (all in relation to hand length; p<0.05). The same was true for handgrip strength and length of the 2nd finger only for female subjects. Female players differed from controls in having higher (p<0.05) dominant handgrip strength in relation to hand length, whereas no such difference was found in male players.

Discussion

Somatic dimensions and morphological characteristics play an important role in determining the success of an athlete [13]. Quite naturally, the interest in anthropometric characteristics and body composition of athletes from different competitive sports has increased tremendously over the last decades. All ball games require comprehensive abilities including physical, technical, mental and tactical [27,30].

In this study, a significant difference in handgrip strength was found only between female players and controls. This could be due to regular physical exercise and practice of players that could be more pronounced in the female than in male subjects. Both in male and female softball players, the partition of R^2 into the contributions of individual independent variables revealed that body height (18%), hand width (11%), body mass (8%) and hand length (5%) significantly contributed to the total variance (44%) of handgrip strength. It was also reported that strong correlations existed between handgrip strength and height, weight, BMI and all the five hand anthropometric characteristics studied. In fact, all the flexor muscles of hand and forearm responsible for grip strength are closely related anatomically, physiologically and biomechanically to each other to perform the task, showing close affinity to each other. It was reported earlier that handgrip strength strongly correlated with various anthropometric characteristics [2,15-19], males attaining stronger handgrip than their female counterparts [2]. Right and left handgrip strength was positively correlated with body mass, body height and body surface area [6].

The data presented here carry immense practical applications. To excel the performance of the players as well as to avoid sport-specific injuries, the sports authorities can use the data to arrange gender-specific training programmes. As softball players require a significant amount of upper body muscle balance due to the specificity of the forearm activity, specific muscle(s) of hand and arm would be strengthened for specific purposes of the game. The data might be useful in future investigation on player selection and talent identification in the game. This would call, however, for a study on national level players in order to validate these correlations.

References

1. Barut C., P.Demirel, S.Kiran (2008) Evaluation of hand anthropometric measurements and grip strength in basketball, volleyball and handball players. *Anatomy* 2:55-59.

2. Benefice E., R.Malina (1996) Body size, body composition and motor performances of mild-to-moderately undernourished Senegalese children. *Ann.Hum.Biol.* 23:307-321.

3. Bohannon RW. (1997) Reference values for extremity muscle strength obtained by handheld dynamometer from adults aged 20 to 79 years. *Arch.Phys.Med.Rehab.* 78:26-32.

4. Brylinskyl J., M.J.C.F.Melanie (1992) The effect of using a weighted softball on pitching velocity, wrist strength and handgrip. *J.Strength Cond.Res.* 6:170-173.

5. Budoff J.E. (2004) The prevalence of rotator cuff weakness in patients with injured hands. *J.Hand Surg.* 29:1154-1159.

6. Chatterjee S., B.J.Chowdhuri (1991) Comparison of grip strength and isometric endurance between the right and left hands of men and their relationship with age and other physical parameters. *J.Hum.Ergol.* 20:41-50.

7. Foo L.H. (2007) Influence of body composition, muscle strength, diet and physical activity on total body and forearm bone mass in Chinese adolescent girls. *Br.J.Nutr.* 98:1281-1287.

8. Fry A.C., M.D.Ciroslan, C.D.Fry, C.D.LeRoux, B.K.Schilling (2006) Anthropometric and performance variables discriminating elite American junior men weightlifters. *J.Strength Cond.Res.* 20:861-866.

9. Giardina D., H.Leslie, L.Raridon, D.Zimmer (1997) Relationship of grip strength and forearm size to bat velocity in college female softball players. *IAHPERD J.* 30(2). http://www.iowaahperd.org/journal/j97s_baseball.html

10. Jeejeebhoy K.N. (1998) Nutritional assessment. *Gastroentrol.Clin.North Am.* 27:347-369.

11. Jurimae T., J.Hurbo, J.Jurimae (2009) Relationship of handgrip strength with anthropometric and body composition variables in prepubertal children. *J.Copmar.Hum.Biol.* 60:225-238.

12. Kaur N., S.Koley (2010) An association of nutritional status and hand grip strength in female laborers and sedentary women of Jalandhar, Punjab, India. *Anthropologist* 12:237-243.

13. Keogh J. (1999) The use of physical fitness scores and anthropometric data to predict selection in an elite under-18 Australian rules football team. *J.Sport Sci.Med.* 2:125-133.

14. Koley S., A.P.Singh (2009) An association of dominant hand grip strength with some anthropometric variables in Indian collegiate population. *Anthropol.Anz.* 67:21-28.

15. Koley S., N.Kaur (2009) A Study on handgrip strength and some anthropometric variables in younger and older female labourers of Jalandhar, Punjab, India. *Int.J.Biol.Anthropol.* 3(2). http://www.ispub.com/journal/the_internet_journal_of_biological_anthropology/volume_3_number_2_59/article/a-study-on-handgrip-strength-and-some-anthropometric-variables-in-younger-and-older-female-laborers-of-jalandhar-punjab-india.html

16. Koley S., M.K.Yadav (2009) An association of hand grip strength with some anthropometric variables in Indian cricket players. *Facta Universitatis, Series: Phys.Educ.Sports* 7:113-123.

17. Koley S., N.Kaur, J.S.Sandhu (2009) Association of handgrip strength and some anthropometric traits in female laborers of Jalandhar, Punjab, India. *J.Life Sci.* 1:57-62.

18. Koley S., J.Singh, J.S.Sandhu (2010) Anthropometric and physiological characteristics on Indian inter-university volleyball players. *J.Hum.Sport Exerc.* 5:389-399.

19. Lohmann T.G., A.F.Roche, R.Martorell (1988) Anthropometric Standardization Reference Manual. Human Kinetics Books, Champaign IL.

20. Nwuga V. (1975) Grip strength and grip endurance in physical therapy students. *Arch.Phys.Med.Rehab.* 56:296-299.

21. Pieterse S., M.Manandhar, S.Ismail (2002) The association between nutritional status and hand grip strength in older Rwandan refugees. *Eur.J.Clin.Nutr.* 56:933-939.

22. Poliquin C. (2006) The Poliquin International Certification Program Theory II Manual. East Greenwich RI. Pp 2-42.

23. Richards L., B.Olson, P.Palmiter-Thomas (1996) How forearm position affects grip strength. *Am.J.Occup.Therapy* 50:133-139.

24. Ross C.H., B.Rösblad (2002) Norms for grip strength in children aged 4–16 years. *A.Paediatr.* 91:617-625.

25. Samson M.M., B.I.Meeuwsen, A.Crowe, J.E.Dessens, SA.Duursma, H.J.Verhaar (2000) Relationships between physical performance measures, age, height and body weight in healthy adults. *Age and Ageing* 29:235-242.

26. Stupnicki R., P.Tomaszewski, K.Milde (2007) Contributions of age, body height and body mass to the total variance of an example physical fitness variable. *Papers Anthropol.* 16:266-272.

27. Terbizan D.J., M.Waldera, P.Seljevold, D.J.Schwigert (1996) Physiological characteristics of masters women fastpitch softball players. *J Strength Cond.Res.* 10:157-160.

28. Tsunawake N., Y.Tahara, K.Moji, S.Muraki, K.Minowa, K.Yukawa (2003) Body composition and physical fitness of female volleyball and basketball players of the Japan inter-high school championship teams. *J.Physiol.* (*Anthropol.Appl.Hum. Sci.*) 22:195-201.

29. Watters D.A., AA.Haffejee, I.B.Angom, K.J.Duffy (1985) Nutritional assessment by hand grip dynamometry. *S.Afr.Med.J.* 68:585-587.

30. Werner S.L., G.J.Deryk, J.A.Guido, M.E.Brunet (2006) Kinematics and kinetics of elite windmill softball pitching. *Am.J Sports Med.* 34:597-603.

31. Yasuo G., T.Daisaku, M.Nariyuki, S.Junya, O.Toshihiko, M.Masahiko, M.Yashiyuki (2005) Relationship between grip strength and surgical results in rotator cuff tears. *Shoulder Joint* 29:559-562.

Physical activity of male and female adolescents living in a town and a city in the context of public health recommendations

Władysław Mynarski, Agnieszka Nawrocka, Michał Rozpara, Wiesław Garbaciak

The Jerzy Kukuczka Academy of Physical Education in Katowice, Poland

Summary

Study aim: To assess the physical activity of male and female adolescents from Poland living in a town (Czechowice-Dziedzice) and in a city (Katowice).
Material and methods: The research involved 431 high school students aged 16-18 years (249 from Czechowice-Dziedzice and 182 from Katowice). Physical activity was measured by the short form of the International Physical Activity Questionnaire (IPAQ). The volume of the different levels of physical activity was calculated in units of MET min/wk.
Results: The total volume of weekly physical activity was higher among high school students living in a town (Czechowice-Dziedzice) than students living in a city (Katowice). Only 31.5% of the students met the criteria for recommended physical activity.
Conclusions: The level of physical activity varies by place of residence. Students living in towns are more physically active than youth living in cities. Most high school students (64%) included in the research can be considered to be insufficiently physically active.

Key words: Physical activity – IPAQ – Environmental factors – Health recommendations

Introduction

Long-term epidemiological studies have demonstrated the relationship between the deficiency of physical activity (hypokinesia) and premature mortality or the incidence of many diseases [15,27]. However, despite large amounts of newly presented scientific evidence about the benefits of regular physical activity, the awareness of the role of reasonable effort in both maintaining physical health and in preventing and treating lifestyle diseases remains insufficient. The low percentage of Poles who satisfy the recommended physical activity as suggested by the American College of Sports Medicine (ACSM), the American Heart Association (AHA), and the World Health Organization (WHO) [6,12] substantiate this conclusion.

Experts have recognized the decline in physical activity of children and adolescents as a growing problem [34]. Regular physical exercise plays a fundamental role in normal, balanced psychophysical development. Meanwhile, the younger generation frequently becomes a "victim" of technological progress. They spend more time at the computer, while their mobile phone replaces traditional ways of spending time with peers. These behaviours reduce the physical activity of children and adolescents to a minimum during their spare time. The result is an increasing number of children and young people with postural defects and obesity. The latter, according to World Health Organization, has grown to the size of being considered a global epidemic [33].

Physical activity is determined by, among other factors, place of residence. Many authors highlight the greater levels of activity of rural and small towns residents, arguing that the higher level of physical activity is a result of, among other things, work performed on farms and gardens, as well as commuting – to get to school, the bus, shops – on foot or by bicycle, which is referred to as "active transport" [14] or "active commuting" [19].

Czechowice-Dziedzice, with a number of residents that is almost 10 times fewer than Katowice, can be considered a town. Within the town's administrative boundaries are located administrative units (town councils) that lack high schools. Thus, over 50% of the students from Czechowice-Dziedzice commute to school by bus or train, or need to go to school on foot. In cities with well developed public transportation systems, it is much easier to get to school. A significant share of the so-called "school transport" in the physical activity of children and adolescents has been confirmed in numerous scientific studies in countries with school commuting systems organized better than Poland's. [8,14,30]. This allows for the

Author's address Prof. Władysław Mynarski, Chair of Tourism and Recreation, The Jerzy Kukuczka Academy of Physical Education, Mikołowska 72a, 40-065 Katowice, Poland

assumption that active forms of commuting to school (active commuting) play an important part in physical activity undertaken by young Polish people residing in villages and towns who attend secondary schools.

In research on the subject of physical activity, comparisons between the actual parameters of physical activity and the recommended parameters are rare. The lack of such comparisons allowed the research problem at the centre of this study to be defined. The aim of this study is thus to compare the parameters of physical activity of male and female adolescents aged 16-18 years who live in a town (Czechowice-Dziedzice) and in a city (Katowice) in the context of the amount of physical activity recommended to maintain health. The following research questions were formulated:

1. What is the level of high, moderate, and low physical activity among male and female adolescents who live in a town and in a city?
2. What is the total weekly physical activity of male and female adolescents in a town and a city?
3. What percentage of the researched students met the criteria for minimum and optimum recommended physical activity needed for a healthy life?

Material and Methods

The survey study included a total of 431 subjects. The research was conducted in 2009 among 182 high school students enrolled in Paderewski General Education Lyceum number 1 in Katowice (included 87 boys and 95 girls), and in 2010, among 249 students of the Staszic Technical and General Education School Complex of Czechowice-Dziedzice (143 boys and 106 girls). In the study, participating students included first- and second-year high school students, aged 16-18 years, who regular attended physical education classes. The selection of schools was intentional. The lyceum in Katowice is located in the centre of the city, and the students were residents of the city. The school of Czechowice-Dziedzice was chosen from among three schools with lyceum-type classes, as its students were mostly from out of town. Participation in the study was voluntary.

In the assessment of physical activity, the short version of the international physical activity questionnaire (IPAQ) was used [1,3]. The collected information about physical activity was supplemented with the measurement of the subjects' body height and mass, and calculation of body mass index (BMI). Respondents completed the IPAQ alone in the presence of a trained interviewer, who explained all the emerging doubts about the interpretation of the questions contained in the questionnaire.

The level of weekly physical activity (measured in units METmin/wk), which was described as high, moderate and low intensity, was determined by multiplying the number of days in which the activity was done in a week, the average length of the activity's duration in one day, and metabolic equivalent of the task (MET, metabolic equivalent of work = 1kcal/kg/h [11]). The MET value of 3.3 was adopted for low intensity effort (AF3), MET value 4 for moderate (AF2), and MET value 6 for high (AF1). In the latter case MET value 8 was assumed per IPAQ instruction. In this work, it was reduced to MET value 6 in accordance with a solution adopted by other authors [16,29] connected with the propensity of youth to overestimate high intensity efforts [3,25]. The total weekly physical activity of subjects was determined by summing its level in the aforementioned ranges of intensity (AF4).

The level of weekly physical activity of respondents was interpreted on the basis of selected criteria of physical activity recommended for children and adolescents from 5 to 18 years old. The latest standards of physical activity recommended for optimal health indicate a need to do daily moderate (4.0 MET) or vigorous (6.0 MET) physical activity (MVPA) with a cumulative daily duration of not less than 60 minutes [10,31,33]. A moderate to vigorous intensity of physical activity that lasts at least 30 minutes per day is considered a daily minimum for children and young people [17].1

The statistical analysis of the collected results was performed using the Statistica 9.1 software and Microsoft Excel. The significance of differences in the mean results of physical activity in male and female adolescents from Czechowice-Dziedzice and Katowice was evaluated using Student's t-tests or the Mann-Whitney U test. The proportion of male and female adolescents who met the criteria for minimum and optimum desired physical activity to maintain health was calculated and compared using Chi-square test. The level of $\alpha = 0.05$ was considered significant.

Results

Analysis of the parameters of the respondents' somatic build indicates the diversity of gender and place of residence (Table 1). The female students from Katowice were on average shorter and heavier than their peers from Czechowice-Dziedzice, as was reflected in the higher ($p<0.01$) values of their body mass index (BMI). The differences in somatic build among male individuals were minor. In most cases, the mean values and dispersion values of BMI results show that the body build of the studied adolescents was normal.

The analysis of physical activity of the compared groups of secondary school youth from Czechowice-Dziedzice and Katowice was limited to an assessment of frequency per week, as well as daily and weekly levels, as categorized in three ranges of effort intensity.

Table 1. Somatic characteristics (mean ± SD) of male (M) and female (F) adolescents from a town (T) and a city (C)

Variable	FT (n=106)	MT (n=143)	FC (n=95)	MC (n=87)
Body height (cm)	166,3 ± 5,7	177,8 ± 6,9	163,8 ± 5,6**	177,4 ± 6,6
Body mass (kg)	56,9 ± 8,7	70,3 ± 11,5	57,9 ± 10,0	72,2 ± 12,9
Body Mass Index (kg/m²)	20,6 ± 2,7	22,1 ± 2,8	21,5 ± 3,4**	22,8 ± 3,5

** Significantly (p<0.01) different from FT group

Table 2. Frequency and daily volume (mean ± SD) of physical activity in male (M) and female adolescents (F) classified within 3 ranges of intensity

Intensity	FT (n=106)		MT (n=143)		FC (n=95)		MC (n=87)	
	Frequency of physical activity (days/week)							
AF 1	76	2,84 ± 1,47	127	3,39 ± 1,22	67	2,55 ± 1,10	80	3,08 ± 1,29
AF 2	98	3,41 ± 1,95	137	4,01 ± 1,81#	76	3,19 ± 1,64	74	3,19 ± 1,80#
AF 3	106	6,42 ± 0,99	143	6,46 ± 0,94	95	6,37 ± 1,31	86	6,31 ± 1,15
	Daily volume of physical activity (min.)							
AF 1	76	44,7 ± 19,1	127	59,4 ± 25,0	67	45,4 ± 22,3	80	42,9 ± 20,3###
AF 2	98	56,3 ± 32,2	137	67,4 ± 34,8	76	46,9 ± 28,7*	74	47,5 ± 23,9###
AF 3	106	84,1 ± 33,6	143	82,0 ± 33,7	95	67,8 ± 34,0***	86	63,9 ± 37,1###
AF 4	106	168,8 ± 65,2	143	199,5 ± 64,2	95	140,2 ± 63,9***	86	143,1 ± 51,9#

Legend: T – Town; C – City; AF 1 – High physical activity; AF 2 – Moderate physical activity; AF 3 – Low physical activity; AF 4 – Total physical activity; Numbers in columns pertain to number of subjects meeting criteria for respective physical activity intensities; Significantly different from FT group:*p<0.05; ***p<0.001; Significantly different from MT group: #p<0.05; ###p<0.001

The male and female secondary school students who lived in Czechowice-Dziedzice were, on average, more often physically active per week. Most days of the week, the surveyed students undertook only physical activity of low intensity, regardless of gender and place of residence (Table 2). The boys declared participation in physical activities of high and moderate intensity more often than the girls. Also, the average daily duration of physical activity in the evaluated ranges of intensity was higher for individuals from the town (Table 2).

The level of weekly physical activity in each of the evaluated ranges of intensity was higher for adolescents from Czechowice-Dziedzice. Statistically significant inter-group differences were found in all cases with the exception of high intensity activities of the girls from Czechowice-Dziedzice in relation to their peers from the city (Fig. 1). In all compared groups, low intensity activity had the largest share of the total volume of weekly physical activity, while moderate efforts had the smallest share. The boys declared greater amounts of activity of moderate and high intensity than the girls did; an inverse relationship was found for efforts of low intensity.

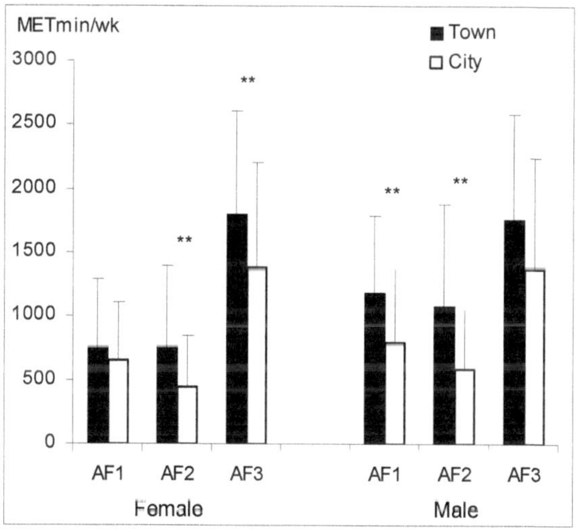

Fig. 1. Mean (± SD) weekly volume of physical activity of male and female adolescents; classified within 3 ranges of intensity

For explanation of symbols see Table 2; *** p<0.01

Greater amounts of activity of students from Czechowice-Dziedzice in certain ranges of intensity were reflected in total volume of weekly physical activity (Fig. 2).

The secondary school students from Katowice presented a significantly lower level of weekly physical activity. A particularly significant difference, on average 1271 METmin/wk, was observed between the boys, while between the girls it was smaller, 629 METmin/wk. In both cases, these differences proved to be statistically significant ($p<0.01$; Fig. 2).

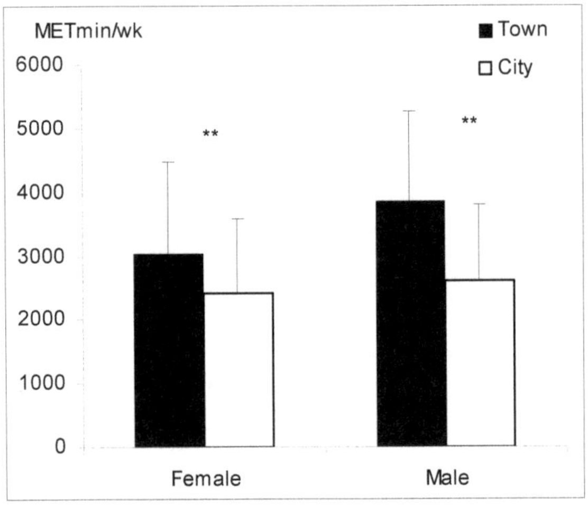

Fig. 2. Mean (± SD) total volume of weekly physical activity of male and female adolescents
*** $p<0.01$

The current standards of physical activity recommended for health emphasise that to keep or improve their health, children and adolescents must do exercise of moderate or high intensity. In our study, a significant proportion of the girls did not meet this recommendation. The volume of their total weekly physical activity was a result of undertaking mainly efforts of low intensity. A much larger share of efforts of moderate and high intensity was observed for the boys (Fig. 1).

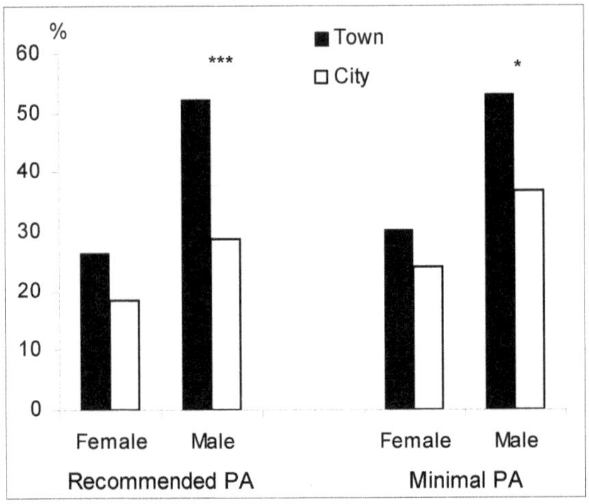

Fig. 3. Percentages of the male and female adolescents meeting recommended [10,31,33] and minimal [17] physical activity (PA) standards
*** $p<0.01$

The assessment of physical activity parameters of the surveyed subjects indicates a significantly higher proportion of sufficiently active male adolescents among these living in a town (Fig. 3). Undertaking daily physical effort of intensity ≥ 4 MET was observed in 41.6% of the students from Czechowice-Dziedzice (53.1% boys, 30.2% girls) and 30.4% of the students from Katowice (36.8% boys, 24.0% girls). Yet only for 39.4% of respondents from Czechowice-Dziedzice and 23.0% from Katowice, however, the cumulative duration per day was not less than 60 minutes.

Discussion

The recommendations on necessary physical activity for children and young people are much stricter than for adults due to a developing organism's greater need for movement activities. Numerous publications highlight the positive impact of movement activities on the physical, mental, and social development of the young generation. The same publications also warn of the decline in participation of youth in extracurricular physical activities [7]. The results of the last report of the Health Behaviour in School-Aged Children (HBSC, 2010) are particularly alarming. According to the authors, only 10.3% of students aged 16-18 years (17.9% male students, 4.2% female students) undertook efforts of moderate or high intensity for at least an hour on a daily basis. In other studies of a nationwide sample of Polish youth, 65% of the evaluated respondents did not present the recommended level of physical activity [5]. According to Stankiewicz *et al.* [28], 30.7% of these young people declared daily physical efforts. Such an unsatisfactory result was confirmed by the high school students from Czechowice-Dziedzice and Katowice. It was found that only 36% of the studied adolescents reached the minimal physical activity levels recommended for health, while only 31.5% reached the optimal physical activity levels recommended for health. It should be stressed that it was the claimed physical activity of the young people that was analysed (surveys); hence, the actual level was probably even lower, because research results show the tendency of youth to overestimate their physical efforts. It applies especially to physical activity of high intensity [3,4,25]. Biernat *et al.* [4] point out that discrepancies between the actual level of physical activity and the declared level could be prevented by the proper training of interviewers. In light of the experience of the authors of this paper, even such an essential measure may be ineffective in surveys of the physical activity of youth. Increasingly lower levels of fitness and physical efficiency of today's adolescents quite often make students regard their efforts of moderate intensity as being highly intensive. However, it does not mean that their caloric expenditure exceeds 6 kcal/kg/h (6 MET).

Many researchers highlight the sexual dimorphism in physical activity that shows boys undertake recommended physical efforts of moderate and high intensity more often than girls, and this is reflected in the boys' higher total volume [21,22]. In our study we also reported the higher volumes of moderate and intensive efforts of the boys. As a result, and similar to the opinions of other authors [9,18,23], a higher percentage of male secondary school students met the recommendations for physical activity assumed to have healthy effects.

One of the crucial factors differentiating participation of children and adolescents in physical activities is their place of residence [20,13]. This was also reflected in the results of this study, according to which the percentage of both male and female adolescents who fulfilled the criteria of minimal and optimal physical efforts recommended for health was much larger in Czechowice-Dziedzice than Katowice. The lower levels of physical activity of residents of urban areas has also been addressed by Bergman *et al.* [2], Sandercock *et al.* [26] and Wojtyła-Buciora and Marcinkowski [32].

In light of the high percentages of insufficiently physically active adolescents observed in this research, the results of other studies on teenagers' self-evaluation of physical activity levels seem interesting. In research by Stankiewicz *et al.* [28], in which 69.3% of adolescents did not attain recommended physical activity, only 10% of the respondents considered themselves insufficiently physically active. In another study, the percentage of respondents unsatisfied with their physical activity level was 20% [32]. This shows the low awareness of young people regarding the need of an organism for physical effort, and indicates the need for development of healthy behaviour among students, especially the habit of regular physical activity.

To summarise the above results of the study, it should be noted that secondary school students living in a town (Czechowice-Dziedzice) presented higher levels of physical activity than their peers living in a city (Katowice) in all ranges of effort intensity. The physical activity of boys was characterised by the prevalence of efforts of high and moderate intensity. Girls dominated the physical activity forms of low intensity efforts. Thus it confirmed the results of many previous observations conducted in Poland and abroad.

The most important cognitive conclusion of this research is a finding that in light of the latest recommended standards of physical activity for children and adolescents aged 5-18 years, 36.0% of secondary school students from Czechowice-Dziedzice and Katowice reached the recommended minimal level of physical activity, while 31.5% reached the optimal level. This indicates a justified and urgent need for intensification of actions intended to promote healthy lifestyles, with a particular emphasis on physical activity and its continuous monitoring among all children, young people, and adults. A key role in this process is played by scholastic physical education, in which the main objective should be to prepare a student for a life of physical activity. Some countries promote the idea contained in the slogan "lifetime sports", which assumes that a purpose of scholastic physical education is to help students find the movement forms (sports) that they will do throughout their lives.

References

1. Bauman A., F.Bull., T.Cheyl, C.L.Craig, B.E.Ainsworth, J.F.Sallis, H.R.Bowles, M.Hagstromer, M.Sjostrom, M.Pratt (2009) The International Prevalence Study on Physical Activity: results from 20 countries. *Int.J Behav.Nutr.Phys Act.*, 6-21.
2. Bergman P., A.M.Grjibovski, M.Hagströmer, A.Bauman, M.Sjöström (2008) Adherence to physical activity recommendations and the influence of socio-demographic correlates – a population-based cross-sectional study. *BMC Publ.Health*, 8-367.
3. Biernat E., R.Stupnicki, A.K.Gajewski (2007) Międzynarodowy Kwestionariusz Aktywności Fizycznej (IPAQ) wersja polska. *Wych.Fiz.Sport*, 51:47-54.
4. Biernat E. R.Stupnicki, B.Lebiedziński, L.Janczewska (2008) Assessment of physical activity by applying IPAQ questionnaire. *Phys.Educ.Sport*, 52:46-52.
5. Cabak A., B.Woynarowska (2004) Physical activity of youths aged 11-15 years in year 2002 in Poland and other countries. *Phys.Educ.Sport*, 48:361-366.
6. Centrum Badania Opinii Społecznej (2003) O aktywności fizycznej Polaków. Warszawa.
7. Charzewska J., B.Wajszczyk, E.Chabros, M.Rogalska-Niedźwiedź (2006) Aktywność fizyczna w Polsce w rożnych grupach według wieku i płci. In: M.Jarosz (ed.) Otyłość, żywienie, aktywność fizyczna, zdrowie Polaków. Instytut Żywności i Żywienia, Warszawa, pp. 311-340.
8. Cooper R. A.L.Andersen, N.Wedderkopp, A.Page, K.Froberg (2005) Physical activity levels of children who walk, cycle, or are driven to school. *Am.J.Prev.Med.*, 29:179-184.
9. De Cocker K., Ch.Ottevaere, M.Sjöström, L.Moreno, J.Wärnberg, J.Valtueña (2010) Self-reported physical activity in European adolescents: results from the HELENA (Healthy Lifestyle in Europe by Nutrition in Adolescence) study. *Pub.Health Nutr.*, 14.246-254.
10. Department of Health and Aging (2005) Australia's Physical Activity Recommendations for Children and Young People.
11. DiLoreto C., C.Fanelli, P.Lucidi, G.Murdolo, A.DeCicco, N.Parlanti, A.Ranchelli, C.Fatone, C.Taglioni, F.Santeusanio, P.De Feo (2005) Make your diabetic patients walk. Long-term impact of different amounts of physical activity on type 2 diabetes. *Diabetes Care*, 28:1295-1302.
12. Drygas W., M.Kwaśniewska, D.Szcześniewska, K.Kozakiewicz, J.Głuszek, E.Wiercińska, B.Wyrzykowski, P.Kurjata (2005) Ocena poziomu aktywności fizycznej dorosłej populacji Polski. Wyniki Programu WOBASZ. *Kardiologia Polska*, 63:636-640.

13. Dyck V., G.Cardon, B.Deforche, I.Bourdeaudhuij (2011) Urban-rural differences in physical activity in Belgian adults and the importance of psychosocial factors. *J.Urban Health*, 88:154-167.

14. Faulkner G.E., N.R.Buliungb, P.K.Florac, C.Fusco (2009) Active school transport, physical activity levels and body weight of children and youth: A systematic review. *Prev.Med.*, 48: 3-8.

15. Fogelholm M. (2010) Physical activity, fitness and fatness: relations to mortality, morbidity and disease risk factors. A systematic review. *Obes.Rev.*, 11:202-221.

16. Haskell W.L., I.M.Lee, R.P.Pate, K.E.Powell, S.N.Blair, B.A.Franklin, C.A.Macera, G.W.Heath, P.D.Thompson, A.Bauman (2007) Physical activity and public health: updated recommendation for adults from the American College of Sports Medicine and the American Heart Association. *Med.Sci.Sports Exerc.*, 39:1423-1434.

17. Health Canadian Society for Exercise Physiology (2005) Canada's Physical Activity Guide for Children and Youth.

18. Kołoło H., J.Mazur, K.Mikiel-Kostyra, M.Guszkowska (2010) Determinanty aktywności fizycznej młodzieży. *Med.Wiek Rozw.*, 24:310-318.

19. Lee M.C., M.R.Orenstein, M.J.Richardson (2008) Systematic review of active commuting to school and children's physical activity and weight. *J.Phys.Activ.Health*, 5:930-949.

20. Liu J., K.Bennett, N.Harun, J.C.Probst (2008) Urban-rural differences in overweight status and physical inactivity among US children aged 10-17 years. *J.Rural Health*, 24:407-415.

21. Mitáš J., J.Nykodým, K.Frömel (2009). Physical activity and sedentary behavior in 14-15 year old students with regard to location of school. *Acta Univ.Palacki.Olomuc.Gymn.*, 39:7-11.

22. Mynarski W., W.Garbaciak, H.Stokłosa, G.Grządziel (2007) Sprawność fizyczna ukierunkowana na zdrowie (H-RF) populacji Górnego Śląska. AWF, Katowice.

23. Patnode C., A.Lytle, D.Erickson, J.Sirard, D.Barr-Anderson, M.Story (2010) The relative influence of demographic, individual, social, and environmental factors on physical activity among boys and girls. *Int.J.Behav.Nutr.Phys.Act.*, 7-79.

24. Health Behavior in School-aged Children (HBSC) Survey (2010).

25. Rozpara M., W.Mynarski, K.Czapla (2008) Szacowanie kosztu energetycznego aktywności fizycznej na podstawie badań kwestionariuszem IPAQ. In: W.Mynarski (ed.). Teoretyczne i empiryczne zagadnienia rekreacji i turystyki. AWF, Katowice, pp. 257-281.

26. Sandercock G., C.Angusa, J.Barton (2010) Physical activity levels of children living in different built environments. *Prev.Med.*, 50:193-198.

27. Schnohr P., P.Lange, H.Scharling, J.S.Jensen (2006) Long-term physical activity in leisure time and mortality from coronary heart disease, stroke, respiratory diseases and cancer. The Copenhagen City Heart Study. *Eur.J.Cardiovasc.Prev.Rehab.*, 13:173-179.

28. Stankiewicz M., M.Pieszko, A.Śliwińska, S.Małgorzewicz, Ł.Wierucki, T.Zdrojewski, B.Wyrzykowski, W.Łysiak-Szydłowska (2010) Obesity, knowledge of diet and healthy behaviors in children and adolescents from small towns and villages – results of Polish Project of 400 Cities. *Endokrynol.Otył.Zab.Przem.Mat.*, 6: 59-66.

29. Suchomel A., D.Sigmundová, K.Frömel (2008) The role physical activity in the lifestyle of the inhabitants of the Liberec region. *Hum.Movement*, 9:19-26.

30. Tudor-Locke C., Y.Hatano, R.P.Pangrazi, M.Kang (2008) Revisiting "How many steps are enough". *Med.Sci.Sports Exec.*, 40:537-543.

31. United States Department of Health and Human Services (2005) Dietary Guidelines for Americans.

32. Wojtyła-Buciora P., J.Marcinkowski (2010) The opinion of high school students and their parents concerning physical activity. *Probl.Hig.Epidemiol.*, 91: 644-649.

33. World Health Organization (2010) Global Recommendations On Physical Activity For Health.

34. Woynarowska B. (2007) Edukacja zdrowotna. PZWL, Warszawa.

Health potential of female candidates to the professional military service

Alicja Kaiser [1], Marek Sokołowski [2]

[1] Wielkopolska Higher School of Tourism and Management, Poznań; [2] University School of Physical Education, Poznań, Poland

Summary

Study aim: To assess health and social characteristics of female candidates for professional officers and non-commissioned officers of Polish Army.
Material and methods: All female students of officer and non-commissioned officer Military Academies (16 each) were studied in 2009. Two questionnaires were applied in the study: IPAQ (short) for assessing the level of physical activity of the respondents and a specially designed questionnaire for assessing social situation, perceived health and pro-health behaviours.
Results: The influence of the society on the respondents' decision to join the army is significantly higher among NCOS students than in the group of OS respondents ($p<0.05$). OS students perceive their health better than their NCOS mates ($p<0.05$). Among students' pro-health behaviours that were assessed in the research, the most advantageously presented is their physical activity. NCOS students are more resilient mentally ($p<0.01$), yet their inclination to make use of health service is much lower ($p<0.01$).
Conclusions: The modern educational trends in health promotion call for modifying the existing military school curricula by including health education issues so that the superiors acquire not only commanding skills but become also exemplary health educators.

Key words: Female soldiers – Health behaviours – Physical activity

Introduction

System changes in Poland, which started in 1989, included armed forces and the participation of women in them. Like in case of men, female subjects in armed forces have to be in good health, be resistant psycho-emotionally and be physically fit. Therefore, those issues have been under a regular monitoring in Poland and in other countries as well [3,4,8,9,16]. The health potential of soldiers includes also issues related to the lifestyle, the health behaviours, health-directed training and education are thus the matter of studies [7,11,15]. Armed forces are a specific and important community, regarding the educational issues. Armed forces are regarded as a totalitarian organisation, whose community is fairly isolated from the outer population; all daily activities of military community take place in a restricted region under steady supervision. The lifestyle of subordinates depends, to quite an extent, on their superiors and the officers and non-commissioned officers are thus responsible for shaping health behaviours by their educational activities and by setting a good example. The aim of this study was thus to determine the health-related characteristics of female candidates for officers and non-commissioned officers.

Material and Methods

Two groups of female students of Armoured Land Forces Academies in Wrocław (officer school; OS) and in Poznań (non-commissioned officer school; NCOS), n – 16 each, volunteered to participate in the study conducted in 2009. Two questionnaires were applied by hall interviews: IPAQ (short) [1,2, 22] for assessing the level of physical activity of the respondents and a specially designed questionnaire for assessing the perceived health and related issues, physical fitness, dietary habits, demographic data, etc. That questionnaire contained 32 items and was validated by a preceding pilot study.

The data were assessed by applying the chi-square function in logarithmic form [19]. The level of $p \leq 0.05$ was considered significant. Whenever no significant differences between groups were noted, the results of both groups combined were shown.

Author's address Dr Alicja Kaiser, Departament of Tourism, Wielkopolska Higher School of Tourism and Management in Poznań, Św. Marcin St. 40, 61-807 Poznań, Poland

Results

The results are presented in Tables 1 – 7. All students of officer school had higher education, most of them came from medium-size or big towns and were older than their mates from the NCO school ($p<0.05$). No significant differences were found in other demographic variables (Table 1). When interviewed, they were asked about military traditions in their families; most NCOS students had family members in the army or working for the army in contrast to only few OS students who reported having them ($p<0.05$). Only 8 of all 32 subjects had neither relatives nor friends associated with the army.

Table 1. Numbers of female students of military officer schools responding to demographic questions

Variable	OS n = 16		NCOS n = 16
Mean age (years)	28		21
BMI		21.9 (18 – 29)	
Education of respondents			
Secondary	0		9
Higher	16		7
Mother's education			
Primary		3	
Vocational		13	
Secondary		12	
Higher		4	
Father's education			
Primary		4	
Vocational		14	
Secondary		8	
Higher		6	
Residence			
Village	3		8
Town, up to 10 000 inhabitants		1	
Town, 10 – 100 000 inhabitants		9	
Town, above 100 000 inhabitants	8		3
Economic status			
Very good		3	
Good		19	
Moderate		10	
Bad		0	
Family members in the army	6		12

Legend: OS – Officer school; NCOS – Non-commissioned officer school; The numbers were reported for each school separately only when significantly different ($p<0.05$)

The OS students rated their health status significantly ($p<0.05$) higher than their NCOS mates. No significant between-group differences were found with respect to the perceived physical fitness or to the engagement in physical activities as determined by IPAQ questionnaires (Table 2). The motives of undertaking motor activities are presented in Table 3. The predominant reason for practicing motor activities was keeping fit. It should be noted that OS students declared health maintaining/improving significantly ($p<0.05$) more frequently than their NCOS mates, the latter ones indicating also relaxing from stress, not mentioned by any OS subject.

Table 2. Perceived health and physical fitness of female students of military officer schools

Variable	OS n = 16		NCOS n = 16
Perceived health			
Very good	11		5
Good	5		11
Perceived fitness			
Very good		19	
Good		10	
Moderate		3	
Physical activity by IPAQ			
High		15	
Sufficient		14	
Insufficient		3	

For explanations see Table 1

Table 3. Numbers of female students of military officer schools responding to questions related to motives of undertaking motor activities (multiple choice answers)

Motivation	OS n = 16		NCOS n = 16
Keeping fit		22	
Relaxing from stress	0		7
Pleasant leisure		6	
Good results in fitness tests		15	
Attractive body shape		5	
Health maintaining/improving	9		3
Fashion		3	

For explanations see Table 1

As follows from Table 4, motor activities were not the dominant form of leisure activities. No between-group differences were noted in various leisure activities with one exception: significantly ($p<0.05$) more OS students declared reading books and magazines compared with their ONCS mates.

Some questions pertained to the mode of nutrition. No significant between-group differences were found regarding the numbers of meals consumed daily; overall,

13 subjects declared having more than 3 meals a day, 16 – having 3 meals and only 3 had less than 3 meals. The declared frequencies of consuming various food products are presented in Table 5. Among the beneficial dietary habits were frequent consumptions of fruit and vegetables, dominance of poultry over beef/pork meat, dairy products, drinking mineral water every day and avoiding sweet beverages. Among the unfavourable ones were very low consumption of fish, low consumption of wholemeal bread (mainly OS subjects; $p<0.05$), too high a consumption of animal fats and frequent consumption of sweets.

Table 4. Numbers of female students of military officer schools responding to questions related to the forms of leisure activities (multiple choice answers)

<table>
<tr><th>Forms of leisure activities</th><th>OS
n = 16</th><th>NCOS
n = 16</th></tr>
<tr><td>Hobbies</td><td colspan="2">16</td></tr>
<tr><td>Meeting friends</td><td colspan="2">13</td></tr>
<tr><td>Various motor activities</td><td colspan="2">10</td></tr>
<tr><td>Sleeping</td><td colspan="2">5</td></tr>
<tr><td>Reading books, magazines</td><td>8</td><td>3</td></tr>
<tr><td>Computer, TV-watching</td><td colspan="2">3</td></tr>
</table>

For explanations see Table 1

Table 5. Consumption of various food products (mean numbers of days per week) as declared by female students of military officer schools

<table>
<tr><th>Product</th><th>OS
n = 16</th><th>NCOS
n = 16</th></tr>
<tr><td>Milk</td><td colspan="2">3.3</td></tr>
<tr><td>Milk products</td><td colspan="2">3.3</td></tr>
<tr><td>Plant fats</td><td>3.6</td><td>2.2</td></tr>
<tr><td>Animal fats</td><td colspan="2">3.7</td></tr>
<tr><td>White bread</td><td>5.3</td><td>4.3</td></tr>
<tr><td>Wholemeal bread</td><td>1.8</td><td>2.4</td></tr>
<tr><td>Cured pork meat</td><td>3.3</td><td>2.3</td></tr>
<tr><td>Cured poultry meat</td><td colspan="2">2.8</td></tr>
<tr><td>Beef meat</td><td>2.0</td><td>2.7</td></tr>
<tr><td>Poultry</td><td colspan="2">3.3</td></tr>
<tr><td>Fish</td><td colspan="2">1.1</td></tr>
<tr><td>Potatoes</td><td colspan="2">4.4</td></tr>
<tr><td>Grains, rice</td><td colspan="2">1.7</td></tr>
<tr><td>Leguminous plants</td><td colspan="2">4.4</td></tr>
<tr><td>Vegetables, salads</td><td colspan="2">5.9</td></tr>
<tr><td>Fruit</td><td>1.9</td><td>1.5</td></tr>
<tr><td>Fruit/vegetable juice</td><td colspan="2">4.8</td></tr>
<tr><td>Mineral water</td><td colspan="2">4.3</td></tr>
<tr><td>Coca-cola, Pepsi, Fanta, etc.</td><td colspan="2">6.6</td></tr>
<tr><td>Sweets</td><td colspan="2">1.1</td></tr>
</table>

For explanations see Table 1

When asked about the use of stimulants, 23 out of 32 subjects declared being non-smokers, 17 of which used to smoke but were no addicts. The smokers declared smoking about 10 cigarettes a day for at least 8 years. Also 23 subjects used alcoholic beverages only occasionally and in small quantities, 3 subjects – regularly or in larger quantities, the other ones abstained from alcohol altogether.

The NCOS students exhibited much higher ($p<0.01$) psycho-emotional resistance than their OS mates (Table 6). The most common ways to cope with an increased nervousness were meeting friends, next motor activities, shopping or visiting cinema. No subject mentioned being helpless or taking medicines in stressful situations. On the other hand, the NCOS students cared less for their health compared with their OS mates (Table 7) – more of them ignored symptoms of health disorders and only less than half of them declared performing preventive examinations ($p<0.01$). With respect to other ways of dealing with health disorders mentioned in Table 7, or to visiting dentists both when needed or for preventive reasons, no between-group differences were noted.

Table 6. Incidence of increased nervousness as declared by female students of military officer schools

Frequency	OS n = 16	NCOS n = 16
Seldom or at times	7	14
Frequently	9	2

$p<0.01$; For other explanations see Table 1

Table 7. Managing various health disorders and the necessity of prophylaxis as declared by female students of military officer schools

<table>
<tr><th>Response</th><th>OS
n = 16</th><th>NCOS
n = 16</th></tr>
<tr><td>Ignoring them</td><td>3</td><td>8</td></tr>
<tr><td>Self-administered therapy</td><td colspan="2">11</td></tr>
<tr><td>Seeking advice in the web</td><td colspan="2">11</td></tr>
<tr><td>Going by friends' advice</td><td colspan="2">9</td></tr>
<tr><td>Visiting the physician</td><td colspan="2">10</td></tr>
<tr><td>Preventive examinations</td><td>14</td><td>7</td></tr>
</table>

For explanations see Table 1

Discussion

When analysing the social and educational factors associated with the female students of an officer school and a non-commissioned officer school, some significant differences could be detected. All OS students had higher education in contrast to about half of the NCOS students; moreover, more OS students resided in big towns and less in villages compared with the NCOS ones. The latter had also a stronger family background regarding military activities and traditions.

When assessing health attitudes of the female soldiers, the current principles of health promotion and specificity of the military environment as a total institution had to be considered. Thus, women who wanted to meet the requirements of military service had to strengthen their health potential by adjusting their health behaviours; the presented data show they managed that task. Among the health behaviours, the engagement of all the subjects studied in motor activities was remarkable compared with the Polish population. The level of physical activity as determined by IPAQ was comparable to that reported by other authors for military communities [6,12,13,17] or for physical education female students [18]. However, some behaviours ought to be modified, like e.g. shaping preventive attitudes, especially among the NCOS students who often neglected them. This tallies with the effects of longitudinal observations in student communities, although female students were superior in that respect to the male ones [14,20]. On the other hand, OS students proved inferior to their NCOS mates with respect to managing stressful situations. Problems in that respect were also reported for university female students in Poland and abroad [5,10,21]. Inasmuch physical education curricula contain a number of health-directed activities introduced in Poland in 2009, no obligatory classes in health education and promotion exist in officer or NC-officer schools for land forces. The presented results are thus pointing to the indispensability of adjusting the existing curricula. Physical education in military schools aims at shaping a high physical fitness but its educational role ought to be expanded and include the health-directed issues to a greater extent.

Army, as a total institution, offers both benefits and drawbacks with regards to the modern health education. Since the lifestyle of subordinates depends largely on the attitudes and behaviour of their superiors, the latter may positively or negatively affect the health behaviours of the subordinates. Since health education is an interactive process, the "order-execution" principle ought to be replaced by partnership to the necessary extent, i.e. the superior should create conditions for making health-directed choices. In conclusion, the modern educational trends in health promotion call for modifying the existing military school curricula by including health education issues so that the superiors acquire not only commanding skills but become also exemplary health educators.

References

1. Biernat E., R.Stupnicki (2005) An overview of internationally applicable questionnaires designed for assessing physical activity. *Phys.Edu.Sport,* 49:32-42.

2. Craig C.L., A.L.Marshall, M.Sjöström, A.E.Bauman, M.L.Booth, B.E.Ainsworth, M.Pratt, U.Ekelund, A.Yngve, J.F.Sallis, P.Oja (2003) International physical activity questionnaire: 12-country reliability and validity. *Med.Sci.Sports Exerc.,* 35(8):1381-1395.

3. Dyrstad S.M., R.Soltvedt, J.Halle (2006) Physical fitness and physical training during Norwegian military service. *Mil.Med.,* 171:736-741.

4. Faff J., P.Satora, K.Stasiak (2002) Changes in the aerobic and anaerobic capacities of army recruits during their military training are related to the initial level of physical fitness of the subjects. *Biol.Sport.,* 19:251-265.

5. Hermon D.A., G.Davis (2004) College student wellness: a comparison between traditional and nontraditional age students. *J.Coll.Counsel.,* 7: 32-39.

6. Kaiser A., M.Sokołowski, (2009). Health and social issues of women in the army. In: M.Sokołowski (ed.) Contemporary tasks, problems and perspectives of physical education in the army, Polish Scientific Physical Education Association Section of Physical Education in the Army, Warsaw, pp. 313-322.

7. Kalina R.M., B.J.Barczyński (2009) Permanent health-related training of regular soldiers – conditions and assumptions. In: M.Sokołowski (ed.) Contemporary tasks, problems and perspectives of physical education in the army. Polish Scientific Physical Education Association Section of Physical Education in the Army, Warsaw, pp. 323-331.

8. Klukowski K., K.Mazurek (2007) Physical performance of women in the light of military service requirements. In: M.Sokołowski (ed.) Biosocial effects of military service as a basis for further improvement of future physical education and sports programmes. Wyd. AWF Poznań, pp. 67-74.

9. Knapik J.J., M.A.Sharp, S.Darakjy, S.B.Jones, K.G. Hauret, B.H.Jones, (2006) Temporal changes in the physical fitness of US Army recruits. *Sports Med.,* 36(7): 613-634.

10. LaFountaine J, M.Neisen, R.Parsons (2006) Wellness factors in first year college students. *American J.Health Stud.,*21 (4): 214-218.

11. Laudańska-Krzemińska I., A.Kaiser (2009) Lifestyle of regular army applicants - a difficult beginning or a good start? In: M.Sokołowski (ed.) Contemporary tasks, problems and perspectives of physical education in the army. Polish Scientific Physical Education Association Section of Physical Education in the Army, Warsaw, pp. 323-331.

12. Lenart D. (2010) Physical activity vs. morpho-functional development of women (english abstract). In: J.Łuczak, S.Bronowicki (eds.) Zdrowotne aspekty aktywności fizycznej Wyd. Wielkopolska Wyższa Szkoła Turystyki i Zarządzania w Poznaniu, Poznań, pp. 245-253.

13. Mierzejewski, R. (2008) Evaluation of the level of the land forces solders' physical activity on the base of the International Physical Activity Questionnaire (IPAQ) (english abstract). In: E.Szczepanowska, M.Sokołowski (eds.) Aktywność fizyczna i odżywianie się jako uwarunkowania promocji zdrowia Wyd. Wielkopolska Wyższa Szkoła Turystyki i Zarządzania w Poznaniu, Poznań, pp. 225-232.

14. Popay J., M.Bartley, I.Plewis (1992) Gender Inequalities in Health: Social Position, Affective Disorders and Minor Physical Morbidity. *Soc.Sci.Med.,* 36 (1): 21-32.

15. Rasińska R., M.D.Głowacka, A.Głowacka-Rębała (2011) Educational determinants in shaping soldiers' health attitudes. In: A.Kaiser, A.Tomczak (eds.), Physical activity and health promotion in the military environment. Polish Scientific Physical Education Association Section of Physical Education in the Army, Warsaw, pp.235-246.

16. Sokołowski M. (2004) Type of body build and motor ability of candidates for professional military sevice. *Ceska Antropologie,* 54:183-184.

17. Sokołowski, M., M.Mrozkowiak, A.Kaiser (2009) International physical activity questionnaire (IPAQ) as a tool to assess the potential regular soldiers. In: M.Sokołowski (ed.) Contemporary tasks, problems and perspectives of physical education in the army. Polish Scientific Physical Education Association Section of Physical Education in the Army, Warsaw, pp. 349-355.

18. Sokołowski M., A.Kaiser, A.Cepulenas (2010) Physical activity of female students of the University School of Physical Education in Poznań on the basis of IPAQ- educational and social perspectives. *Ugdymas Kuno Kultura Sportas*, 3:90-95.

19. Stupnicki R. (2008) Analysis and Presentation of Questionnaire Data. University of Physical Education Editions, Warsaw.

20. Verbrugge L.M. (1985) Gender and Health: An update on hypotheses and evidence. *J.Health Soc.Behav.,* 26 (3):156-182.

21. Von Bothmer M.I., B.Fridlund (2005) Gender differences in health habits and in motivation for healthy lifestyle among Swedish university students. *Nurs.Health.Sci.* 7(2):107-18.

22. www.ipaq.ki.se/downloads.htm.

Changes in physiological and biomechanical variables in women practicing the Power Yoga system

Anna Mróz[1], Krzysztof Buśko[2,3], Bożena Wit

[1] Department of Physiology and [2] Department of Anthropometry, The Jozef Pilsudski University of Physical Education in Warsaw, [3] Institute of Sport, Warsaw, Poland

Summary

Study aim: To investigate changes in selected indices of anaerobic capacity, the ability to maintain body balance and the height of elevating body's centre of mass, and maximum power output in lower limbs during countermovement jump (CMJ) after 6 months of participation in yoga classes in Ashtanga Vinyasa system (Power Yoga).
Material and methods: The study included 24 untrained women who volunteered to participate in a half-year experiment. The analysis focused on 12 women who participated in the classes until the experiment ended. The Wingate test was used to evaluate anaerobic capacity. In order to measure the functional state of vestibular organ the authors used a stabilographic method. Measurements of power output in the lower limbs and the height of elevation of the centre of mass in CMJ jumps were carried out using a dynamometric platform.
Results: The 6 months of training in the Power Yoga system considerably improved the height of CMJ jumps from 0.276 ± 0.048 m to 0.308 ± 0.038 m ($p<0.05$). These changes were not accompanied by significant increases in maximum power output (1286 ± 200 W and 1327 ± 2134 W before and after, respectively; $p>0.05$).
Conclusions: Practicing Power Yoga does not induce changes in the anaerobic capacity and the functional state of the vestibular organ in women.

Key words: Anaerobic capacity – Body balance – Power Yoga – Women

Introduction

There is a growing popularity of different types of recreational activity today. Decisions concerning the choice of a particular form of activity are usually made intuitively, without consideration of actual results for the body. The decision is often driven by current fashion. One of the most fashionable forms of physical activity today is Ashtanga Vinyasa (Power Yoga).

Power Yoga was popularized by American author Beryl Bender Birch [3]. She developed a methodology that allows almost everybody to perform vigorous series of exercise. The exercises in the Power Yoga system are of a more dynamic character compared to classical yoga [9]. They are practiced in attractive, spectacular systems. There are also dynamic transitions between the sequences of exercises performed to the rhythm of respiration. A specific type of respiration is used during the whole Power Yoga training session. It consists of performing a strong, profound inhalation through the nose and a strong extended expiration through the mouth. This method of respiration results in increased respiratory volume, more efficient respiratory cycle, and increased oxygen uptake [19]. Moreover, when performing individual exercises during a training session, the practitioner frequently changes the body position with respect to the ground. The person adopts 'reversed positions', i.e. vertical position with the head down.

The literature abounds in studies that have discussed the effects of practicing different yoga styles. Practicing yoga systems has been shown to improve muscle and joint elasticity, to strengthen muscle strength (with particular focus on static strength) [6,13,18], to cause body mass reduction [15], and to change body composition [2,15]. Yoga training has also been shown to increase aerobic power [1,16,17] and to decrease anaerobic power [1]. However, only the work of Buśko and Rychlik [6] concerned Power Yoga .

The aim of the present study was to investigate the changes in selected indices of anaerobic capacity, ability to maintain body balance and the height of elevation of the centre of mass, and maximum power output of lower limbs in counter movement jump (CMJ) after 6 months of participation in yoga classes in Ashtanga Vinyasa system (Power Yoga).

Author's address Dr Anna Mróz, Department of Physiology, University of Physical Education, Marymoncka 34, 00-968 Warsaw, Poland

Material and Methods

24 untrained women volunteered to participate in a half-year experiment of Power Yoga training, the analysis focused on the results obtained from the 12 women (mean age 24.2 ± 5.8 years) who participated in the classes until the experiment ended. At the beginning of the experiment their body height and body mass were 168.4 ± 6.3 cm and 60.0 ± 6.9 kg, respectively, and did not change significantly after 6 months of training. The Power Yoga classes were scheduled for 1 to 1.5 hours, 3 times a week, for 6 months. Throughout the experiment, the women did not participate in other classes of recreational and physical exercise nature and they had never practiced yoga before. The women were informed about the aim of the experiment and expressed their written consent to participate in the measurements; the study was approved by the Bioethical Commission of Scientific Research at the Institute of Sport in Warsaw, Poland.

The subjects followed a training regime based on the Power Yoga system. The classes were guided by a professional Power Yoga coach. During the classes, the participants performed a standard set of exercises at their own speed, controlled by the number of breaths. A training session was divided into several stages that differed in the body positions adopted for individual *asanas*. In terms of difficulty, the exercise sets were dedicated to beginner yoga practitioners. Mean values of heart rate throughout the duration of the whole training session ranged from 110 to 140 bpm. The following Power Yoga exercises were performed:

Initial Exercises: Two dynamic cycles of exercises with a duration of approximately 12 minutes, performed according to the individual rate of respiration, changing consecutively from one position to another. In each cycle, in one head-down position, the movement was stopped for a period of 5 deep breaths. The whole procedure was repeated 5 times. The aim of this procedure was to warm up the body and to prepare it for the next exercises.

Standing Positions: A series of static stretching exercises aimed at strengthening in particular the muscles of the lower limbs took approximately 15 minutes. In all the exercises, the body weight was supported on the feet. The subjects remained in each position for a period of 5 deep breaths (10 to 20 s). The transitions between the positions occurred by means of dynamic but short movements and jumps. Each exercise, including the elements of entry and exit from the position, began and ended in a basic stance. The character of exercise was static. The intensity of exercise was increased gradually.

Sitting Positions: A series of varied static exercises that took approximately 30 minutes started from a sitting position on the floor with legs stretched, which represented a counterpart to the basic standing position. The subjects remained in each position for a period of 5 deep breaths (10 to 20 s, depending on their respiratory rate). The elements of initial exercises were cyclically repeated between the exercises in order to maintain body warm-up. During a cycle of sitting positions, the exercise intensity was maintained at a relatively constant, thought higher, level compared to standing exercises.

Head-Down Exercises: These exercises were included in a cycle of static positions maintained for a longer time (from 10 to 25 breaths) in order to gently end the exercises. They began with a deep front bend, followed by a shoulder stand, headstand, and a cycle of positions with legs crossed. These exercises took approximately 15 minutes.

Final Exercises: They were the last position of the final sequence. In this position, the subjects lifted their hips up off the ground with legs crossed and remained supported with their hands only. They tried to perform this intensive exercise for as long as possible, performing from 25 to 100 deep breaths. This was the last intensive exercise before final relaxation.

Rest: A deep relaxation ended each session. It consisted in lying on the back. Relaxation time was approximately 10 minutes.

The Wingate test was used for evaluation of anaerobic capacity [20]. It consisted of performing a standard warm-up on a cycle ergometer followed by a 5-minute rest, maximum 30-second exercise with individual load in consideration of body weight of a subject. The load amounted to 7.5% of body weight (BW). Monark 824 E cycle ergometer (Sweden) connected with IBM PC Pentium computer with MCE v. 4.0 ("JBA" Zb. Staniak, Poland). The sensors were fixed on a flywheel that covered the distance of 6 m during one pedal rotation. The subjects, after adjustment of the appropriate height of the saddle and handlebar, performed the sitting tests without standing on pedals, starting the exercise from an immobilized position, with the feet attached to pedals with belts. Standard conditions were met during the exercise and the subjects received verbal encouragement to achieve a maximum pedalling frequency and maintain it as long as possible. MCE v. 4.0 software was used for measuring and computation of: mean power output (P_m), maximum power output (P_{max}), and fatigue index (FI) [7].

Stabilographic method was used for evaluation of the functional state of vestibular organ. The authors used for the purpose a 400×400×55 mm platform with strain gauge sensors that recorded the forces applied on the ground. The subjects stood on the platform and were asked to maintain a stable upright position for the duration of the measurement. The point of pressure of the feet on the ground was recorded as a dynamic parameter that changed its position in time. Posturo software was used for determining the following indices:

– mean radius [mm]: mean value obtained from the sum of consecutive distances from the centre of the system,

– sway area [mm^2]: the sum of triangles formed by 2 consecutive deviations ,

– total length [mm]: total length of the feet pressure point pathway in the test.

The experiment was repeated for 3 times for 30 s each time. The first measurement was performed when a subject stood on the platform with eyes open; the second one was performed with eyes closed and the third with the feedback. In the latter case, the subject stood on the measurement platform in front of a screen located at the distance of 5 m. The central area of the screen displayed a square (0.5×0.5 cm) and the point of pressure of the person studied. The subjects were asked to control the point so that it remained within the square's boundaries (feedback) on the screen.

Measurements of the power output in lower limbs and the height of elevation of the centre of body mass during CMJ were carried out using a dynamometric platform with Kistler amplifier. The amplifier was connected by means of an analogue-digital converter with an IBM PC computer and MVJ v. 1.0 software ("JBA" Zb. Staniak, Poland). The use of a physical model, where the whole body mass of a person who jumped vertically from the dynamometric platform, was reduced to a point to which vertical components of external forces are applied (body's force of gravity and vertical component of platform reaction forces). Based on the recorded ground reaction forces, the authors obtained the following parameters of the jump: maximum power output (P_{max}), mean power output (P_m), maximum height of elevation (h) and lowering (k) of the centre of mass before the jump [5]. Each person performed 2 maximum vertical jumps from a standing position, which was preceded by the body's pre-movement towards the ground (CMJ). The analysis was based on the jump with the greatest value of height of elevation of the centre of body mass.

The paired t-test or repeated measures analysis of variance (ANOVA) followed by Scheffé's test (*post hoc*) were used in data analysis. All the calculations were carried with the use of STATISTICA package (StatSoft, USA); the level of significance was set at α=0.05.

Results

Table 1 presents mean values of indices obtained in the Wingate test. Maximum power output, mean power output, and fatigue index did not change significantly after a 6-month Power Yoga programme. The results obtained during the measurements that encompassed changes in basic stabilographic indices (mean radius, sway area, and total length) did not show statistical difference after the period of 6 months of practicing Power Yoga (Table 2).

Table 1. Mean values (±SD) of the relative mean power output (P_m), relative maximum power output (P_{max}) and fatigue index (FI) obtained before the experiment and after 6-month Power Yoga training (n = 12)

Variable	Before	After
P_m (W/kg)	5.70 ± 0.78	5.75 ± 0.61
P_{max} (W/kg)	6.84 ± 1.04	6.83 ± 0.82
FI (%)	14.00 ± 6.32	13.25 ± 5.58

Table 2. Mean values (±SD) of stabilographic indices in studied women (n = 12) obtained before the experiment and after 6 months of Power Yoga training

Variable	Before	After
Mean radius (mm)		
Eyes Closed	9.83 ± 3.39	9.03 ± 2.73
Eyes Open	9.43 ± 4.42	8.45 ± 2.98
Feedback	4.50 ± 0.97	4.23 ± 0.85
Sway Area (mm^2)		
Eyes Closed	714.6 ± 285.8	691.1 ± 225.3
Eyes Open	874.1 ± 467.3	760.6 ± 253.3
Feedback	574.8 ± 250.1	530.8 ± 348.6
Total Length (mm)		
Eyes Closed	242.0 ± 44.9	254.4 ± 33.8
Eyes Open	315.7 ± 70.2	311.8 ± 58.1
Feedback	386.2 ± 114.7	362.6 ± 117.4

Table 3. Mean values (±SD) of variables characterising countermovement jump performance in studied women (n = 12) obtained before the experiment and after 6 months of Power Yoga training

Variable	Before	After	R (%)
P_{max} (W)	1286.1 ± 200.1	1326.8 ± 213.6	3.4
P_{max}/BM (W/kg)	21.51 ± 4.29	21.96 ± 4.07	2.8
P_m (W)	720.0 ± 153.9	30.9 ± 133.0	3.7
P_m/BM (W/kg)	12.10 ± 3.16	12.12 ± 2.52	3.2
h (m)	0.276 ± 0.048	0.308 ± 0.038*	13.0

Legend: P_{max} – Maximum power output; P_m – Mean power output; BM – Body mass; h – Height of elevation of the centre of body mass; R – percentage change with respect to before value; * Significantly ($p<0.05$) different from respective value recorded before the experiment.

Mean values obtained during counter-movement jumps (CMJ) among the women studied are presented in Table 3. Maximum power output developed in CMJ jumps did not change after the 6-month Power Yoga training (1286 ± 200 W and 1327 ± 2134 W before and after, respectively; $p>0.05$). Significant ($p<0.05$) changes were found only in height of elevation of the centre of body mass, which improved by 13%.

Discussion

The data concerning the effect of yoga exercise on physical capacity are ambiguous. Tran *et al.* [21] found that practicing yoga as the only form of physical activity did not result in changes in the level of physical capacity. Furthermore, Balasubramanian *et al.* [1] demonstrated an increase in maximum oxygen uptake and reduction in anaerobic capacity in a group of students after 6 weeks of yoga training. These authors suggested that participation in yoga classes caused a conversion of fast-twitch tissues into slow-twitch tissues. In our study, no significant changes in anaerobic capacity were found after a 6-month Power Yoga programme. These results are consistent with previous research discussed in a study by Balasubramanian *et al.* [1].

The effect of yoga training on changes in balance has not been widely researched in the literature yet. However, the authors who attempted to measure this effect found beneficial changes. Chen *et al.* [8], after a 4-week participation of women in Silver Yoga classes, demonstrated a significant improvement ($p<0.05$) in balance and mobility range in shoulder joints. The yoga training discussed in the present study did not cause significant changes in basic stabilographic indices. It is difficult to explain this fact since apart from the strength and flexibility components, performing asanas in standing or reversed positions contains a balance-related component. It was expected that the exercises should improve the ability to maintain balance.

There is also some inconsistency in the results obtained for changes in the height of elevation of the centre of body mass and power developed during counter-movement jump (CMJ), drop jump (DJ), and squat jump (SJ) that occurred after different types of training [4,11,14]. In a study by Harris *et al.* [12], strength training did not improve jumping ability measured in CMJ jumps, whereas power training (i.e. training with the load of 30% of maximum isometric force) improved jumping ability in CMJ jumps. Diallo *et al.* [10] demonstrated that 10 weeks of plyometric training caused a significant increase in maximum power output measured for CMJ, DJ, and SJ jumps in footballers. However, no reports are available in the literature concerning changes in the height of elevation of the centre of body mass and maximum power output measured for CMJ, DJ, or SJ after Hatha Yoga training. In our study, Power Yoga training did not affect maximum power output and mean power output during CMJ jumps; the respective improvements being 3.4% and 3.7%. A significant increase of 13.0% was observed for the height of elevation of the centre of body mass. Yoga exercises have a nature of isometric training combined with stretching and dynamic transitions between individual asanas. This is likely to have caused the improvement in jumping ability, which could have increased as a result of enhanced neuromuscular coordination.

Summing up, a 6-month training programme in the Power Yoga system significantly increased the height of elevation of the centre of body mass in CMJ jumps but, no significant changes in maximum power output were found. It also seems that practicing Power Yoga does not affect changes in anaerobic capacity in women and the functional state of the vestibular organ.

References

1. Balasubramanian B., M.S.Pansare (1991) Effect of yoga on aerobic and anaerobic power of muscles. *Indian J.Physiol. Pharmacol.*, 35(4):281-282.

2. Bera T.K., M.V.Rajapurkar (1993) Body composition, cardiovascular endurance and anaerobic power of yogic practitioner. *Indian J.Physiol.Pharmacol.*, 37(3):225-228.

3. Birch B.B. (1995) Power Yoga. Fireside, New York.

4. Bruhn S., N.Kullmann, A.Gollhofer (2004) The effects of a sensorimotor training and a strength training on postural stabilization, maximum isometric contraction and jump performance. *Int.J.Sports Med.*, 25 (1):56-60.

5. Buśko K., Nowak A. (2008) Changes of maximal muscle torque and maximal power output of lower extremities in male judoists during training. *Hum.Mov.*, 9(2):111-115.

6. Buśko K., R.Rychlik (2006) Changes of the maximal muscle torque in women training Power Yoga (Astanga Vinyasa). *Hum.Mov.*, 7(2):168-177.

7. Buśko K., B.Wit, R.Borys (2002) Selected physiological variables during the preparatory period in junior rowers. *Phys. Educ.Sport*, 46 (3):375-385.

8. Chen K.M., W.S.Tseng (2008) Pilot-testing the effects of a newly-developed silver yoga exercise program for female seniors. *J.Nurs.Res.*, 16:37-46.

9. Cowen V.S., T.B.Adams (2007) Heart rate in yoga asana practice: a comparison of styles. *J.Bodywork Mov.Ther.*, 11:91-95.

10. Diallo O., E.Dore, P.Duche, E.Van Praagh (2001) Effects of plyometric training followed by a reduced training programme on physical performance in prepubescent soccer players. *J.Sports Med.Physiol.Fitness*, 41(3):342-348.

11. Fowler N.E., Z.Trzaskoma, A.Wit, L.Iskra, A.Lees (1995) The effectiveness of a pendulum swing for the development of the leg strength and counter-movement jump performance. *J.Sports Sci.*, 13:101-108.

12. Harris G.L., M.H.Stone, H.S.O'Bryant, C.M.Proulch, R.L.Johnson (2000) Short-term performance effects of high power, high force, or combined weight-training methods. *J.Strength Cond.Res.*, 14(1):14-20.

13. Hart C.E., B.L.Tracy (2008) Yoga as steadiness training: effects on motor variability in young adults. *J.Strength Cond.Res.*, 22(5):1659-1669.

14. Kyröläinen H., J.Avela, J.M.McBride, S.Koskinen, J.L.Andersen, S.Sipilä, T.E.Takala, P.V.Komi (2005) Effects of power training on muscle structure and neuromuscular performance. *Scand.J.Med.Sci.Sports*, 15(1):58-64.

15. Madhavi S., P.S.Raju, M.V.Reddy, N.Annapurna, B.K.Sahay, D.G.Kumari, K.J.Murthy (1985) Effect of yogic exercises on lean body mass. *J.Assoc.Physicians India*, 33 (7):465-466.

16. Raju P.S., S.Madhavi, K.V.Prasad, M.V.Reddy, M.E.Reddy, Sahay B.K., K.J.Murthy (1994) Comparison of effects of yoga & physical exercise in athletes. *Indian.J.Med.Res.*, 100:81-86.

17. Raju P.S., K.V.Prasad, R.Y.Venkata, K.J.Murthy, M.V.Reddy (1997) Influence of intensive yoga training on physiological changes in 6 adult women: a case report. *J.Altern.Complement. Med.*, 3(3):291-295.

18. Raub J.A., (2002) Psychophysiologic effects of hatha yoga on musculoskeletal and cardiopulmonary function: a literature review. *J.Altern.Complement. Med.*, 8(6):797-812.

19. Sarang P.S., S.Telles (2006) Oxygen consumption and respiration during and after two yoga relaxation techniques. *Appl. Psychophysiol.Biofeedbeck*, 31:143-153.

20. Skiner A., O.Bar-Or (1996) The Wingate Anaerobic Test. Human Kinetics, USA.

21. Tran M.D., R.G.Holly, J.Lashbrook, E.A.Amsterdam (2001) Effects of hatha yoga practice on the health-related aspects of physical fitness. *Prev.Cardiol.*, 4:165-170.

Generation changes over the period of 1986-2006 in the physical fitness of boys aged 7-19 from eastern Poland at particular stages of education

Jerzy Saczuk, Agnieszka Wasiluk, Mirosław Zalech

The Jozef Pilsudski University of Physical Education in Warsaw, Faculty of Physical Education and Sport in Biala Podlaska, Poland

Summary

Study aim: To assess the size of secular trends in the physical fitness of boys from eastern Poland taking into consideration stages of education.

Material and methods: The physical fitness results of boys aged 7-19 years living in eastern regions of Poland were analyzed: 3188 students were examined in 1986 while in 2006 the research included 10 810 boys. In both examinations (1986 and 2006), the level of motor abilities was measured according to the guidelines of the International Physical Fitness Test. The individual results of children and youth examined in 2006, which took into account calendar age, were converted into points on a T scale, with means and standard deviations from 1986 accepted as norms. On the basis of the obtained point values and taking into account stages of education (7-9 – integrated teaching, 10-12 – primary school, 13-15 – lower-secondary school, 16-18 – upper-secondary school), arithmetic means and dispersion values concerning motor abilities in the groups were calculated. Individual results in motor abilities of every subject were used to define quantitative generation changes. Differences between the means obtained in 1986 and 2006, as well as between the fractions of boys qualified for respective fitness category in both examinations, were assessed.

Results: Over the 2-decade period the boys from eastern Poland slightly improved their results only as far as sit-ups are concerned (1.47 points), while the level of bent arm hang, handgrip, 50 m run, and shuttle run 4×10 m remained the same. In contrast, negative changes were observed in the long run (4.44 points), the sit-and-reach test (4.47 points), and the standing broad jump (3.74 points). The greatest decline in motor abilities was noted amongst schoolchildren from integrated education classes (2.69 points); whereas the smallest decline was noted in adolescents from lower secondary schools (0.60 points).

Conclusions: The changes noted in physical fitness indicate that in the context of health the revision of the Act on Physical Culture from 2002, which reduced the number of school's physical education classes, is a debatable issue.

Key words: Physical fitness – Boys – Generation changes – Eastern Poland

Introduction

At present, the acceleration of the maturation of children and adolescents, as well as the increase in their body height and body mass, has been observed globally [1,3–5, 11,14,20]. It is noteworthy that greater increases are observed in body mass compared to in body height, which affects the increase in the value of the BMI and, consequently leads to an increase in the numbers of girls and boys with overweight and obesity [2,9,23]. So tangible changes have not been observed in the physical fitness of children and adolescents. In Europe and beyond, declines have been reported in the level of selected motor abilities of children and youth, as documented by, inter alia, Malina *et al.* [10], Lewis *et al.* [8], Molinre-Urdiales *et al.* [12], Runhaar et al. [16], and Smopokos *et al.* [21]. These authors have claimed that the rate of generation changes in the basic somatic traits, maturation, and physical activity depended on the socioeconomic status of their country or region and on the living standards of their populations.

A similar tendency for change in the described developmental variables has been observed in Poland. An in-depth analysis of environmental factors made it possible to conclude that the environment itself is subject to transformations at a different rate in different regions of the country. Hence, the time variability of somatic traits and the variable rate of biological maturation in different regions and social environments has been confirmed in studies by Łaska-Mierzejewska and Olszewska [7], Przewęda and Dobosz [15], Saczuk and Wasiluk [19], and others.

Author's address Dr Jerzy Saczuk, Faculty of Physical Education and Sport, Akademicka 2, 21-500 Biała Podlaska, Poland

An overview of literature indicates that the course of changes in the physical fitness of children and adolescents is different in various regions of the country. After the observed positive trends, the earliest decrease in the results of motor tests was noted by authors who made their observations in economically developed regions. In turn, on the basis of the national research, the aforementioned changes were noted only in the last decade of the last century [15]. In view of the above, it would seem interesting to monitor trends and the rate of changes in the level of motor abilities of young inhabitants of regions with the lowest economic indices. Therefore, the objective of this study was to determine values of generation changes in physical fitness of boys from eastern Poland at different stages of their development and to establish the size of the population affected by generation changes in the level of motor abilities.

Material and Methods

In 1986, research was undertaken to assess the physical fitness of 3188 boys inhabiting eastern regions of Poland. In 2006, the same observations were conducted with 10 810 boys in the same regions, within statutory research of the University of Physical Education in Warsaw. The detailed information on the number of boys from different educational stages in particular observation periods is provided in Table 1.

Table 1. The number of boys examined in 1986 and 2006

Stage of education	1986	2006	Total
Integrated education (7-9 years)	513	1261	1774
Primary school (10-12 years)	912	3477	4389
Lower-secondary school (13-15 years)	939	3000	3939
Upper-secondary school (16-19 years)	824	3072	3896
Total	3188	10 810	13 998

In both surveys (1986 and 2006), motor abilities were evaluated according to the guidelines of the International Physical Fitness Test [6] through the following tests: 50 m run, shuttle run 4×10 m (SHR), long run (LOR) at a distance of 600 m (up to 12 years of age) or 1000 m (over 12 years of age), standing broad jump (SBJ), bent arm hang (BAH), sit-ups (SUP), handgrip (HGR), and the sit-and-reach test (SAR). In order to determine generation changes in physical fitness, all individual results of children and adolescents evaluated in 2006 were converted into points on a T scale, with means and standard deviations from 1986 accepted as norms. In these calculations, the calendar age of study participants was taken into consideration. On the basis of the obtained point values, the arithmetic means and dispersion values concerning motor abilities in the groups took into account stages of education (7-9 – integrated education, 10-12 – primary school, 13-15 – lower-secondary school, and 16-19 – upper-secondary school). In turn, individual results in motor abilities of every subject were used to define quantitative generation changes. Taking the values of mean±1SD from 1986 as the norm, the individual physical fitness results of each participant from both observation periods were classified into the following groups:

- group I (below the norm) – boys who achieved results below the standard score (up to 39.99 points);
- group II (norm) – boys who achieved results within the range of standard score (from 40.0 to 60.0 points);
- group III (above the norm) – boys who achieved results above the standard score (over 60.0 points).

The above criteria was established assuming that on the T point scale the mean of reference group accounted for 50 points; standard deviation, for 10 points. The percentage of boys within a given age category for particular motor abilities and for overall fitness were calculated. Differences between the results in each group indicate in how many boys from 2006 the level of the described motor abilities changed as compared to the results of 1986.

The significance of differences between mean values from 1986 and 2006 was verified with the Student's t-test for independent variables. In turn, the significance of differences between the number of boys assessed in 2006 and classified to groups resulting from standard scores of the population evaluated in 1986 was determined with the chi-square test [22]. In all analyses, the level of significance was set at $\alpha = 0.05$.

Results

From 1986 to 2006, the level of physical fitness in boys attending schools in the eastern regions of Poland declined, which can be seen in both the physical fitness results and in the calculations of overall fitness (Fig. 1). The greatest negative changes were found in the students of integrated education. A statistically significant decrease was observed in the long run – by 6.72 points; handgrip – by 4.37 points; sit-and-reach – by 4.10 points; bent arm hang – by 3.70 points; and standing broad jump – by 3.77 points. In contrast, a similar level of results in both study periods analyzed was noted in the 50 m run, the 4×10 m shuttle run, and sit-ups.

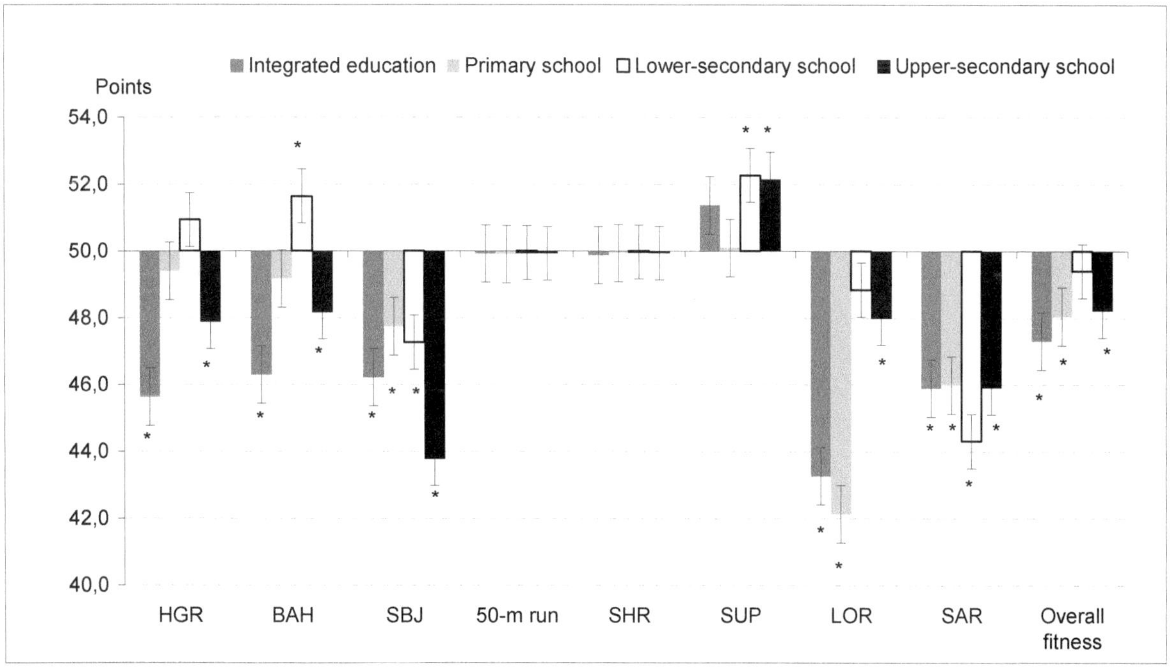

Fig.1. Results of motor abilities of boys examined in 2006, standardized against the results from 1986 (means±SD expressed in T-scale points)

Legend: HGR – Handgrip; BAH – Bent-arm hang; SBJ – Standing broad jump; SHR – 4×10m shuttle run; SUP – Sit-ups; LOR – Long run; SAR – Sit-and-reach; * Significantly ($p<0.05$) different from the results obtained in 1986

Over the 2 decades analyzed in the study, a smaller decrease in the level of physical fitness was observed in the boys from primary schools. Statistically significant differences were noted in long run (7.87 points), sit-and-reach test (4.00 points), and standing broad jump (2.25 points). In the other motor abilities, results from 1986 and 2006 were at similar levels, and the differences observed were not statistically significant. In turn, in the case of boys attending lower-secondary schools in eastern Poland and evaluated in 2006, the level of physical fitness was similar to that of the boys examined in 1986. It should be emphasized that this was not a uniform picture of changes in all motor abilities. The investigated schoolboys achieved better results in sit-ups (2.27 points) and bent arm hang (1.65 point), and worse results in sit-and-reach test (5.68 points) and standing broad jump (2.73 points).

In turn, in the oldest group of boys, results that were higher than in 1986 were only noted in sit-ups (2.16 points) In the case of the 50 m run and the shuttle run 4×10 m, small, insignificant differences were observed between the results. In the case of the other motor abilities, worse results were recorded in: standing broad jump – by 6.22 points; stand-and-test – by 4.09 points; handgrip – by 2.12 points; long run – by 2.00 points; and bent arm hang – by 1.83 points.

Results concerning the overall level of physical fitness make it possible to conclude that in 2006, the number of boys who achieved results above the standard score decreased by 1.8%; the number of boys achieving results within the standard score range, – by 9.2%. In contrast, the number of boys who achieved results lower than the standard score increased by 11.1%. The above differences were statistically significant. The analysis of particular motor abilities demonstrated the most beneficial changes occurred with sit-ups, where the percentage of boys achieving results above the standard score increased by 5.5%; the percentage of boys with results within the standard score decreased by 4.9%; the percentage of boys with results lower than the standard score decreased by 0.6%. In contrast, the greatest negative changes were observed in the sit-and-reach test. In the first 2 groups analyzed, a decrease in the number of boys examined in 2006 by 6.2% and 15.4%, respectively, was noted, whereas the number of boys achieving the worst results increased by 21.6%. In the case of the other motor abilities, analyses demonstrated fewer and not always significant differences (Table 2).

Discussion

Economic development observed in many European countries and around the world contributes to the lifestyle changes of entire societies, since the development of civilization influences human lifestyles. Apart from the positive aspects, it also has a negative impact on the human body. Driving children and adolescents to schools located

Table 2. Difference between fractions of boys examined in 2006 and in 1986, classified according to fitness result

Variable	Below SS (<39.9 pts)	Within SS (40.0-60.0 pts)	Above SS (> 60.0 pts)
HGR	1.83*	-2.42*	0.60
BAH	19.18*	-17.01*	-2.15*
SBJ	16.85*	-15.04*	-1.79*
50-m run	16.32*	-9.44*	-6.87*
SHR	3.52*	-2.73*	-0.77
SUP	-0.55	-4.92*	5.50*
LOR	9.77*	-6.78*	-2.97*
SAR	21.56*	-15.38*	-6.17*
OF	11.06*	-9.21*	-1.83*

Legend: SS – Standard score; HGR – Handgrip; BAH – Bent-arm hang; SBJ – Standing broad jump; SHR – 4×10m shuttle run; SUP – Sit-ups; LOR – Long run; SAR – Sit-and-reach; OF – Overall fitness; * Significant difference ($p<0.05$)

near their residences, allowing young people to devote too much time to watching television and DVDs, or to using computers and other inventions of contemporary technology reduces their physical activity [9,21,24]. Hence, nowadays, a decrease in the level of some motor abilities of both girls and boys is being observed in Poland and other countries [15,18]. Reasons behind the decreasing physical fitness of children and adolescents are being sought in, among other things, reduced physical activity and preferences for more and more sedentary lifestyles. It affects a growing number of children and adolescents with excessive body mass, which in turn is reflected in their physical fitness. It is common knowledge that boys with overweight and obesity achieve worse results in motor ability tests [17]. These processes do not proceed at a constant rate, but are modified by the environment in which the subjects live [13,15]. The problem of the decline in physical fitness observed globally in children and youth has been noted in the areas of eastern Poland as well [17]. The negative generation changes in the level of motor abilities did not proceed with equal intensity in all age categories. In the case of boys attending lower-secondary schools in eastern Poland and examined in 2006, no decrease was noted in physical fitness compared to the results reported 20 years earlier, but only changes in its structure were observed. However, at the other educational stages a significant decline was reported in the test results. It is alarming that the greatest decrease in physical fitness results was observed in boys in the youngest age category. Hence, the introduction of physical education classes led by teachers of integrated education and not by graduates of the University of Physical Education, as is observed in many schools, is disputable.

It is noteworthy that the negative generation changes did not affect all tests of the International Physical Fitness Test. In some motor abilities, the boys examined in 2006 achieved better results than the boys evaluated 20 years earlier (trunk muscle strength), and in the case of some tests the results noted in the 2 examinations were alike (50 m run, shuttle run 4×10 m, and in 2 age categories – handgrip strength). The generation changes in the motor abilities of boys from eastern Poland may reflect their adaptation to the changing environment. Analysis of the overall physical fitness proves that the described differences were observed in 11.1% of the boys. The highest percentage of the boys showed negative changes in sit-and-reach test, whereas the greatest positive changes were observed in trunk muscle strength.

On the basis of the study results, the following conclusions and observations may be formulated: 1) The changes noted in physical fitness indicate that in the context of health the revision of the Act on physical culture from 2002, which reduced the number of a school's physical education classes, is a debatable issue, 2) In the first 3 years of primary school, physical education classes should be taught by graduates of the University of Physical Education and not by integrated knowledge teachers, since the biggest negative changes in motor abilities were observed in this age group, 3) The content of physical education classes at all education levels should be verified in order to increase the level of these motor abilities that underwent the biggest negative generation changes.

References

1. Bizhen W., Y.Jicheng (2005) Secular growth changes in body height and weight in children and adolescents in Shandong, China between1939 and 2000. *Ann.Hum.Biol,.* 5:650-665.

2. Celi F., V.Bini, G.De Gorgi, D.Molinari, F.Faroni, G.Di Stefano, M.L.Bacosi, M.G.Serioli, G.Contessa, A.Falorni (2003) Epidemiology of overweight and obesity among children and adolescents in three provinces of central Italy, 1993-2001: study of potential influencing variables. *Eur.J.Clin.Nutr.* 57:1045-1051.

3. Chodick G., M.Huerta, R.D.Balicer, N.Davidovitch, I.Grotto (2005) Secular trends in age at menarche, smoking, and oral contraceptive use among Israeli girls. *Prev.Chronic Dis.* 2: A12.

4. Jovanović H., Ž.Prebeg, I.Stanić, G.Vuletić (2003) Impact of war on growth patterns in school children in Croatia. *Coll. Antropol.* 2:573-579.

5. Kac G., M.Auxiliadora De Santa Cruz Coelho, G.Velasquez-Melendez (2000) Secular trend in age at menarche for women born between 1920 and 1979 in Rio de Janeiro, Brazil. *Ann.Hum. Biol.,* 4:423-428.

6. Larson L.A. (1966) An international research program for the standardization of physical fitness tests. *J.Sports Med.Phys. Fitness,* 4:259-261.

7. Łaska-Mierzejewska T., E.Olszewska (2007) Anthropological assessment of changes in living conditions of the rural population in Poland in the period 1967-2001. *Ann.Hum.Biol.* 3:362-376.

8. Lewis N., J.Dollman, M.Dale (2007) Trends in physical activity behaviours and attitudes among South Australian youth between 1985 and 2004. *J.Sci.Med.Sport,* 6:418-427.

9. Lobstein T., N.Rugby, R.Leach (2005) Obesity in Europe – 3 International Obesity Task Force March 15, Brussels.

10. Malina R.M., C.Bouchard, O.Bar-Or (2004) Growth, maturation and physical activity. 2 edition. Champaign, IL: Human Kinetics.

11. Marques-Vidal P., G.Madeleine, R.Romain, A.Gabriel, P.Bovet (2008) Secular trends in height and weight among children and adolescents of the Seychelles, 1956-2006. *BMC Public Health.* 8:166-176.

12. Moliner-Urdiales D., J.R.Ruiz, F.B.Ortega, D.Jiménez-Pavón, G.Vicente-Rodriguez, J.P.Rey-López, D.Martínez-Gómez, J.A.Casajús, M.I.Mesana, A.Marcos, M.J.Noriega-Borge, M.Sjöströmb, M.J.Castillo, L.A.Moreno (2010) Secular trends in health-related physical fitness in Spanish adolescents: The AVENA and HELENA Studies. *J.Sci.Med.Sport,* 13:584-588.

13. Nelson M.C., D.Neumark-Stzainer, P.J.Hannan, J.R.Sirard, M.Story (2006) Longitudinal and secular trends in physical activity and sedentary behaviour during adolescence. *Pediatrics.* 6:1627-1634.

14. Padez C., M.A.Rocha (2003) Age at menarche in Coimbra (Portugal) school girls: a note on the secular changes. *Ann.Hum. Biol.* 5:622 632.

15. Przewęda R., J.Dobosz (2005) Growth and physical fitness of Polish youths. University of Physical Education Editions. Warsaw.

16. Runhaar J., D.C.M.Collard, H.C.G.Kemper, W.van Mechelen, M.Chinapaw (2010) Motor fitness in Dutch youth: Differences over a 26-year period (1980-2006). *J.Sci.Med.Sport,* 13:323-328.

17. Saczuk J., D.Olszewska, A.Wasiluk, J.Olszewski (2011) Physical fitness of boys with overweight and obesity living in the eastern provinces of Poland. *Pol.J.Public Health.* 4:350-354.

18. Saczuk J., A.Wasiluk (2009) Secular trend in the physical fitness of rural girls from eastern regions of Poland in respect of generation gaps of their urban peers. In: H. Popławska (ed.) Somatic development, physical fitness and health status of rural children and adolescents. Josef Pilsudski University of Physical Education Faculty of Physical Education, Biala Podlaska. pp. 277-288.

19. Saczuk J., A.Wasiluk (2010) Changes in the somatic and fitness variables in girls over two decades. *Biomed.Hum.Kinet.,* 2:102-105.

20. Silva P. (2005) Menarche and Lifestyle. WMJ. 104:65-69.

21. Smpokos E.A., A.Linardakis, A.Papadaki, Ch.Lionis, A.Kafatos (2012) Secular trends in fitness, moderate-to-vigorous physical activity, and TV-viewing among first grade school children of Crete, Greece between 1992/93 and 2006/07. *J.Sci.Med. Sport,* 15:129-135.

22. Stupnicki R. (2008) Analysis and Presentation of Questionnaire Data. University of Physical Education Editions. Warsaw.

23. Wang Y., C.Monteiro, B.M.Popkin (2002) Trends of obesity and underweight in older children and adolescents in the United States, Brazil, China, and Russia. *Am.J.Clin.Nutr.,* 75:971-977.

24. Żak S., J.Szopa (2001) Effects of diversified motor activity on the level of motor fitness in children and youth from Cracow (Poland). *J.Hum.Kinet.* 6:47-58.

Seasonal variation of American Indian children's school-day physical activity

Timothy A. Brusseau[1], Pamela H. Kulinna[2], Tiffany Kloeppel[3], Matthew Ferry[4]

[1] University of Utah, [2] Arizona State University, [3] Montclair State University, [4] George Mason University, USA

Summary

Study aim: To examine the pedometer steps taken during the school-day by American Indian children during all four seasons.

Material and methods: Participants included third-sixth grade children (n = 157) aged 9.6±1.07 (boys) and 9.7±1.2 (girls) attending school from one Southwestern US American Indian community. Children had a mean BMI of 23.9±7.7 with 70% being classified as overweight or obese. Children wore a pedometer (Yamax Digiwalker SW-200) for 20 days (5 days per season).

Results: Children accumulated 4762±1544 (boys) and 4408±1194 (girls) steps/day across the four seasons with the highest totals occurring during the Fall (4899, males; 4796, females) and the lowest totals during the Winter (4463, males; 4043, females). Repeated measures ANOVA showed no significant differences in daily school-day steps across seasons. Children classified as normal weight averaged 5146±1688 steps/day, overweight children averaged 5020±1333 steps/day, and obese children accumulated 4275±1123 steps/day.

Conclusions: PA stayed relatively consistent across seasons in this sample of children. However, children were the least active during Winter months. With 70% of the current sample being classified as overweight and with American Indian children at greater risk for numerous hypokinetic diseases there is a clear need for additional school-day PA opportunities.

Key words: Indigenous populations – Pedometer – Step Counts – Youth – Health

Introduction

Schools have been identified as an essential component of physical activity (PA) promotion in youth [33] and have been called upon to take on more leadership in this endeavor [31]. Most children regularly attend school [21] and with this understanding, many researchers have developed and implemented PA interventions and/or programming while youth are at school [13,39]. PA surveillance has been identified as an important component of global action against physical inactivity; if physical activity is important it must be measured [23]. When evaluating school-based intervention programs it is essential to have baseline or expected PA values for youth while at school.

Studies have begun to describe typical school-day PA in youth [1,22,27] and the contributions of the school-day to overall daily PA levels [3,6,7,11,30,42]. Children appear to accumulate between 2900-7600 steps/day at school accounting for 35-47% of their total daily steps. Table 1 shows school-day steps and daily contributions of school-day PA to overall PA from previous pedometer research. Additionally, two accelerometer based studies have suggested that children accumulate 30-44% of their total daily activity throughout the school-day [16,18].

Numerous researchers have suggested that it is important to understand the role that seasons play on youth PA as temperature and weather patterns can influence PA levels [2,8,17,19,25,35,45]. Furthermore, it has been suggested that a better understanding of seasonal differences may help prioritize intervention programs or school resources to meet the needs of the low active students [3]. Previous examinations of seasonal impact on youth PA have primarily found that children are more active when the weather is warmer and allows for outdoor activity and have mostly examined total daily physical activity [2,4,19,25,35,45]. Most recently, research findings suggested that seasons (Fall and Winter) played a role in out of school PA but had no impact on school-day PA [3]. Only one previous study has examined seasonal impact on school-day PA [3] and included PA during the Fall and Winter months in Southeastern US elementary aged children. With most children attending school and a growing number of school-based PA interventions, it is imperative for the researchers and practitioners developing the interventions/ programming to have a more complete understanding of seasonal influences on school-day PA to ensure appropriate allocation of resources during the low activity seasons.

Author's address Dr. Timothy A Brusseau, Department of Exercise and Sport Science, University of Utah, 250 S 1850 E Rm 205; Salt Lake City, UT USA 84112

Table 1. School day step counts and contributions to overall daily physical activity (PA)

Autor	Male Steps	Female Steps	Contribution to Daily PA	Location	Season	Sample (n)
Loucaides and Jago [27]	6979	5078	N/A	Cyprus	Winter	5-6th Grade (104)
Cox *et al.* [11]	7594	6070	47%	New Zealand	Spring	5-11 Years (91)
Barfield *et al.* [1]	4464	3796	N/A	USA	N/A	2nd-5th Grade (71)
Brusseau *et al.* [6]	4779	4027	35-38%	USA-American Indian Community	Fall	5-6th Grade (77)
Johnson *et al.* [22]	4237	4042	N/A	USA-American Indian Community	N/A	8-12 Years (176)
Beighle *et al.* [3]	3925 3816	2976 2956	35-38% 40-42%	USA-Southeast	Fall Winter	3rd-5th Grade (112)
Brusseau *et al.* [7]	5042	4124	36-37%	USA-Southwest	Fall	4-5th Grade (829)
Morgan *et al.* [30]	3800	2900	40%	USA-Southwest	N/A	8-11 Years (389)
Tudor-Locke *et al.* [42]	6832	4895	40%	USA-Southwest	Spring	6th Grade (81)

This information is of upmost importance for American Indian youth who are at a greater risk for hypokinetic diseases and obesity when compared to other US youth [5,24,36,40,47]. For example, a recent study found that 67% of American Indian children were classified as overweight or obese [6]. Therefore the purpose of this study was to examine the pedometer steps taken by American Indian children during all four seasons; Summer, Fall, Winter, and Spring throughout the school-day.

Material and Methods

Participants: Participants included 157 American Indian children (77 males and 80 females) in grades 3-6 at one elementary school in a Southwestern US American Indian Community. The only requirement for inclusion was that children had to be ambulatory. Children were aged 9.64±1.1 (9.6±1.07 boys; 9.7±1.2 girls) years and had a BMI of 23.9±7.7 with 70% being classified [32] as overweight (>85% BMI) or obese (>95% BMI) and 96% of parents reported that their children were of American Indian descent. University Review Board, Tribal Council, school principals, and teachers approved the research design. Parental consent and informed assent were provided by all participants.

Instruments: The Yamax Digiwalker SW-200 pedometer (Yamax, Tokyo, Japan) was used to measure PA. This pedometer has been validated for measuring PA in pediatric populations [20,29,38]. Prior to data collection, batteries were changed and both shake tests [46] and step tests [44] were completed to ensure the instrument accurately measured steps. Anthropometrics were measured without shoes and with light clothing on a calibrated digital scale (Seca 882 Digital BMI Scale; Hanover, MD) and stadiometer (Seca 214 Portable Stadiometer; Hanover, MD). BMI was calculated using the formula kg/m^2. A demographic form completed by parents provided the child's grade, gender, and ethnic background.

Procedures: All children had previous experience wearing a pedometer before participating in this study. Prior to data collection, students were reminded how the pedometer worked, the appropriate location to wear (on the waist above the right knee) the monitor, and all children completed a step test to ensure accuracy. The students wore their pedometer from Monday to Friday during school hours for four separate weeks (aligning with the four seasons). Research team members and classroom teachers reminded the youth to put their pedometer on each morning when they arrived at school. At the end of each school day, research team members and the classroom teacher reminded youth to leave their pedometers on their desks. When students left school for the day, research team members recorded step counts for each student and reset the pedometer to "zero." This process was repeated for each of the 20 days of data collection. This protocol is consistent with previous studies using pedometers [3,22].

Data were collected four times during the school year to align with the four traditional seasons (August, November, February and April). Table 2 illustrates the weather differences across the four data points.

Table 2. Average temperature and precipitation during each season in the Southwest US

Season	Temperature (°F)		Precipitation
	High	Low	(Inches)
Summer (August)	104	76	1.14
Fall (November)	75	47	0.77
Winter (February)	71	41	1.03
Spring (April)	85	54	0.33

Data Treatment and Analysis: Following established procedures [34] a minimum of two days of data were required to be included in analyses. A valid day was defined as a day where the children wore the pedometer the entire school-day. Means for steps/day were computed for each season as well as an overall steps/day average. Repeated Measures ANOVA was utilized to compare differences across seasons. *T*-tests and ANOVA's (followed by Bonferroni tests) were used to examine differences across gender and BMI; the level of significance was set at $\alpha = 0.05$

Results

Repeated measures ANOVA showed no significant differences ($p = 0.07$) in daily school-day steps across seasons, across seasons by gender ($p = 0.44$), or across seasons by BMI category ($p = 0.54$), suggesting that seasonal differences were similar. Figures 1 and 2 shows the steps/day across each season by gender and by BMI category, respectively.

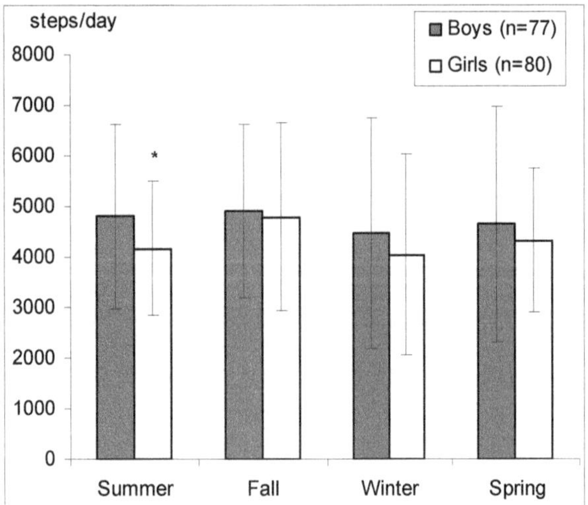

Fig. 1. Steps/day by season and gender (mean±SD)

* Significantly ($p<0.05$) different from respective value in boys

Children accumulated 4762±1544 (boys) and 4408±1194 (girls) steps/day across the four seasons with t-test results indicating that boys and girls took a statistically similar number of in-school steps ($p = 0.11$). Individual t-tests indicated that the only season that boys were significantly more active than girls was during the Summer ($p<0.05$).

Children classified [32] as normal weight averaged 5146±1688 steps/day, overweight children averaged 5020±1333 steps/day, and obese children accumulated 4275±1123 steps/day. Normal weight children accumulated the greatest steps/day in the Summer and Spring. Overweight children were the most active during the Fall and Winter. ANOVA results ($F_{2,128} = 6.19$; $p<0.01$) suggested significant differences in daily steps by BMI. Bonferroni *post hoc* tests indicated that the significant differences ($p<0.01$) were between the normal and obese groups. Individual season ANOVA's by BMI indicated that there were only differences during the Summer (Normal and Obese; $p<0.01$) and Fall (Overweight and Obese; $p<0.05$).

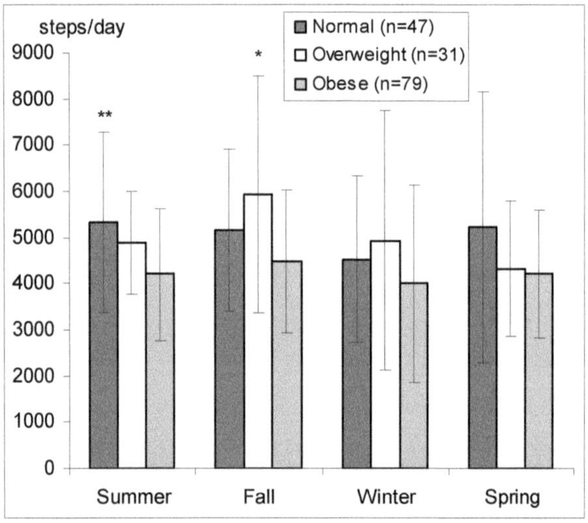

Fig. 2. Steps/day by season and BMI category (mean±SD)

Significantly different from respective value in obese children: *$p<0.05$; $p<0.01$

Discussion

This is the first known study designed to examine the seasonal differences in school day PA (across all 4 seasons). This study supports previous findings [3] suggesting that school-day PA (Fall and Winter) is not influenced by the seasons. These findings, however, are not supported by studies examining total daily activity throughout the different seasons [4,14,17,19,25,35,45]. Although not significant, children did accumulate their greatest step totals during the Fall (4899, males; 4796, females) and their lowest totals during the Winter (4463, males; 4043, females), suggesting a 9% and 16% decrease in steps/day for boys and girls, respectively in the Winter. Beighle *et al.* [3] found that activity performed outside of school-day dropped significantly during the Winter months, making school-day PA even more essential. The current finding is especially interesting because temperatures during the Fall and Winter seasons were not drastically different (Table 2), precipitation is typically a non-issue, and both would be considered mild when compared to other regions of the country/world.

Children in the current study had physical education twice per week (30 minutes each) and had a daily lunch-time recess that typically led to about 15-20 minutes of free play opportunities. By simply adding an extra 15 minute recess during the Winter months (or during any season), previous research suggests there would be opportunities for an extra 900-1250 steps/school-day [7]. Similarly, research examining the impact of classroom based PA has suggested that activity breaks can add over 900 steps/day [15]. It would appear that by adding a second recess opportunity and classroom activity breaks, there is potential to add an additional 1800-2100 steps/day.

The daily step averages in the current sample are consistent (or greater) with most other US school day studies [3,12] and these students were also generally more active than other American Indian children [6,22]. The current sample, however, lags behind (Δ=-1200-1800 steps/day, boys; Δ=-600-1600 steps/day, girls) international studies of children's school-day PA levels [11,27]. By adding an extra recess and classroom based physical activity breaks, it seems reasonable that the current sample of children could accumulate similar steps to the international children throughout the school-day. Importantly, research has suggested that the short-term cognitive benefits of physical activity during the school-day adequately compensates for time spent away from other academic areas [41].

Approximately 50% of the current sample was classified as obese. These children accumulated nearly 1000 less steps/day during the school-day compared to non-obese children during the warmer seasons (Summer/Spring). When the weather cooled down (Fall/Winter), however, the differences dropped to only 300-400 steps/day. Similarly, overweight children were less active than normal weight children during the Summer and Spring and more active during the Fall and Winter. These findings suggest that overweight and obese children may be less inclined to participate in PA when the temperatures are warmer. Perhaps, if possible, allowing these children to choose indoor and/or temperature controlled activities may encourage greater participation in PA.

A recent study examined the efficacy of four interventions to increase both school and total day PA [26]. The schools targeted PA through structured recess, classroom activity breaks, and daily physical education, and found that school designed programming was able to increase school day step counts from 900-1700 steps when the teachers and administrators committed to increasing PA opportunities.

Although, seasonal differences appear to be minimal when children are in school, there is a continued need to develop programming and PA opportunities at school. Studies have begun to accumulate demonstrating the positive relationship that school PA can have on behavior, attentiveness, and performance at school [9,10,37]. For example, teachers from the Southwest US reported that physical activity in the classroom gave students something to be excited about, and students who didn't always participate in class activities enjoyed it. Furthermore, many teachers saw a distinct increase in attentiveness after physical activity, and used it to wake students up or take a break to refresh the students for more reading and math [10].

There are some notable limitations to this study. First, the study was conducted with only one group of children living in an American Indian community. Similar work with a more diverse sample of children is warranted for more generalizable findings. This study was also conducted in the Southwest US and in a desert community. Temperatures were regularly over 100°F in the Summer and almost never dropped below freezing in the Winter. A sample with more traditional seasons may be more representative of US children. For example, August is often considered a high outdoor activity month in much of the country and in this community the warmest month of the year (temperatures regularly over 100°F, therefore, perhaps limiting PA opportunities. Lastly, spring levered pedometers, although the most widely used pedometer in the pediatric literature [43] have been shown to underestimate steps in overweight and obese adults [12], something that is important to consider when 70% of the current sample are classified as overweight or obese (perhaps future studies could use piezoelectric pedometers of accelerometers to confirm findings).

In conclusion, PA stayed relatively consistent across seasons in this sample of American Indian children. However, children were the least active during Winter months and this sample had fewer steps than children living internationally accumulated within the school-day. With 70% of the current sample being classified as overweight and at a greater risk for numerous hypokinetic diseases, there is a clear need for additional school day physical activity opportunities.

References

1. Barfield J.P., D.A.Rowe, T.Michael (2004) Interinstrument consistency of the Yamax Digi-Walker in elementary school children. *Meas.Physl.Educ.Exer.Sci.* 8:109-116.
2. Beighle A., B.Alderman, C.F.Morgan, G.LeMasurier (2008) Seasonality in children's pedometer measured physical activity levels. *Res.Q.Exer.Sport.* 79:256–260.
3. Beighle A., H.Erwin, C.F.Morgan, B.Alderman (2012) Children's in-school and out-of-school physical activity during two seasons. *Res.Q.Exerc.Sport.* 83:103-107.

4. Belanger M., K.Gray-Donald, J.O'Laughlin, G.Paradis, J.Hanley (2009) Influences of weather conditions and seasons on physical activity in adolescents. *Ann.Epi.* 19:180-186.

5. Broussard B.A., A.Johnson, J.H.Himes, et al. (1991) Prevalence of obesity in Native American Indians and Alaska Natives. *Am.J.Clin.Nutr.* 53:1535S-1542S.

6. Brusseau T.A., P.H.Kulinna, C.Tudor-Locke, M.Ferry (2012) Daily physical activity patterns of children living in an American Indian community [published online ahead of print]. *J.Phys.Act.Health.*

7. Brusseau T.A., P.H.Kulinna, C.Tudor-Locke, M.Ferry, H.van der Mars, P.W.Darst (2011) Pedometer determined segmented physical activity patterns of fourth- and fifth- grade children. *J.Phys.Act.Health.* 8:279-286.

8. Carson V., J.C.Spence, N.Cutumisu, N.Boule, J.Edwards (2010) Seasonal variation in physical activity among preschool children in a northern Canadian city. *Res.Q.Exerc.Sport.* 81: 392-399.

9. Centers for Disease Control and Prevention. The association between school-based physical activity, including physical education, and academic performance. http://www.cdc.gov/healthyyouth/health_and_academics/pdf/pa-pe_paper.pdf. Accessed October, 15, 2012.

10. Cothran D.J., P.H.Kullina, A.Garn (2010) Classroom teachers and physical activity integration. *Teach.Teach.Educ.* 26:1381-1388.

11. Cox M., G.Schofield, N.Greasley, G.S.Kolt (2006) Pedometer steps in primary school aged children: A comparison of school-based and out-of-school activity. *J.Sci.Med.Sport.* 9:91–97.

12. Crouter S.E., P.L.Schneider, D.R.Bassett (2005) Spring-levered vs. piezo-electic pedometer accuracy in overweight and obese adults. *Med.Sci.Sports.Exerc.* 37:1673-1679.

13. Demetriou Y., O.Honer (2012) Physical activity interventions in the school setting: A systematic review. *Psych.Sport.Exerc.* 13:186-196.

14. Duncan J.S., W.G.Hopkins, G.Schofield, E.Duncan (2008) Effects of weather on pedometer-determined physical activity in children. *Med.Sci.Sport.Exerc.* 40:1432-1438.

15. Erwin, H.E., A.Beighle, C.F.Morgan, M.P.Nolan (2011) Effect of a low-cost, teacher-directed classroom intervention on elementary students' physical activity. *J.Sch.Health.* 81:455-461.

16. Fairclough S.J., A.Beighle, H.Erwin, N.D.Ridgers (2012) School day segmented physical activity patterns of high and low active children [epub ahead of print). *BMC.Pub.Health.*

17. Fisher A., J.J.Reilly, C.Montgomery, L.Kelly, A.Williamson, D.M.Jackson, J.Y.Paton, S.Grant (2005) Seasonality in physical activity and sedentary behavior in young children. *Ped.Exerc. Sci.*17:31–40.

18. Gidlow C.J., T.Cochrane, R.Davey, H.Smith (2008) In-school and out-of-school physical activity in primary and secondary school children. *J.Sport.Sci.* 26:1411–1419.

19. Goran M.I., T.R.Nagy, B.A.Gower, et al. (1998) Influence of sex, seasonality, ethnicity, and geographic location on the components of total energy expenditure in young children: Implications for energy requirements. *Am.J.Clin.Nut.* 68:675-682.

20. Hart T.L., T.A.Brusseau, P.H.Kulinna, J.J.McClain, C.Tudor-Locke (2010) Evaluation of low-cost, objective instruments for assessing physical activity in 10-11-year old children. *Res.Q. Exerc.Sport.* 82:600-609.

21. Hofferth S.L., J.F.Sandberg (2001) How American children spend their time. *J.Mar.Fam.* 63:295–308.

22. Johnson T.G., P.H.Kulinna, P.W.Darst, R.P.Pangrazi (2007) School day physical activity patterns of Pima children in two communities. *Res.Q.Exerc.Sport.* 78:364-368.

23. Kohl H.W., C.L.Craig, E.V.Lambert, S.Inoue, J.R.Alkandari, G.Leetongin, S.Kahlmeier (2012) The pandemic of physical inactivity: Global action for public health. *LANCET.* 380:194-305.

24. Kriska A.M., A.Saremi, R.L.Hanson (2003) Physical activity, obesity, and the incidence of type 2 diabetes in a high-risk population. *Am.J.Epidemiol.* 158:669-675.

25. Kristensen P.L., L.Korsholm, N.C.Moller, N.Wedderkopp, L.B.Anderson, K.Froberg (2007) Sources of variation in habitual physical activity of children and adolescents: The European youth heart study. *Scan.J.Med.Sci.Sport.* 18:298-308.

26. Kulinna P.H., T.A.Brusseau, D.J.Cothran, C.Tudor-Locke (2012) Changing school physical activity: An examination of individually school designed programs. *J.Teach.Phys.Edu.* 31: 113-130.

27. Loucaides C.A., R.Jago (2006). Correlates of pedometer-assessed physical activity in Cypriot elementary school children. *J.Phys.Act.Health.* 3:267-276.

28. Mattocks C., S.Leary, A.Ness, K.Deere, J.Saunders, J.Kirkby, S.N.Blair, K.Tilling, C.Riddoch (2007) Intraindividual variation of objectively measured physical activity in children. *Med.Sci. Sport.Exerc.* 39:622-629.

29. McKee D.P., C.A.G.Boreham, M.H.Murphy, A.M.Nevill (2005) Validation of the Digiwalker pedometer for measuring physical activity in young children. *Ped.Exerc.Sci.* 17:345-352.

30. Morgan C.F., R.P.Pangrazi, A.Beighle (2003) Using pedometers to promote physical activity in physical education. *JOPERD.* 74:33–38.

31. National Association for Sport and Physical Education. (2008) Comprehensive school physical activity programs (Position statement). Author, Reston, VA. http://www.aahperd.org/naspe/standards/upload/Comprehensive-School-Physical-Activity-Programs2-2008.pdf. Accessed October, 15, 2012.

32. Ogden C.L., R.J.Kuczmarski, K.M.Flegal, Z.Mei, S.Guo, R.Wei, L.M.Grummer-Strawn, L.R.Curtin, A.F.Roche, C.L.Johnson (2002) Centers for Disease Control and Prevention 2000 growth charts for the United States: improvements to the 1977 National Center for Health Statistics version. *Pediatics,* 190:45-60.

33. Pate R.R., M.G.Davis, T.N.Robinson, E.J.Stone, T.L.McKenzie, J.C.Young (2006) Promoting physical activity in children and youth: A leadership role for schools: A scientific statement from the American Heart Association Council on Nutrition, Physical Activity, and Metabolism (Physical Activity Committee) in collaboration with the Councils on Cardiovascular Disease in the Young and Cardiovascular Nursing. *Circulation.* 114:1214–1224.

34. Rowe D.A., M.T.Mahar, T.D.Raedeke, J.Lore (2004) Measuring physical activity in children with pedometers: Reliability, reactivity, and replacement of missing data. *Pediatr.Exerc. Sci.*16:343-354.

35. Rowlands A.V., D.R.Hughes (2006) Variability of physical activity patterns by type of day and season in 8–10-year old boys. *Res.Q.Exerc.Sport,* 77:391–395.

36. Salbe A.D., C.Weyer, R.S.Lindsay, P.A.Tatranni (2002) Assessing risk factors for obesity between childhood and adolescence: II. Energy metabolism and physical activity. *Pediatics,* 110:299-306.

37. Sallis J.F., T.L.McKenzie, B.Kolody, M.Lewis, S.Marshall, P.Rosengard (1999) Effects of health-related physical education on academic achievement: Project SPARK. *Res.Q.Exerc.Sport,* 70:127-134.

38. Schneider P.L., S.E.Crouter, O.Lukajic, D.R.Bassett (2003) Accuracy and reliability of 10 pedometers for measuring steps over a 400-m walk. *Med.Sci.Sport.Exerc.* 35:1779–1784.

39. Strong W.B., R.M.Malina, C.J.Blimkie, S.R.Daniels, R.K.Dishman, B.Gutin, A.C.Hergenroeder, A.Must, P.A.Nixon, J.M.Pivarnik, T.Rowland, S.Trost, F.Trudeau (2005) Evidence based physical activity for school-age youth. *J.Pediatr.* 146: 732–737.

40. Styne D.M. (2010) Childhood obesity in American Indians. *J.Pub.Health.Man.Prac*. 16:381-387.
41. Taras H (2005) Physical activity and student performance at school. *J.Sch.Health*. 75:214-218.
42. Tudor-Locke C., S.M.Lee, C.F.Morgan, A.Beighle, R.P.Pangrazi (2006) Children's pedometer determined physical activity patterns during the segmented school day. *Med.Sci.Sport.Exerc.* 38:1732–1738.
43. Tudor-Locke C., J.J.McClain, T.L.Hart, S.B.Sisson, T.L. Washington (2009) Expected values for pedometer-determined physical activity in youth. *Res.Q.Exerc.Sport*. 80:164-174.
44. Tudor-Locke C., J.E.Williams, J.P.Reis, D.Pluto (2002) Utility of pedometers for assessing physical activity: Convergent validity. *Sport.Med* 32:795-808.
45. Uitenbroak, D.G (1993) Seasonal variation in leisure time physical activity. *Med.Sci.Sport.Exerc.* 25:755-760.
46. Vincent S.D., C.L.Sidman (2003) Determining measurement error in digital pedometers. *Meas.Phys.Educ.Exerc.Sci.* 7:19-24.
47. Zephier E., J.H.Himes, M.Story (1999) Prevalence of overweight and obesity in American Indian school children and adolescents in the Aberdeen area: A population study. *Int.J.Obesity.* 23:28-32.

Nutritional habits of female university students in relation to self-perception of body

Edyta Suliga [1], Iwona Wronka [2], Romana Pawlińska-Chmara [3]

[1] Institute of Public Health, Jan Kochanowski University, Kielce, [2] Department of Anthropology, Institute of Zoology, Jagiellonian University, Krakow, [3] Department of Biotechnology and Molecular Biology, Opole University, Opole, Poland

Summary

Study aim: To determine whether the self-assessment of body mass has an impact on the nutritional behaviour of young women.
Material and methods: The material was gathered in cross-sectional research of 1129 female university students. The measurements of body height, body mass, and waist and hip circumference were taken. Each person completed a questionnaire concerned the nutritional habits, recreational physical activity, and self-perception of body mass. In this work, only the data of 925 students with BMI between 18.5 and 24.9 were included.
Results: Of the participants, 2.8% of the students assessed their body mass as too low, 75.4% as correct, and 21.8% as too high. Students assessing their body mass as too low featured the lowest values of BMI and waist circumference, whereas those with a body mass assessment of too high featured the highest values of BMI. Those students with a body mass assessment as too high followed a diet and skipped meals far more frequently, consumed breads and sweets far less frequently, and drank more liquids daily than students who assessed their body mass as correct. No differences were found in the frequency of recreational physical activity in relation to self-perception of body mass.
Conclusions: BMI values above population average, even if they fit within the norm, are regarded by the students as too high. The self-assessment of body mass as too high results in undertaking efforts aimed at reducing body mass.

Key words: Body mass perception – BMI – Nutritional habits – Physical activity

Introduction

In Poland, as in many other European countries, the prevalence of obesity and overweight, as well as average relative body mass, is on the increase [4,5,9,18,20]. Simultaneously, the mass media has created a contrasting image that promotes slimmer and slimmer models and actresses, thus creating an even wider gap between an ideal and an average figure [1,19]. Many women compare their body mass not to standards recommended by professionals but to norms set by celebrities. That leads to overestimation and stimulates the pursuit for a slimmer figure.

Among young people, in particular young females, the concern over one's own image is ever so evident. In Western culture, appearance makes a very significant image factor. No wonder, then, that so many young women conform to the demands of fashion. However, diets that are often designed along homemade recipes with no professional supervision may have adverse effects on the health for those who, while being neither overweight nor obese, are determined to lose weight anyway. Many studies show that the phenomenon of groundless dieting is on the increase among people with non-excessive body mass [6,11,13]. It has been proven that the decision of whether or not to go on a diet is frequently based not on actual body mass but rather on a perception of it being excessive [1,11,13]. Misperception of overweight constitutes one of the important factors affecting unhealthy behavior and thereby health in general. The aim of this study was to determine whether the self-assessment of body mass has an impact on the nutritional behavior of young women.

Material and Methods

The material for this study has been gathered in cross-sectional research of female students at Jagiellonian University in Cracow, Jan Kochanowski University in Kielce, and the University of Opole. In total, 1129 students took part in the research. In this work, the data of 925 students with correct body mass (BMI = 18.5-24.9 kg/m^2) were included. This constitutes 81.9% of the total. Measurements of body height, body mass, waist (WC) and hip circumference (HC) were taken and two

Author's address Prof. Edyta Suliga, Institute of Public Health, Jan Kochanowski University, Al. IX Wieków Kielc 19, 25-317 Kielce, Poland.

indices, i.e. Body Mass Index (BMI) and waist-to-hip ratio (WHR), were calculated

Each person completed a questionnaire. The questions posed in the questionnaire concerned the frequency of main meals (breakfast, lunch, dinner, and supper) and specified food consumption. In addition, the information concerning leisure-time physical activity and smoking was collected. In the final part of the questionnaire, the students were asked whether they considered their body mass as too low, correct or too high, and whether they would like to change their body mass.

The Shapiro-Wilk test was applied to determine normality of the distribution of variables; the Levene's test was used to asses homogeneity of variances. To evaluate the differences in terms of anthropometrical parameters between groups of a varied body mass self-assessment, the Kruskal-Wallis test followed by multiple comparisons of mean ranks for all groups was used. The selection of a non-parametric test resulted from the lack of homogeneity of variances between sub-groups. The significance of differences in the meal frequency, frequency of eating specified foods, and physical activity in leisure-time were estimated by using of the chi-square test. The level of $\alpha = 0.05$ was considered significant.

Results

A total of 26 (2.8%) students assessed their body mass as too low, 697 (75.4%) assessed it as correct, and 202 (21.8%) assessed it as too high. Table 1 presents anthropometrical data (mean ± SD) according to student assessment of body mass. The self-perception of body mass is actually linked with real body mass, waist and hip circumference, Body Mass Index (BMI), and waist-to-hip ratio (WHR). Students assessing their body mass as too low featured the lowest values of the analyzed parameters, whereas those with the body mass assessment as too high featured the highest values of the analyzed parameters. It is worth noting, though, that the average BMI and the waist circumference values in the group of students who overestimated their body weight were nowhere near the limits defining overweight, i.e. 25 kg/m^2 for BMI and 80 cm for waist circumference (Table 1).

Of the students who perceived their body mass as too high, 78.80% declared their wish to have lower body mass. Within a group that assessed their body mass as correct, this wish was expressed by only 10.9% of women, whereas a mere 1.3% want to have higher body mass. In the group of students who regarded their body mass as too low, not one person expressed the desire to have lower body mass, whereas 88.5% of them want to have higher body mass.

Further analysis investigated whether the perception of body mass had an influence on lifestyle. A comparison was made between two groups, namely between the students with correct body mass assessment and those who assessed their body mass as too high. Due to an insignificant number of students assessing their body mass as too low, the group was not included in the analysis.

Within the group that assessed their body mass as too high, the percentage of those on a weight-reducing or vegetarian diet equaled 23.8%, whereas among other students it equaled 8.3%. The difference was statistically significant ($p<0.001$). frequencies of daily main meal consumption are presented in Table 2. Students assessing their body mass as too high much less frequently declared that they have breakfast, lunch and supper every day and much more frequently declared they seldom have those meals than students who assessed their body mass as correct (Table 2). In the case of supper, the difference was particularly evident. Almost double the number of students who assessed their body mass as too high declared to rarely have this meal.

Table 1. Anthropometrics characteristic of surveyed female students (mean ± SD)

Variable	Group 1 (n = 26)	Group 2 (n = 697)	Group 3 (n = 202)
Body height (cm)	163.1 ± 6.97	166.1 ± 5.82	163.6 ± 5.72
Body mass (kg)	52.4 ± 4.37	57.3 ± 5.32***	60.9 ± 5.73*** ###
Body Mass Index	19.5 ± 0.77	20.8 ± 1.23***	22.1 ± 1.50*** ###
Waist circumference (cm)	65.7 ± 5.26	70.4 ± 5.45***	73.4 ± 6.95*** ###
Hip circumference (cm)	90.0 ± 1.82	93.3 ± 5.03***	96.7 ± 6.79*** ###
Waist to hip ratio	0.73 ± 0.06	0.76 ± 0.06	0.77 ± 0.08*

Legend: Group 1 - Students who perceive their body mass as too low; Group 2 - Students who perceive their body mass as correct; Group 3 - Students who perceive their body mass as too high; Significantly different from group 1: *p<0.05; ***p<0.001; ### Significantly (p<0.001) different from group 2:

Table 2. The frequency (%) of consuming the main meals of a day among surveyed female students

Meal	Group 2 (n = 697)	Group 3 (n = 202)
Breakfast		
Every day	75.0	66.3*
2-6 time/week	13.9	19.3*
Rarely	11.0	14.4*
Lunch		
Every day	53.4	43.6***
2-6 time/week	30.0	39.1***
Rarely	8.2	17.3***
Supper		
Every day	62.1	44.1***
2-6 time/week	25.2	34.2***
Rarely	12.6	21.8***
Snack		
Every day	57.4	50.5
2-6 time/week	21.1	21.1
Rarely	21.5	21.5

Legend: Group 2 - Students who perceive their body mass as correct; Group 3 - Students who perceive their body mass as too high Significantly different from group 1: *p<0.05; ***p<0.001.

Table 3. The frequency (%) of consuming specified foods among surveyed female students

Products	Group 2 (n = 697)	Group 3 (n = 202)
White bread		
Every day	49.6	35.2***
2-6 time/week	20.1	26.7***
Rarely	30.3	38.1***
Whole grain bread		
Every day	29.1	20.3*
2-6 time/week	29.3	33.2*
Rarely	41.6	46.5*
Sweets		
Every day	15.9	6.4***
2-6 time/week	38.4	33.7***
Rarely	45.6	59.9***
Fruits		
Every day	35.4	40.1
2-6 time/week	42.5	36.1
Rarely	22.1	23.7
Vegetables		
Every day	26.8	28.7
2-6 time/week	44.6	44.1
Rarely	28.6	27.2

For explanations of symbols see Table 2

Table 3 presents the consumption frequencies of selected food products such as those commonly considered as "fattening," i.e. breads, sweets and soft drinks, and those recommended as weight-reducing, i.e. fruit, vegetables, and mineral water. The students who assessed their body mass as too high less frequently consumed breads, white bread in particular, and sweets. No differences were found regarding the frequencies of fruit and vegetable consumption (Table 3).

Students who overestimated their body mass drank higher amounts of liquids daily than those with the body mass assessed as correct (8.4 vs. 5.9 glasses; p<0.001). In the group that assessed their body mass as too high, a higher intake of water was observed (2.5 vs. 1.6 glasses; p<0.05), though with a lower intake of sweet and soft drinks (0.4 vs. 0.7; p<0.05). Among students who perceive their body mass as correct 24.1% declared participation in recreational activity twice a week, 39.0% – once a week and 36.9% rarely or never. Among students who perceive their body mass as too high the respective percentages were 23.8, 40.1 and 36.1%; the differences being non-significant. Moreover, no significant between-group differences were found with respect to declared smoking, on average about 17% of studied subjects declared that they smoke.

Discussion

From this analysis, it emerged that the students made the assessment of how correct their body mass is by comparing themselves to the media-promoted "ideal figure" rather than to the WHO recommendations. BMI values above the population average, even if they fit within the norm, were regarded by surveyed students as too high. According to data published in subject literature, the incorrect self-assessment of body weight is commonplace among women [6,14]. Research carried out among university students in seven European countries, i.e. Bulgaria, Denmark, Spain, Lithuania, Germany, Poland and Turkey, shows that 20% of women with BMI equal to 20 kg/m^2 describe their own figure as "a bit too fat" or "too fat"; among women with BMI equal to 22.5 kg/m^2, it soars to 60% [14]. This problem is also noticeable in younger age groups [8].

The relationship between the self-perception of body weight and nutritional behavior and recreational physical activity has been the subject of numerous analyses [1,10,12,17]. For overweight people, the underestimation of their body mass does not provide a positive impulse for taking up actions aimed at reducing it. Whereas for people with correct body mass, the overestimation may prompt the decision to go on a diet, oftentimes an incorrect one or one that some doctors describe as "extreme." It may cause nutritional deficiency and consequently electrolytic disorders, heart problems, sleep disorders, depression, lower self-esteem, delayed growth and puberty, and disturbed menstruation [3,7,15]. Long-term dieting may result in the development of eating disorders such as anorexia and bulimia [13].

In the surveyed group, a relationship between nutritional habits and the self-assessment of body mass has been determined. The perception of body mass as too high prompts undertaking activities aimed at reducing it, namely reducing the number of meals (mainly evening meals), reducing the intake of products regarded as fattening (breads, sweets), and increasing the amount of water drunk daily. This suggests that students who assess their body mass as too high undertake efforts towards losing weight following dieting guidelines found over the Internet. They simply try to eat less by limiting the number of meals daily, although with no attention paid to the quality of the diet. For example, the consumption of fruit and vegetables in the group is much lower than the recommended daily intake. Similar results were obtained in other studies out of which a disturbing fact has emerged: that when it comes to the control of body mass very often irrational actions (skipping meals, eliminating certain foodstuffs, and restrictive diets) win over rational actions (undertaking physical activity, balancing meal contents) [1,2, 10,12,16,17]. Moreover, such behavior is frequently caused not by necessarily possessing excessive body mass in reality but by perceiving themselves as overweight.

Summing up, the obtained results indicate that misperception of weight status is common in young women. BMI values above population average, even if they fit within the norm, are regarded by the students as too high. Because self-perception of body mass is a key determinant of weight management and nutritional habits, many female students who are not overweight but who perceive themselves as such are likely to undertake efforts aimed at reducing body weight. This may lead to an increase in the prevalence of underweight. What is more, overestimation of body weight is associated with unhealthy eating behavior. These findings highlight the importance of appropriate dietary counseling and education in order to understand medical definitions of overweight for young women. There needs to be tailored strategies focused on preventing both extremes of BMI: overweight and underweight.

References

1. Anton S.D., M.G. Perri, J.R.Riley (2000) Discrepancy between actual and ideal body images: Impact on eating and exercise behaviors. *Eat.Behav.*, 1:153-160.

2. Boschi V., M.Siervo, P.D'Orsi, N.Margiotta, E.Trapanese, F.Basile, G.Nasti, A.Papa, O.Bellini, C.Falconi (2003) Body composition, eating behaviour, food-body concerns and eating disorders in adolescent girls. *Ann.Nutr.Metab.*, 47: 284-293.

3. Boutelle K., D.Neumark-Sztainer, M.Story, M.Resnick (2002) Weight control behaviors among obese. overweight and non overweight adolescents. *J.Pediatr.Psychol.*, 27:531-540.

4. Chrzanowska M., A.Suder (2010) The extent of overweight index in children and adolescents from Cracow. Poland (1971-2000). *Homo,* 61:453-458.

5. Chrzanowska. M., S.Kozieł, S.J.Ulijaszek (2007) Changes in BMI and the prevalence of overweight and obesity in children and adolescents in Cracow. Poland. 1997–2000. *Econ.Hum.Biol.*, 5: 370–378

6. Currie C., O.Samdal, W.Boyce, B.Smith (2001) Health behaviour in school-aged children: a World Health Organization Cross-National Study. Research protocol for the 2001.02 survey. University of Edinburgh. Edinburgh.

7. Daee A., P.Robinson. M.Lawson. J.A.Turpin. B.Gregory. J.D.Tobias (2002) Psychologic and physiologic effects of dieting in adolescence. *South.Med.J.*, 95:1032-1041.

8. DeLee M.L., T.L.Hughes, J.A.Miller, A.Hipwell, L.A.Theodore L.A (2009) Prevalence of eating disturbance and body image dissatisfaction in young girls: an examination of the variance across racial and socioeconomic groups. *Psychol.Sch.*, 46:767–775.

9. Finucane M.M., G.A.Stevens, M.Cowan, G.Danaei, J.Lin, Ch.J.Paciorek, G.M.Singh, H.R.Gutierrez, Y.Lu, A.N.Bahalim, F.Farzadfar, L.M.Riley, M.Ezzati (2011) National. regional. and global trends in body-mass index since 1980: systematic analysis of health examination surveys and epidemiological studies with 960 country-years and 9-1 million participants. *Lancet,* 377:557-567.

10. Kapka-Skrzypczak L., B.Bergier, J.Diatczyk, J.Niedźwiecka, P.Biliński, A.Wojtyła (2012) Dietary habits and body image perception among Polish adolescents and young adults – a population based study. *Ann.Agric.Environ.Med.*, 19:299-308.

11. Kurdak H., N.Bozdemir, E.Saatci, P.Ozturk, S.Ozcan, E.Akpinar (2010) Self-perceived body weight status and weight-control behaviors of high school students in a Southern City of Turkey. *Coll.Antropol.*, 34:1295–1302.

12. Lowry R., D.A.Galuska, J.E.Fulton, H.Wechsler, L.Kann, J.L.Collins (2000) Physical activity. food choice. and weight management goals and practices among US college students. *Am.J.Prev.Med.*, 18:18–27.

13. Makino M., M.Hashizume, M.Yasushi, K.Tsuboi, L.Dennerstein (2006) Factors associated with abnormal eating attitudes among female college students in Japan. *Arch.Womens Ment. Health*, 9:203–208.

14. Mikolajczyk R.T., A.E.Maxwell, W.El Ansari, Ch.Stock, J.Petkeviciene, F.Guillen-Grima (2010) Relationship between perceived body weight and body mass index based on self- reported height and weight among university students: a cross-sectional study in seven European countries. *BMC Pub.Health* 10:1-11.

15. Oksuz E. (2008) Unhealthy body perception among Turkish youths: socioeconomic status and social comparisons. *Coll. Antropol.*, 32:5–13.

16. Putterman E., W.Linden (2004) Appearance versus health: Does the reason for dieting affect dieting behavior? *J.Behav. Med.*, 27:185–204.

17. Rahman M., A.B. Berenson (2010) Self-perception of weight and its association with weight-related behaviors in young, reproductive-aged women. *Obstetrics Gynecol.*, 116:1275-1280.

18. Saczuk J., A. Wasiluk (2010) Changes in the somatic and fitness variables in girls over two decades. *Biom.Hum.Kinetics,* 2:102–105.

19. Seifert T. (2005) Anthropomorphic characteristics of centerfold models: Trends towards slender figures over time. *Int. J.Eat.Disord.*, 37:271–274.
20. Żądzińska E., I.Rosset, S.Kozieł, T.Nawarycz, B.Borowska-Strugińska, W.Lorkiewicz, L.Ostrowska-Nawarycz, A.Sitek (2012) Frequency of under- and overweight among children and adolescents during the economic transition in Poland. *Homo*, 63:216–232.

Effects of vertical, horizontal, and combination depth jump training on long jump performance

Dalwinder Singh [1], Sukhwinder Singh [2]

[1] Department of Physical Education, Panjab University, Chandigarh, [2] University College, Dhilwan, Barnala, India

Summary

Study aim: To assess the effects of vertical, horizontal, and combination depth jump training programs on the performance of the running long jump by male athletes.
Material and methods: A total of 80 physical education students ranging in age between 18-21 years with mean depth jump performance of 44.3 ± 5.13 cm from a 45 cm high box were purposively selected to act as subjects. The subjects were randomly assigned to vertical depth jump training (VD), horizontal depth jump training (HD), the combination of both (CD), and a control group (CG). Each week, experimental groups performed 6 sets (10 repetitions per set) twice a week for 10 weeks of depth jump training from a height of 20 cm, which progressed to 40 cm according to the step method. Running long jump (RLJ) was measured before and after 10 weeks. Analysis of covariance, with pre-test scores as a covariate, was applied to compare scores. A pairwise comparison was done by using the Scheffe's *post-hoc* test.
Results: The average increase of RLJ performance in groups VD (0.17 m) and CD (0.23 m) was significantly different ($p<0.05$) than in group CG (0.05 m). Improvement in group HD (0.12 m) was not significantly different than in group CG; moreover, no significant difference existed between training groups.
Conclusions: A combination of both vertical and horizontal depth jumping is required for long jumpers, with a higher proportion of vertical depth jumping.

Key words: Plyometrics – Step Progression – Depth jumping – Long Jump

Introduction

Depth jump training is the common and most-researched forms of plyometric drills. Depth jumping requires athletes to drop from a height and, upon landing, immediately perform a jumping movement [23]. Depth jumps use the athlete's body weight and gravity to exert force against the ground [8]. An elevated surface is required for this exercise. The landing surface should be forgiving yet resilient; grass gymnastic flooring or cushioned turf will work well. The depth jump is a shock method exercise and comes in the final portion of the training continuum. Therefore, progression into this drill is a must, as well as progression within it. Implement the shock method by using an elevated platform and a drop or fall to the takeoff surface. The key is to initiate a rhythm of landing. The landing is the precise phase we are negotiating in order to create a performance that is as efficient as possible. This requires handling the surprise of landing and subsequent takeoff in as optimal an execution as possible. This aspect makes the depth jump elite in its strength, speed, and quickness. It also can be a source of problems if you do not progress into it properly [19].

In practical terms, the task of determining the proper depth jump height centers on the ability to achieve maximal elevation of the body's center of gravity after performing a depth jump. If the height is too great for the strength of the legs, then the legs spend too much time absorbing the impact of the landing and cannot reverse the eccentric loading quickly enough to take advantage of the serial elastic component of muscle and the stretch reflex phenomenon. The result is a slow jump dependent on strength and devoid of power. Coach and athlete should work on finding the proper height: one that lets the athlete maximize the height jumped plus achieves the shortest amortization phase [8]. Countermovement vertical jump height has been used as a test protocol to measure successful depth jump performance. An athlete is made to carry out a standing high jump after flexing his legs and the maximum height is reached with his hand on a graduated board (Vertical Jump Test). The highest reading of 3 jumps is registered. The athlete is made to carry out the same operation, landing on the same point from a height that is progressively higher by 20-40-60 centimeters and from each different height of fall. The subsequent jump is read off of the graduated board. The value of the greater

Author's address Prof. Dalwinder Singh, Department of Physical Education, Panjab University, Sector 14, Chandigarh, U.T. - 160014, India

height reached in the subsequent jump (after landing), which should be higher than that of the jump from level '0' (standing jump), determines the optimum height of fall for that particular athlete at that moment of the training process [26].

By using boxes of different heights or a stair-step apparatus, the athlete drops from levels between 12 and 42 centimeters onto grass or a firm but resilient mat. Upon landing, the athlete immediately jumps upward, reaching or surpassing the mark placed on the wall during the Vertical Jump Test. The athlete continues to move to a higher drop until he or she can no longer attain the same height as in the vertical jump. Allow 1 or 2 minutes of rest between each trial for the muscle systems to recover. The point of the depth or drop height when the athlete attained maximum vertical (rebound) height is the approximate height to train for in this type of plyometric exercise [19]. There are 2 major categories of depth jumping for the purpose of achieving maximum vertical height or horizontal distance after taking off. One type of exercise is performed by stepping off the box and dropping to land on both feet. Try to anticipate the landing and spring up as quickly as possible. Keep the body from "settling" on the landing and make the ground contact as brief as possible. The second category is performed by stepping off the box and dropping to land on both feet. Upon landing, immediately jump as far forward as possible, again landing on both feet [8]. The idea behind plyometrics is simple: exploit the muscles' cycle of lengthening and shortening to increase power [7]. The mechanisms thought to contribute to greater power output during a drop jump are the stretch reflex [14], storage and use of elastic energy [4,13], and potentiation of the contractile machinery [2]. Power is an essential component for successful performance in many sports. Power represents the amount of work a muscle can produce per unit of time. An increase in power gives the athlete the possibility of improved performance in sports in which the improvement of the speed-strength relationship is sought [15]. The principle stimulus in power training is performing a movement dynamically linked with the force magnitude that is taking place in the same exertion. For instance, during sprinting an athlete's force of leg propulsion is 3.5 times that of his or her body weight, but the force used to throw a javelin is much smaller. Thus, the force of acceleration is the main stimulus for power training. In acyclic sports (i.e., jumping events), power is the determinant ability for achieving a good result. On the other hand, in cyclic sports (i.e., sprinting), power is brought into action repetitively and rapidly. Consider these general characteristics of sports requiring power, and then reflect them in a strength training program [3].

Effectiveness of depth jump training in improving acyclic power [6,16,22] and cyclic power [25] is well-known fact. The present study researched its effects on running long jump performance (combination of both cyclic and acyclic activities). The long jump is a contest that determines how far a competitor can jump horizontally after a running start [21]. Therefore, the purpose of this study was to investigate the influence of vertical depth jump training, horizontal depth jump training, and the combination of both vertical and horizontal depth jump training on running long jump performance of college level male athletes by employing depth jumping from optimal dropping height.

Material and Methods

Subjects: Purposive sampling technique was used to select 80 male physical education students ranging in age between 18 to 21 years. Their mean age, body height, and body mass was 19.9±0.8 years, 172.6±4.4 cm and 66.1±2.6 kg, respectively. They were medically fit to undergo the type of training program and completed an informed consent form prior to participate in the present study. They were tested for proper execution of depth jump performance (mean 44.3±5.1 cm) from dropping height of 45 cm. The university's joint research board approved all procedures for the study.

Study protocol: Studied subjects were randomly assigned to 3 experimental groups and 1 control group. Group VD (n=20) trained with vertical depth jumping on Monday and Thursday; group HD (n=20) trained with horizontal depth jumping on Tuesday and Friday; group CD (n=20) trained with vertical depth jumping on Wednesday and horizontal depth jumping on Saturday throughout 10 weeks of training having identical intensities and volumes. Group CG (n=20) served as the control group. All subjects were attending classes according to the college curriculum, except the training session. Running long jump performance was measured for subjects of each group before and after the 10-week period. Participants were part of an instruction session before the pre-test to ensure proper technique and comprehension of the testing process. Testing was demonstrated by the trained athlete. To ensure uniformity in the testing conditions, the subjects were tested in the morning sessions by the same testers, under the supervision of the investigator.

Procedures: A pilot study was conducted to determine the training intensity and progression of load. The investigator randomly selected 10 out of the 80 participants. They were tested for vertical jump performance and depth jump performance from heights of 10, 20, 30, 40, 50, and 60 centimeters. Investigators found the initial increase in attained height with maximum performance (i.e., 48.64 cm) from 20 cm dropping height and depth jump performance remained greater than vertical jump test performance (i.e. 46.25 cm) up to 40 cm dropping height (Fig. 1).

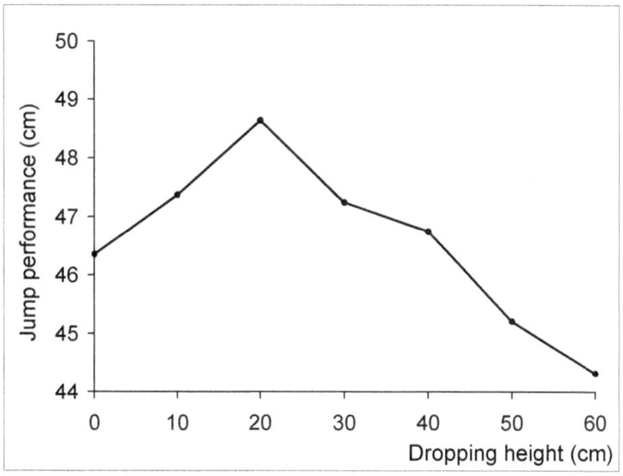

Fig. 1. The mean vertical and depth jump performance in pilot study

Dropping height of 20 cm, from which depth jump performance was maximum and higher than vertical jump performance, was the initial training intensity [8,19,26]. All participants were trained twice a week for 10 weeks, performing 6 sets of 10 repetitions per session [10]. A period of 15 seconds of rest-walk was given for recovery between repetitions [20]; 1.5-2 minutes of slow jogging for 220 m was given for recovery between sets [24]. Dropping height progressed according to the step method from the height with maximum depth jump performance (20 cm) up to the height from which performance was remained higher than vertical jump performance (40 cm) during the 10-week period of training (Table 1).

Table 1. Progression of dropping height (DH) during experiment

Week	I	II	III	IV	V	VI	VII	VIII	IX	X
DH (cm)	20	25	30	25	30	35	30	35	40	35

Training was administered by dividing 20 participants into 4 groups, with 5 subjects per group. After warm up, they were trained simultaneously at 4 stations. Rest-walk between repetitions was given by placing a cone 11 m and 12.1 m ahead of the dropping height for vertical and horizontal depth jump training, respectively. Slow jog between sets was given by placing another cone 220 m from first cone. Subjects participated in cool-down program after training.

To measure running long jump performance, a takeoff area of 2.16 m length (it was the average standing broad jump performance of 10 subjects tested for this purpose) was marked by spreading lime on the surface of the runway from the jumping pit, to identify the takeoff mark. The subject was asked to perform a long jump after a sprint start by taking off from the takeoff area to jump as far as possible. The distance between the landing spot near the takeoff area and takeoff mark in the takeoff area was measured. Three trials were given and performance was recorded to the nearest 0.01 m below the distance measured, if the distance measured was not a whole centimeter. Best performance was considered as the score.

Data analysis: Analysis of covariance was applied to find significance of differences among groups. The pretest scores were used as the covariate and post-test scores, adjusted for covariance, were the dependent measures. When significant F value was encountered, a pair-wise comparison was done by using the Scheffe's post-hoc test to identify significant differences between groups. The level of significance was set at $\alpha = 0.05$.

Results

The mean and standard deviation values for running long jump performance obtained from pre-test and posttest scores of 3 experimental groups (VD, HD, and CD) and control group (CG) are presented in Figure 2.

Analysis of covariance with pre-test scores as a covariate showed significant differences ($F_{3,75}$ =82.43; $p<0.001$) in running long jump performance of all the 4 groups. Post-hoc analysis revealed a significant ($p<0.05$) difference between groups VD and CG (mean difference equal to 0.17 m); CD and CG (mean difference equal to 0.24 m). The differences between groups HD and CG, as well as between all training groups were not significant.

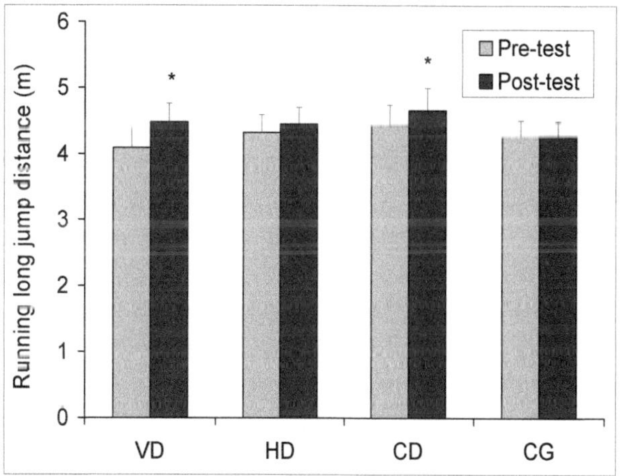

Fig. 2. The mean and standard deviation values for running long jump performance obtained in studied groups during pre- and post-test

Legend: VD – Vertical depth jumping; HD – Horizontal depth jumping; CD – Combination of vertical depth jumping and horizontal depth jumping; CG – Control group. * Significantly ($p<0.05$) different from CG

Discussion

After the 10-week period designated for the vertical, horizontal, and combination depth jump training programs, the running long jump performance of 3 experimental groups and the control group showed significant difference. Further, the analysis of data reveals that experimental groups VD and CD were found to be significantly different as compared to the control group, but the paired adjusted final mean for running long jump performance of experimental group HD was not found to be significantly different as compared to the control group. These findings do not find any support from existing literature as reviewed by the investigators; further research may be conducted in this direction. These running long jump performance findings revealed that vertical depth jump training and the combination of vertical and horizontal depth jump training were effective in bringing about a significant training effect. These findings may be attributed to the physiological adaptations such as reduction of the amortization phase, greater cross sectional recruitment, and threshold elevation for the inverse stretch reflex [18]. It is further supported by the fact that plyometric training stimulates chemical, mechanical, and neurological factors that influence the force and stiffness of the contracting muscle [12].

Horizontal depth jump training alone is not effective in bringing about a significant training effect. Thus, it is important to conclude that long jump performance depends upon the ability to raise the body vertically at the time of takeoff after gaining horizontal momentum during the approach run. This finding may be attributed to the results that indicate a negative correlation between jump length and contact time with the takeoff board during the long jump takeoff. In good performances, the center of gravity began to rise immediately after the first touch of the board, while in poorer jumps it remained at about the same height during the early contact phase [5,11]. There appears to be one main possibility for failure of this research to support horizontal depth jumps: the subjects who engaged in the present study were professional physical education students, thus they could have been adapted to the horizontal jumping exercises due to their previous horizontal jump training experience. Thus, horizontal depth jump training did not create the load effect required to produce an extra stimulus. It is already reported that depth jumps did not produce jump increases beyond that of a jumping routine that was a normal part of practice [9].

An increase in running long jump performance of 0.17, 0.12, 0.23, and 0.05 meters was observed in groups VD, HD, CD and CG, respectively; the respective post-training percentage increments being 4, 2.8, and 5.2%. Thus, the trends are in favor of the group CD, it is in line with the suggestion that jumping involves both horizontal and vertical components. It seems to make sense that both horizontal and vertical jump training would contribute to the improvement of jumping performance [8]. A comparison of groups VD and HD showed trends in favor of group VD: it indicates that vertical depth jump training is more effective for improving long jump performance as compared to horizontal depth jump training. It is also worth mentioning that training associated effects on running long jump performance obtained between the paired adjusted final means of 3 experimental groups were not statistically significant. From this prospective of the present study, it does not support in any 1 of the 3 treatments of applied depth jumps as a more effective one.

Dropping height progression of depth jumps applied within the training procedures of previous studies has been varied within wide margins [1,10,17]. It has not been quantified according to the capabilities of subjects under consideration. So another main finding of this study represents the training-associated improvement in long jump performance in experimental groups CD and VD is the application of step method of progression based on the data obtained through vertical and depth jump tests (Fig. 1). But further research is needed in the field to fix optimum step duration, increase in dropping height, and duration of experiment for depth jump training. For determination of these variables of step method we considered general training principles of strength training [3]. These may be considered as limitations of the present study.

Summing up, the combination of both vertical and horizontal depth jumping is required for long jumpers, with a greater proportion of vertical depth jumping. But vertical depth jump training is more effective for improving long jump performance as compared to horizontal depth jump training. Thus, while planning a depth jump training program for long jumpers, coaches and physical educators should include more vertical depth jumping along with horizontal depth jumping.

References

1. Andrew D.P.S. (1999) The effectiveness of three modified Plyometric depth jumps and a periodized weight training program on selected functional tests for power of the lower extremity. University of South Alabama; pp.68.

2. Bobbert M.F., P.A.Huijing, G.J.Van Ingen Schenau (1987) Drop jumping I. The influence of jumping technique on the biomechanics of jumping. *Med.Sci.Sports Exerc.*, 19:332-338.

3. Bompa T.O. (1999) Periodization: Theory and Methodology of Training. Champaign, IL, USA: Human kinetics.

4. Bosco C., P.V.Komi (1979) Mechanical characteristics and fiber composition of human leg extensor muscles. *Eur.J.Appl. Physiol.*, 41:275-284.

5. Bosco C., P.Luhtanen, P.V.Komi (1976) Kinetics of the take-off in long jump. In: Komi P. (ed) Biomechanics VIB. Baltimore, MD: University Park Press, pp. 174-180.

6. Brown M.E., J.L.Mayhew, L.W.Boleach (1986) Effect of plyometric training on vertical jump performance in high school basketball players. *J.Sports Med.Phys.Fitness,* 26:1-4.

7. Chu D.A. (1989) Plyometric exercises with the medicine ball. California: Bittersweet Publishing Company.

8. Chu D.A. (1998) Jumping into plyometrics. Champaign, IL: Human Kinetics.

9. Clutch D., M.Wilton, C.McGown, G.R.Bryce (1983) The effects of depth jumps and weight training on leg strength and vertical jumps. *Res.Q.Eexerc.Sport,* 54:5-10.

10. De Villarreal E.S., J.J.González-Badillo, M.Izquierdo (2008) Low and moderate plyometric training frequency produces greater jumping and sprinting gains compared with high frequency. *J.Strength Cond.Res.,* 22:715-725.

11. Klissouras V., P.Karpovich (1967) Electrogoniometric study of jumping events. *Res.Q.,* 38:41-48.

12. Komi P.V., C.Bosco (1978) Utilization of stored elastic energy in leg extensor muscles by men and women. *Med.Sci.Sports,* 10:261-265.

13. Komi P.V., A.Gollhofer (1997) Stretch reflex can have an important role in force enhancement during stretch-shorten exercise. *J.Appl.Biomech.,* 13:451-460.

14. Komi P.V (1973) Measurement of the force-velocity relationship in human muscle under concentric and eccentric contractions. In: Joki E. (ed), Medicine and Sports. Basel, Switzerland:S. Karger AC, pp. 224-229.

15. Luebbers P.E., J.A.Potteiger, M.W.Hulver, J.P.Thyfault, M.J.Carper, R.H.Lockwood (2003) Effects of plyometric training and recovery on vertical jump performance and anaerobic power. *J.Strength Cond.Res.,* 17:704-709.

16. Matavulj D., M.Kukolj, D.Ugarkovic, J.Tihanyi, S.Jaric (2001) Effects of plyometric training on jumping performance in junior basketball players. *J.Sports Med.Phys.Fitness,* 41:159-164.

17. McClenton, L.S., L.E.Brown, .J.W.Coburn, R.D.Kersey (2008) The effect of short-term VertiMax vs. depth jump training on vertical jump performance. *J.Strength Cond.Res.,* 22:321-325.

18. Pettitt R. (1999) The role of plyometrics in the scope of a periodized training model. *J.Perf.Enhan.,* 1:11-20.

19. Radcliffe J.C., R.C.Farentinos (1999) High-powered Plyometrics. Human kinetics. Champaign, IL.

20. Read M.M., C.Cisar (2001) The influence of varied rest interval lengths on depth jump performance. *J.Strength Cond.Res.,* 15:279-283.

21. Srivastava A.K. (2007) Teach Yourself Long Jump. New delhi-2: Sports Publication.

22. Steben R., A.Steben (1981) The validity of the stretch-shortening cycle in selected jumping events. *J.Sports Med.,* 21: 28-37.

23. Verkhoshansky Y. (1969) Are depth jumps useful? *Yessis Rev.Soviet Phys.Educ.Sports,* 3:75-78.

24. Verkhoshansky Y. (1968) Perspectives in the improvement of speed-strength preparation of jumpers. *Yessis Rev.Soviet Phys. Educ.Sports,* 4:28-34.

25. Young W.B., R.James., I.Montgomery (2002) Is muscle power related to Running Speed with changes of direction? *J. Sports Med.Phys.Fitness,* 42:282-288.

26. Zanon S. (1974) Plieometry in jumping, *Die Lehre der Leichtathletik,* 16:1-13.

Body posture of young female basketball players

Małgorzata Grabara

Department of Recreation, Jerzy Kukuczka Academy of Physical Education, Katowice, Poland

Summary

Study aim: To assess body posture and somatic parameters in young females practicing basketball in comparison with their non-training peers and to state whether there is a relationship between the quality of one's posture and the length and frequency of training.

Material and methods: The study included 32 young female basketball players aged 13-15 years old. The period of basketball practice was 3-4 years for the group aged 13-14 years; the frequency of practice was 3-7 times per week. In the case of the group of 15-year-olds, it was 4-5 years, 4-7 times a week, respectively. The control group consisted of 37 young female subjects in the same age brackets that did not participate in any directed physical activity. Body height was measured with the use of a height meter at medical scales, whereas body mass, fat mass, and total body water mass were defined with the use of Tanita electronic scale. A specialist device using the projection Moiré method (MORA, CQElektronik System, Poland) was used to assess one's body posture.

Results: Body height and water mass were significantly different in the younger group. However, the parameters of body posture differed significantly only in the group of 15-year-olds. The following have been observed: much greater asymmetries in pelvic placement in the transverse plane ($p<0.05$), significantly greater asymmetries of shoulder blades in relation to the transverse plane ($p<0.01$), as well as significantly smaller thoracic kyphosis angle ($p<0.05$) in female basketball players in comparison with the placement of the above parameters in their non-training peers. Moreover, correlations between the frequency of basketball practice and the deflection of the line of spinous processes, torso inclination angle, placement of shoulder blades in the transverse plane and towards the spine, kyphosis angle, and a synthetic index of body posture (i.e. postural symmetry) were noted.

Conclusions: Training basketball may lead to increased occurrence of asymmetry of one's body posture.

Key words: Body posture – Asymmetries – Moiré technique – Young female athletes – Basketball

Introduction

Sport among children and adolescents is a very important stimulator for their development, both motor and physical. A good deal of studies emphasizes the positive influence of physical activity among children and adolescents in all aspects of health [7,12,15,16,19]. Participation in regular sports practice molds the character of a young person, improves one's motor and coordination capabilities, and significantly affects one's physical development and body posture.

Often, however, asymmetrical physical exercise unique to a particular sport may result in the occurrence of abnormal curvatures of the spine, particularly in the period of intensive growth. Some studies show that in many sports, especially those of asymmetric nature, disorders of the statics of the spine; trunk (i.e. torso) asymmetries; as well as disproportions of one's muscle mass occur in the training subjects [4–6]. What is more, attention is paid to the influence of sports practice on the formation of antero-posterior curvatures of the spine [4,10,17,21] Therefore, it is important to take special care of a young athlete, and to bear in mind that training programs should not only aim at the result, but should also foster the harmonious development of a young organism.

The purpose of the work is to evaluate body posture and somatic parameters of young females training basketball in comparison with their non-training peers, and to examine whether a relationship between the quality of one's posture, the length of the training period (in years) and its frequency exists.

Material and Methods

The subjects of the study were 32 young females training basketball (experimental group E) aged 13-14 years (mean = 13.4 ± 0.6 years) and 15 years old (mean = 15.1 ± 0.4 years). The length of the period of basketball

Author's address Dr Małgorzata Grabara, Department of Recreation, Jerzy Kukuczka Academy of Physical Education, Mikołowska Street 72, 40-065 Katowice, Poland

practice for the group of 13-14-year-olds was 3-4 years, with the frequency of 3-7 times a week. For the group of 15-year-olds it was 4-5 years and 4-7 times a week, respectively. The data related to the length of the training period and its frequency was obtained from a questionnaire that was completed by the subjects' parents. The control group (C) included 37 young females who did not undertake any guided physical activity, and who were in the same age brackets (mean =13.3 ± 0.6 and 15.1 ± 0.4 years).

Body height (BH) was measured with the use of medical scales with a height rod (with 5 mm accuracy); body mass (BM), fat mass (FM) and total body water (TBW) were defined with the use of Tanita electronic scale (with 0.1 kg accuracy). On the basis of body height and mass, body mass index (BMI) was calculated.

A specialist device using the projection Moiré technique (MORA, CQElektronik System, Poland) was applied to assess one's posture [13]. Before recording, spinous processes (C_7-S_1), posterior superior iliac spines (M_1, M_2), and lower angles of shoulder blades ($Ł_1$, $Ł_2$) were marked on the subject. The subject was then placed with their back to the recording camera, and the record of the picture of one's posture lasted for about 5 seconds. The short examination time allowed fatigue of postural muscles to be avoided, and at the same time the best record of the subject's placement could be chosen.

In frontal and transverse planes, the analysis included the following:

- torso inclination angle (KNT), specified by the route of the C7-S1 straight line towards the perpendicular;

- deflection of the line of spinous processes towards the straight line C7-S1 (UK; mm);

- symmetry of the shoulders towards each other (KLB; mm);

- symmetry of the shoulder blades evaluated towards each other in the vertical direction (frontal plane) – the UL index, depth symmetry of the shoulder blades in the transverse plane – the UB index, and symmetry of the shoulder blades from the spine (closer-further from the line of spinous processes) – the OL index (mm);

- height symmetry (TT) and width symmetry (TS) of the waist triangles [mm], which are defined by a profile of the torso and the hip line;

- pelvic placement defined by the value of its inclination (frontal plane) – the KNM index, as well as torsion (transverse plane) – the KSM index (mm).

The values of all the above parameters were given as absolute values, obtaining zero deflections from the correct value regardless of the direction of these deflections (right-left, front-back).

In order to specify the total values of deflections from symmetry, a synthetic index of postural symmetry (WSyn) was introduced. The index reflected the placement of particular elements of the posture in the frontal plane and in the transverse one, by pointing deviations from their symmetry [3] (table 1). In the assessment of the placement of shoulder blades and waist triangles, a maximum of 3 points were given for an index with the greatest deflection from symmetry, without adding up the points for individual deflections.

Table 1. Criteria of granting points for the placement of particular elements of body posture for the synthetic index of postural symmetry (WSyn) [3]

Variable	Number of points for the deflections mentioned below						
	< 1	1-2	2.01-3	3.01-5	5.01-10	10.01-15	>15
KNT	0	1	2		3		
UK		0		1	2	3	4
KLB			0		1	2	3
UL*							
UB*			0		1	2	3
OL*							
TT**			0		1	2	3
TS**							
KNM			0		1	2	3
KSM			0		1	2	3
KPT	0	1	2		3		

Legend: KNT – Torso lateral inclination angle (°); UK – Maximum deflection of the spinous process C_7-S_1 (mm); KLB – Symmetry of the shoulders (mm); UL – Height symmetry of the shoulder blades (mm) UB – Depth symmetry of the shoulder blades in the transversal plane (mm); OL – Symmetry of the shoulder blades from the spine (mm); TT – Height symmetry of the waist triangles (mm); TS – Width symmetry of the waist triangles (mm); KNM – Pelvic lateral inclination in the frontal plane (mm); KSM – Pelvic torsion in the transversal plane (mm); KPT – Torso forward inclination angle (°); *, ** - Parameters for the placement of which there are maximum 3 points for the highest-assessed index

In the sagittal plane, the following were taken into consideration:

- the route of the straight line C7-S1 in relation to the vertical axis, determining the torso lateral inclination angle (KPT),
- angular deflection from the perpendicular of the superior thoracic segment (α angle),
- angular deflection from the vertical of the thoracolumbar segment (β angle),
- angular deflection from the perpendicular of the lumbar- sacral segment (γ angle).

While assessing one's posture, the asymmetry direction of the placement of particular parts of the body in female basketball players and non-training young females was analyzed on the basis of deflection values different from zero. Moreover, the percentage of young female athletes with deflections of the examined parameters above 10 mm for the placement of the pelvis, shoulders, and shoulder blades and above 5 mm for deflections of the lines of spinous processes (UK) was calculated.

The results obtained in the course of the computer examination of the posture and somatic parameters in female basketball players and non-training females were compared through t-test for independent samples, Pearson's correlation between the length of the training period and its frequency with regard to the parameters of body posture was calculated. The Statistica software, version 9 (StatSoftInc, USA) was used for statistical analysis, the level of significance was set at $\alpha = 0.05$.

Results

An analysis of somatic indices has shown significant differences of body height (BH) within the group of younger females (Table 2), which may be explained by the specificity of basketball, in which taller athletes can achieve better scores. Besides, in the same age group significantly greater values of total body water in the organism (TBW) were noticed. However, no considerable differences of somatic parameters in females aged 15 years were found.

The trunk (on the basis of the KNT index) was more often inclined to the left in both studied groups (69% basketball players and 70% non-training females). Deflection of the lines of spinous processes from the vertical axis was more often left-sided, both in basketball players (63%), and in the control group (73%), whereas in 22% of the basketball players and 24% of non-training subjects, a deflection value over 5 mm was stated. Deviations exceeding 10 mm were not noted. In total, 59% of basketball players and 70% of the non-training females had their pelvis inclined to the left (on the basis of the KNM index); however, no pelvic asymmetry in the frontal plane exceeding 10 mm was recorded. The majority of the subjects, i.e. 94% of the training females and 81% from the control group, were characterized by the left-sided pelvic torsion (on the basis of the KSM index). It was also noted that 50% of female basketball players were characterized by pelvic asymmetry in the transversal plane of a value exceeding 10 mm, while in the control group, asymmetry of this value was noticed only in 27% of the subjects. In the studied groups, 41% of basketball players and 51% of the non-training females had the left shoulder blade placed more inferiorly (on the basis of the UL index), and deflections greater than 10 mm were noted in 38% of basketball players and in 19% of the non-practicing females. The left shoulder was lowered as compared with the right one in 59% of female basketball players and in 62% of the non-training females, whereas in 16% of the training subjects and in 24% of the non-training ones, the asymmetry value exceeded 10 mm.

All the postural parameters that either define symmetry or the lack of it in the frontal and transverse planes, as well as the synthetic index of postural symmetry in the younger group, did not differentiate the training female subjects from the non-training ones. Within the group of 15-year-old females, considerably greater asymmetries in the pelvic placement in the transversal plane (KSM) and much greater asymmetries of shoulder blades in relation to the transverse plane were noticed, as compared to the arrangement of the aforementioned parameters in the non-training peers (Table 3).

Table 2. Mean values (±SD) of anthropometric variables in young females practicing basketball (E) and in non-training females (C)

Age group	13-14-year-olds		15-year-olds	
Variable	E (n = 16)	C (n = 17)	E (n = 16)	C (n = 20)
Body height (cm)	164.8 ± 6.2 **	158.5 ± 6.8	166.0 ± 6.6	163.5 ± 6.7
Body mass (kg)	54.7 ± 8.9	48.8 ± 8.0	56.0 ± 7.9	54.9 ± 8.2
Body mass index (kg/m^2)	20.1 ± 3.1	19.4 ± 2.6	20.2 ± 1.7	20.5 ± 2.6
Fat mass (kg)	13.1 ± 5.9	10.5 ± 5.3	11.9 ± 4.4	12.6 ± 5.6
Total body water (kg)	30.5 ± 3.0 *	27.9 ± 3.3	32.3 ± 3.4	31.1 ± 3.2

Significantly different from the control group (C): * $p<0.05$; ** $p<0.01$

Table 3. Mean values (±SD) of postural indices in frontal and transverse planes in girls practicing basketball (E) and in non-training females (C)

Age group	13-14-year-olds		15-year-olds	
Variable	E (n = 16)	C (n = 17)	E (n = 16)	C (n = 20)
KNT	1.0 ± 0.7	1.2 ± 0.7	1.1 ± 0.9	1.2 ± 1.0
UK	3.8 ± 2.3	3.6 ± 2.2	4.8 ± 2.7	3.5 ± 1.5
KLB	6.8 ± 5.8	6.2 ± 5.2	7.4 ± 6.2	5.7 ± 5.8
UL	8.0 ± 3.9	7.2 ± 4.3	8.3 ± 6.1	6.0 ± 4.4
UB	15.3 ± 9.4	11.2 ± 7.1	16.2 ± 8.2 **	8.7 ± 7.1
OL	5.2 ± 5.7	8.5 ± 5.1	8.2 ± 4.8	6.1 ± 4.6
TT	11.7 ± 8.3	10.8 ± 10.0	11.7 ± 8.0	11.4 ± 7.2
TS	10.7 ± 7.8	11.3 ± 6.1	9.0 ± 7.1	13.0 ± 7.8
KNM	3.0 ± 2.0	1.9 ± 1.4	2.0 ± 2.0	1.8 ± 1.2
KSM	10.1 ± 5.1	7.9 ± 5.1	11.2 ± 5.1*	7.0 ± 4.8
WSyn	10.0 ± 2.8	9.1 ± 2.8	11.6 ± 2.7	10.0 ± 2.8

Legend: KNT – Torso lateral inclination angle (°); UK – Maximum deflection of the spinous process C_7-S_1 (mm); KLB – Symmetry of the shoulders (mm); UL – Height symmetry of the shoulder blades (mm) UB – Depth symmetry of the shoulder blades in the transversal plane (mm); OL – Symmetry of the shoulder blades from the spine (mm); TT – Height symmetry of the waist triangles (mm); TS – Width symmetry of the waist triangles (mm); KNM – Pelvic lateral inclination in the frontal plane (mm); KSM – Pelvic torsion in the transversal plane (mm); WSyn – Synthetic index of postural symmetry (pts.); Significantly different from the control group (C): * $p<0.05$; ** $p<0.01$

Table 4. Mean values (±SD) of postural indices in the sagittal plane in girls practicing basketball (E) and in non-training females (C)

Age group	13-14-year-olds		15-year-olds	
Variable	E (n = 16)	C (n = 17)	E (n = 16)	C (n = 20)
KPT	1,9 ± 1,5	2,3 ± 1,8	4,0 ± 2,0	3,1 ± 1,8
α angle (°)	14,4 ± 2,7	14,9 ± 5,0	12,4 ± 3,9	14,0 ± 3,8
β angle (°)	14,4 ± 2,3	13,8 ± 2,9	14,9 ± 2,4	16,1 ± 1,9
γ angle (°)	13,2 ± 5,4	13,9 ± 6,0	12,9 ± 7,1	15,2 ± 6,7
Kyphosis ($\alpha+\beta$) angle (°)	28,8 ± 4,3	28,7 ± 6,6	27,2 ± 3,5 *	30,1 ± 4,2
Lordosis ($\beta+\gamma$) angle (°)	27,6 ± 6,0	27,7 ± 6,8	27,8 ± 6,8	31,3 ± 6,7

Legend: KPT – Torso forward inclination angle (°); *Significantly ($p<0.05$) different from the control group;

The form of the spine and the placement of the torso in the sagittal plane within the younger group did not diversify the subject females. Only the thoracic kyphosis angle, defined by the sum of inclination angles of the superior thoracic segment and the thoracolumbar one, was significantly smaller in 15-year-old female basketball players (Table 4).

In order to check whether a potential connection between basketball practice and body posture exists, correlations between the training periods in years, the frequency of practice within a week, and postural indices were estimated. Only young females in training were taken into account in this analysis. The length of the training period had no relation with the quality of one's posture. On the contrary, it has been noticed that there was a relationship ($p<0.05$) between the frequency of basketball practice during the week and the deflection of the lines of spinous processes (r_{UK} = 0.427), torso lateral inclination angle (r_{KNT} = 0.543), the placement of shoulder blades in the transversal plane (r_{UB} = 0.468) or towards the spine (r_{OL} = 0.412), inclination angle of the superior thoracic segment (r_{α} = -0.461), kyphosis angle ($r_{\alpha+\beta}$ = -0.405), and the synthetic index of postural symmetry (r_{WSyn} = 0.550). On the basis of the calculations stated above, it may be stated that frequent basketball practice may lead to increased asymmetry of the posture, including an incorrect placement of the spine in the frontal plane. A correlation between basketball practice and one's body posture in the sagittal plane was noticed in reference to the form of thoracic kyphosis (i.e. flattening, to be more precise).

Discussion

An analysis of somatic parameters did not confirm the facts of lower body mass and smaller percentage of adipose tissue in the female subjects in training, although increased physical activity fosters lesser adiposity [8]. On the other hand, significantly greater body height, as well as significantly greater total body water, has been proven in younger subjects training basketball.

An evaluation of body posture of the young females in training in comparison with their non-training peers only revealed considerable differences in the placement of the shoulder blades and the pelvis in 15-year-old females, and thus characterized by a longer training period and attending training more frequently. The study by Bussey [1] indicates that an asymmetrical placement of the pelvis, which is present in athletes, may be associated with a predominance of work of certain muscle groups responsible for the pelvic placement. However, the observed asymmetry of shoulder blades in the transverse plane may suggest an asymmetrical protrusion of one shoulder blade or a habitual trunk torsion, which results in one shoulder blade being closer than the other.

The observed correlations between postural indices and the frequency of trainings (0.405-0.550) indicate that there is a connection between basketball practice and one's body posture, yet they concern other features of the posture than those significantly different in both compared groups. Studies of various authors [2–6, 9–11,14,17,18, 21,23] point out the influence of sports training on one's body posture; however, depending on the nature of exercises specific for a particular sport, this influence may be both positive and negative.

Team sport games are characterized by both the symmetrical and asymmetrical work of the limbs. Thus, some asymmetrical elements (e.g. a throw to the basket from a layup in case of basketball), performed repeatedly during practice always only on one side, can perhaps lead to an effect of asymmetry of posture.

Zuchetto noticed in her study the occurrence of torso asymmetry in handball players, which she explained among other things by an asymmetrical work of the arms [23]. The study by Hawrylak *et al.* [6], based on the assessment of body posture with regard to its symmetry among university student-athletes, proved that asymmetries in the body occur quite often. The authors also noticed different placement of those asymmetries, which is related to the sport in question. In case of the subjects who trained for team sports, asymmetries over 10 mm were connected with the placement of waist triangles, whereas asymmetries of 5-10 mm were associated with the route of lines of spinous processes. In a comparative study of the posture of volleyball players versus non-training young females, substantially more frequent asymmetries of waist triangles and shoulders were observed in the subjects practicing volleyball [4]. Another study of the posture of female volleyball players mentions a typical posture with asymmetrical shoulder blades, shoulders, and pelvis [18]. Therefore, it follows from the cited studies that asymmetries of one's body posture often appear among those who play team sport games, and that their placement appears to be different. If the values of these asymmetries exceeded 10 mm, one may talk about the deviations (or deflections) from the correct posture. For the sake of linear asymmetry indices (e.g. UK, OL, UL, TT), some authors assume 10 mm or greater deflections as considerable asymmetries, and 5-10 mm deflections as moderate asymmetries [20]. However, it is worth pointing out that not all of the parameters of one's body posture influence postural quality to the same extent. Deflection of the line of spinous processes may upset one's body equilibrium to a larger extent than asymmetrical placement of shoulders or shoulder blades. Although faulty postures associated with scoliosis, specified on the basis of 10 mm or greater deflections of the lines of spinous processes, were not noted in any subject groups, some vestigial side-to-side curves of the spine were found.

Studies of the posture among athletes [5] prove the existence of postural asymmetry. These studies point out that curved lines of spinous processes and an asymmetrical pelvic torsion occur in girls who train much more often than in their non-training peers. In case of runners, the authors explain this fact by the technique of running on a track along with greater strains of the spine during running [5]. On the other hand, a comparison between the posture of gymnasts and non-training females has demonstrated that asymmetries in gymnasts were smaller and occurred more rarely than in their peers, whereas in the sagittal plane, a greater increase of lumbar lordosis was observed in young females with a longer training period [2]. Other researchers drew similar conclusions, namely: the posture of young females doing gymnastics is more often correct than within the group of non-training subjects [14]. An assessment of the posture of young females practicing synchronized swimming and their non-training peers has shown that swimmers are much more frequently characterized by a symmetrical route of lines of spinous processes, shoulders and the pelvis, and their posture in the sagittal plane is more often described as of a very good or good type [11]. This leads to the conclusion that sport training has an impact on the form of the spine in the sagittal plane. It finds evidence in the findings of Wojtys *et al.* [21], who discovered an increase in thoracic kyphosis and lumbar lordosis in athletes doing all sorts of sports. It needs to be noted that an inclination of anteroposterior curvatures of the spine varies in different sportspeople and often results from the specificity of a particular sport. It is also confirmed by the remarks of Lichota *et al.* [9]. In Mrozkowiak's research [13], carried out with the participation of a large group of non-training children and adolescents who were examined from the point of view of their posture with the use of the same measurement technique as in their own study, average values of measurements of the angles of anteroposterior curvatures of the spine were lower than those recorded in the control group in this study.

On the basis of the aforementioned studies, it may be concluded that postural asymmetries also appear in children and the adolescents in training, especially among athletes who practice sports with elements of asymmetrical exercises.

Although postural asymmetry is a very common quality, and a symmetrical structure of the torso is very rare, one should not ignore the signs of an asymmetry of body posture. Often adopted poses of an asymmetrical nature may cause postural deviations, and in case of their consolidation, may lead to deformation [22]. Therefore, frequently performed physical exercises during training, which clearly emphasize the work of one side of the body, may influence the quality of posture.

Summing up, body posture in 13-14-year-old female basketball players and non-training females did not differ significantly. In the group of 15-year-olds who were training basketball, the placement of the shoulder blades and pelvis in the transverse plane was characterized by greater asymmetry, and the angle of thoracic kyphosis had significantly lower value than in the group of their peers. The length of the training period did not show a relationship with the quality of posture. However, it has been stated that more frequent participation in basketball training may contribute to an increase in the asymmetry of shoulder blades, have a negative effect on the placement of the spine in the frontal plane and on the torso inclination angle, and may lead to a decrease in the angle of thoracic kyphosis. On the basis of this study, it cannot be explicitly stated that basketball practice fosters symmetrization.

References

1. Bussey M.D. (2010) Does the demand for asymmetric functional lower body postures in lateral sports relate to structural asymmetry of the pelvis? *J.Sci.Med.Sport*, 13(3):360-364.
2. Grabara M. (2010) Postural variables in girls practicing sport gymnastic. *Biomed.Hum.Kinet.*, 2:74-77.
3. Grabara M. (2012) Analysis of body posture between young football players and their untrained peers. *Hum.Mov.*, 13(2):120-126.
4. Grabara M., A.Hadzik (2009) Postural variables in girls practicing volleyball. *Biomed.Hum.Kinet.*, 1:67-71.
5. Grabara M., A.Hadzik (2009) The body posture in young athletes compared to their peers. *Pol.J.Sports Med.*, 2:115-124.
6. Hawrylak A., T.Skolimowski, K.Barczyk, E.Bieć (2001) Assymetry of trunk in athletes of different kind of sport. *Pol.J. Sports Med.*, 17:232-235.
7. Ischander M., F.Zaldivar, A.Eliakim, E.Nussbaum, G.Dunton, S.Leu, D.Cooper, M.Schneider (2007) Physical activity, growth, and inflammatory mediators in BMI-matched female adolescents. *Med.Sci.Sport Exerc.*, 39(7):1131-138.
8. Jones R.A., A.D.Okely, P.Caputi, D.P.Cliff (2010) Perceived and actual competence among overweight and non-overweight children. *J.Sci.Med.Sport*, 13(6):589-596.
9. Lichota M., M. Plandowska, P.Mil (2011) The shape of anterior-posterior curvatures of the spine in athletes practising selected sports. *Pol.J.Sport Tourism*, 18:112-116.
10. López-Miñarro P.A., J.M.Muyor, F.Alacid (2011) Sagittal spinal and pelvic postures of highly-trained young canoeists. *J.Hum.Kinet.*, 29:41-48.
11. Maćkowiak Z., M.Wiernicka (2010) Body posture in girls aged 13-18 involved in synchronized swimming. *Pol.J.Sports Med.*, 2-3(6):115-122.
12. Menschik D., S.Ahmed, M.H.Alexander, R.W.Blum (2008) Adolescent physical activities as predictors of young adult weight. *Arch.Pediatr.Adolesc.Med.*, 162(1):29-33.
13. Mrozkowiak M. (2007) Determinants of selected parameters of body posture of children and adolescent and their variability in the light of the projection moire (in Polish). ZWKF, Gorzow Wlkp.
14. Sebić L., A.Hadrović, S.Bijelić, V.Kozić (2010) Postural differences between girls who practice and who do not practice rhythmic gymnastics. *Homo Sporticus*, 2:45-48.
15. Strong W.B, R.M.Malina, C.J.Blimkie, S.R.Daniels, R.K.Dishman, B.Gutin, A.C.Hergenroeder, A.Must, P.A.Nixon, J.M.Pivarnik, T.Rowland, S.Trost, F.Trudeau (2005) Evidence based physical activity for school-age youth. *J.Pediatr.*, 146:732-737.
16. Tittlbach S.A., R.Sygusch, W.Brehm, A.Woll, T.Lampert, A.E.Abele, K.Bos (2011) Association between physical activity and health in German adolescents. Eur.J.Sport Sci., 11(4):283-291.
17. Uetake T., F.Ohsuki, H.Tanaka, M.Shindo (1998) The vertebral curvature of sportsmen. *J.Sports Sci.*, 16: 621-628.
18. Vařeková R., I.Vařeka, M.Janura, Z.Svoboda, M.Elfmark (2011) Evaluation of postural asymmetry and gross joint mobility in elite female volleyball athletes. *J.Hum.Kinet.*, 29:5-13.
19. Weinsier R.L., G.R.Hunter, A.F.Heini, M.I.Goran, S.M.Sell (1998) The etiology of obesity: relative contribution of metabolic factors, diet, and physical activity. *Am.J.Med.*, 105:145-150.
20. Wojna D. (2010) Assessment of body posture in young schoolchildren. *Fizjoterapia*, 18(4):27-39.
21. Wojtys E., J.Ashton-Miller, L.Huston., P.J.Moga (2000) The association between athletic training time and the sagittal curvature of the immature spine. *Am.J.Sports Med.*, 28:490-498.
22. Zeyland-Malawka E., E.Pretkiewicz-Abacjew (2006) Symptoms of asymmetry in the posture of children and young people – a threat to a fully efficient locomotor system and to health. Nowiny Lek., 75(4):394-398.
23. Zuchetto A.T. (1991) The effects of training on the development of posture in handball athletes. M. Ed Thesis (In Portuguese). Universidade Federal de Santa Maria.

Effects of stretching exercises on primary dysmenorrhea in adolescent girls

Shahnaz Shahr-jerdy [1], Rahman Sheikh Hosseini [2], Maghsoud Eivazi Gh [3,4]

[1] Department of Physical Education and Sport Sciences, University of Arak, Iran; [2] Tehran University, Tehran, Iran; [3] Physiotherapy Department, Faculty of Rehabilitation Sciences, Tabriz University of Medical Sciences, Iran; [4] Physiotherapy & Rehabilitation Department, Okan University, Tuzla Kampusu Istanbul, Turkey

Summary

Study aim: To assess the effect of one term of stretching exercise on primary dysmenorrhea in high school students.
Material and methods: 179 single girls aged 15-17 years with moderate-to-severe primary dysmenorrhea were selected from 6 high schools located in 2 different city zones. The students were non-athletes and volunteered for the study. The participants were randomly divided into 2 groups: an experimental group (n = 124) and a control group (n = 55). In the intervention group, the subjects were requested to complete an active stretching exercise for 8 weeks (3 days per week, 2 times per day, 10 minutes each time) at home. In the pre-test, all of subjects were examined for pain intensity (10-point scale), pain duration, and the use of sedative tablets in 2 continuous menstruation cycles. The post-test was examined 8 weeks later.
Results: After 8 weeks, pain intensity was reduced from 7.65 to 4.88, pain duration was decreased from 7.48 to 3.86 hours, and use of sedative tablets was decreased from 1.65 to 0.79 tablets in the experimental group ($p<0.05$). In the control group, a significant decline was only noted for pain duration ($p<0.001$).
Conclusions: Stretching exercises are effective in reducing pain intensity, pain duration, and the amount of painkillers used by girls with primary dysmenorrhea.

Key words: Muscle exercise stretching – Dysmenorrhea – Adolescence

Introduction

Primary dysmenorrhea is a difficult menstrual flow in the absence of any pelvic pathology. It is the most common gynecologic problem among adolescent females [7, 9,10,12,20]. Incidence of primary dysmenorrhea was reported to be between 50% and 90% in different societies [4,5,20,24]; its incidence in Iran has been estimated to be between 74% and 84.1% [12,15,27]. It is characterized by lower abdominal pain that potentially could radiate to the back and thigh regions. The pain may be associated with headache, fatigue, nervousness, nausea, vomiting, mood swings, and (rarely) in severe cases syncope [20]. Primary dysmenorrhea reportedly stops spontaneously after 1-3 years; however, sometimes it is possible to continue until childbirth [3,4,11].

The idea that various type of active or passive exercise might help in alleviating pain in primary dysmenorrhea is not a new issue. It is widely thought that exercise reduces the frequency and / or the severity of dysmenorrheal syndrome. Suggestions for primary dysmenorrhea, such the use of stretching exercises [7], sports and regular exercise, are considered to be effective procedures in the prevention and treatment of primary dysmenorrhea. Generally, it seems that exercise therapy may alleviate discomfort associated with dysmenorrhea; however, scientific articles in this area are controversial [21]. The results of various studies have shown that with sport activity, the intensity of symptoms and pain has decreased [17]. Yet at the same time, the frequency of dysmenorrhea in high school girls who were actively involved in sports activities was considerably less than the compared group [13]. Women that participated in heavy sports, as compared with those who occasionally took part in sports, experienced fewer occurrences of symptoms of dysmenorrhea [18]. In some published articles, no correlation was found between physical activity level and dysmenorrhea [14,16,19]. Moreover, after checking with depression and mood swings, they found that sport in some women induce higher levels of symptoms along with menstruation [23].

Several studies have shown that the reduction of dysmenorrhea in women who regularly exercise may be due to effects of hormonal changes on uterine epithelial tissues or an increase in endorphin levels. It appears that exercise has analgesic effects that act in a non-specific way [22,26]. Research in the general population has shown

Author's address Dr. Maghsoud Eivazi Gh, Physiotherapy Department, Faculty of Rehabilitation Sciences, Tabriz University of Medical Sciences, Tavanir-Str, 51576-35411, Valiasr, Tabriz, Iran

that regular exercise can alleviate some types of symptoms including mood transitions, fatigue and abdominal bloating in females with primary dysmenorrhea, but these data are usually empirical and anecdotal rather than evidence based [7]. Results have shown that women who took part in regular, moderate, aerobic exercise had fewer negative effects, such as impaired concentration, pain and behavioral changes, than non-exercisers during period cycles [2]. Primary dysmenorrhea is considered the leading cause of absenteeism from work in young girls [7]. So it seems that this complication is a general problem in young girls, and developing conservative methods to reduce its complications is completely necessary. Since researches have shown contradictory results about the role of exercise therapy in treatment of primary dysmenorrhea [12], there is need for new research about this connection. It was believed that contracted ligamentous bands in the abdominal region were the causative factor for physical compression of nerve pathways and their irritation, so the proposed series of stretching exercise was considered very effective [7–9]. This study was designed to determine the value of stretching exercises in reducing the signs and symptoms of dysmenorrhea in student-aged girls.

Material and Methods

Study design: A research with a quasi-experimental design was performed in 2 groups that were selected from 6 secondary schools in the 2007-2008 scholastic year in Arak, in central Iran. A simple randomized controlled design was used for the allocation of educational districts into intervention or control groups. In Arak, 2 educational districts were sampled that covered all economic and social statuses and were randomly allocated to intervention or control status. A total of 6 schools were randomly selected from the different economic areas of the city. A total of 519 students were screened for the presence of primary dysmenorrheal. Eventually, 179 students aged 15-17 years, single, and non-athletes (without any regular exercise activity) met the inclusion criteria to participate in this project. The selected high schools were divided by simple randomization into experimental group (n = 124; students form 4 high schools) and control group (n = 55; students form 2 high schools with subjects). This meant that in each educational district of a city 2 high schools were assigned as intervention groups and 1 high school as a control group. With purposeful sampling, all participants experienced moderate to severe symptoms of dysmenorrhea. The selection processes of subjects were based on the diagnosis of a specialist with pelvic examination and a thorough history. In some cases of doubt in differentiating primary or secondary dysmenorrhea, sonographic assessment was used. Participants with a history of specific disease, compulsory use of special drugs, or having symptoms such as tingling, itching, discharge, irregular menstruation cycles, or subjects with regular exercise history (3 days per week and a daily average of 30-45 min) were excluded from the study. In the experimental group, the mean age, body height, body mass and age of first menstrual episode was 16 years, 162 cm, 54 kg, 13 years, respectively; in the control group, the mean was 16 years, 161 cm, 53 kg and 12 years, respectively. Additionally, 52.6% had regular exercise occasionally (regular exercise was defined as an exercise performed 3 times a week 30-45 minutes), 37.6% never had any regular exercise, and 9.7% reported performing mostly regular exercise.

All participants were given information written and verbally about the objectives and methods of implementation. Students who agreed to take part in this study were asked to complete a self-administered questionnaire at school in the 2 phases of research that was distributed among subjects with dysmenorrhea pain. Student participation was voluntary after filling out of written consent form. Ethics approval was granted by Arak University.

Methods: The subjects completed a demographic questionnaire that addressed: age, body height, body mass and age at first menstruation; information about levels of exercise activity; amount of analgesic consumption during menstruation; pain intensity assessment by using a visual analogue scale (VAS) during period and a consent form. Meanwhile, subjects were given 2 pre-test questionnaires and asked to answer the questionnaires after the first and second menstrual cycle, and to give information about the most severe pain according the visual analog scale (VAS) [23,26]. The questionnaire used the VAS scale to measure intensity of pain and some questions relating to consumption of analgesics and duration of menstrual pain, which was confirmed in their reliability and validity by the cooperation of 4 gynecologists. Cronbach's α, which determines the internal consistency of items in a survey instrument, was 91%. Based on the VAS scale, those subjects with pain intensity of 4 to 7 were classified as the moderate group. The subjects with a pain score between 7 and 10 were considered to be a severe form of dysmenorrhea. The subjects with pain intensity less 4 were excluded from the research design.

The experimental group was given a questionnaire prior to the stretching exercises, which included 6 stretching exercises in the abdominal, pelvic, and groin regions [25]. The subjects were requested to perform the active stretching exercises for 8 weeks at home (3 days per week and 2 times per day for 10 minutes) Furthermore, they were asked to avoid performing stretching exercises during the period cycle. The correct techniques of performing stretching exercises were explained by a qualified and experienced instructor and were told to do stretching exercises short of the discomfort zone. Furthermore, their performances were controlled from time to time by a physical education teacher in the high school. The subjects completed the questionnaires again after 8 weeks of stretching exercises. The prescribed exercises were as follows:

In the first stretching exercise, the subject was asked to stand behind a chair, bend trunk forward from the hip joint so that the shoulders and back were positioned on a straight line and the upper body was placed parallel to the floor (Fig 1.A). Duration of holding time was 5 seconds; repetition was 10 times.

In the second stretching exercise, the subject was requested to stand 10-20 cm behind a chair, then raise 1 heel off the floor, then repeat the exercise with the other heel alternatively (Fig 1.B). The exercise was performed 20 times.

In the third exercise, the subject was asked to spread their feet shoulder width, place trunk and hands in forward stretching mode, then completely bend her knees and maintain a squatting position (Fig 1.C). Duration of this position was 5 seconds; the subject then raised her body and repeated the same movement 10 times.

In the fourth exercise, the subject was asked to spread her feet wider than shoulder width. Then the subject was asked to bend and touch left ankle with her right hand while putting her left hand in a stretched position above her head, so that the head was in the middle and her head was turned and looked for her left hand (Fig 1.D). This exercise was repeated for the opposite foot with the same method. The exercise was repeated alternatively 10 times for each side of the body.

In the fifth exercise, the subject was asked to lie down in the supine position so that the shoulders, back, and feet were kept on the floor. In this position the knees was bent with the help of her hands and reached to her chin (Fig 1.E). The repetition frequency was 10 times.

In the sixth and last exercise, the subject was asked to stand against a wall and put her hands behind her head and elbows pointed forward in the direction of the eyes (Fig 1.F), then without bending the vertebral column, the abdominal muscle wall was contracted for 10 seconds. This exercise was repeated 10 times.

The control group was asked to complete the same questionnaires in the following 2 menstrual cycles. They were asked to avoid regular physical exercise during this period. After completing the study projects, the stretching exercises that used the same procedures were taught to the control group in the hope of performing these exercises.

Data analysis: Kolmogorov-Smirnov test was used to determine data normality. This test showed that pain intensity pre-test and post-test demonstrated normal scattering. Pain duration variable and data for the amount of consumed medicine were not normally distributed or were discrete values. Thus, the data were analyzed with independent/paired *t*-test or nonparametric U Mann-Whitney/ Wilcoxon tests where appropriate. Differences between fractions were assessed using chi-square test. All analyses were conducted using the SPSS software; the level of significance was set at $\alpha = 0.05$.

Results

The total number of tablets consumed on average during the cycle was 1; the maximum number was 3 tablets per day. In the experimental group, 19.4% of students reported that they did not consume any kind of analgesics, 36.3% took Profen tablets, 10.5% acetaminophen codeine, 11.3% used Mefenamic acid capsules for pain relief, 16.1% took a combination of Profen and Mefenamic acid capsules, and 6.1% consumed non-chemical drugs. In the control group, the respective fractions were 7.3% for analgesics ($p<0.05$), 47.3% Profen tablets, 5.5% acetaminophen codeine, 5.5% Mefenamic acid capsules, 32.7% a combination of Profen and Mefenamic acid capsules ($p<0.05$), and 1.8% for non-chemical medicine.

The majority (49.2%) of students from both the experimental and control group reported pain in the abdomen and low back area, about 30.2% of students irrespective of group experienced pain in the suprapubic, low back, and in the buttocks, 14.5 % reported pain in suprapubic area and 6.1 experienced low back pain. These symptoms were not evaluated following an intervention procedure. The average menstrual cycle length during the study period in the subjects was 6 days in both experimental and control group. Fifty-nine percent of subjects had regular

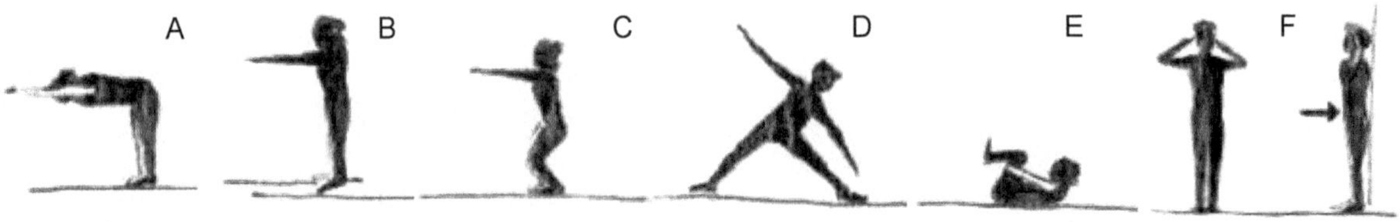

Fig. 1. The active stretching exercises prescribed

menstrual periods; no significant between-group differences were found in this regard.

Of the participants, 38.0% occasionally had regular exercises (regular exercise was defined as an exercise which performed 3 times a week 30-45 minutes); 61.3% of students from the experimental group, and 30.1% from the control group ($p<0.001$) never had any regular exercise; 3.2% and 25.5% respectively ($p<0.001$) reported mostly performing regular exercise.

The descriptive statistics for pain intensity, pain duration, and use of medication recorded in both groups before and after completion of the experiment are presented in Table 1. It was found that following the intervention pain intensity, pain duration, and amount of consumed medications decreased significantly ($p<0.001$) in the experimental group, while in the control group a significant decline was only noted for pain duration ($p<0.001$). Hence, after intervention the mean values for estimated pain intensity were in the control group 2.3 pts higher ($p<0.001$), experienced pain duration was by more than 1 hour longer, and the amount of consumed medications was about 20% higher compared to the experimental group.

Table 1. Mean values (±SD) of studied variables recorded in experimental and control group before and after 8 weeks of intervention

Variable	Experimental Group (n = 124)		Control Group (n = 55)	
	Before	After	Before	After
Pain intensity	7.65 ± 1.94	4.88 ± 1.92***	7.77 ± 1.50	7.16 ± 1.42###
Pain duration (h)	7.84 ± 5.26	3.86 ± 2.50***	5.59 ± 1.33#	4.95 ± 1.28***###
Use of medication (n)	1.65 ± 1.02	0.79 ± 0.69***	1.05 ± 0.72	0.95 ± 0.24###

Legend: *** Significantly ($p<0.001$) different from the respective *Before* value; Significantly different from the respective value in experimental group: # $p<0.05$; ### $p<0.001$;

Discussion

Findings of different studies have shown that therapeutic exercise and physical activity was related with reduced incidence of dysmenorrhea, whereas in some of studies did not demonstrate such a correlation statistically [6]. Results of Israel *et al.* [17] showed that after 12 weeks of aerobic training, the intensity of symptoms decreased. Golub *et al.* [13] expressed that dysmenorrhea in high school girls who were involved in sports and physical activities were less than non-exerciser group. According to Izzo and Labriola [18], women involved in heavy sport activities experienced fewer signs and symptoms of dysmenorrhea in comparison with women who had occasional sport practice. In a few articles, no correlation between levels of physical activity and dysmenorrhea-related symptoms was found [14,16,19]. According to Metheny and Smith [23], after adjusting for depression and mood changes, the level of discomfort due to dysmenorrhea was accompanied by intensity of physical activity. Therefore, the results obtained from their study illustrated that physical activity could lead to improvement of painful dysmenorrhea by reducing depression; however, doing physical activity did not directly effect the reduction of symptoms of dysmenorrhea. Golomb *et al.* [12] studied the effects of exercise therapy on the frequency of dysmenorrhea and premenstrual problems in high school girls for more than 3 years. Their findings showed that 39% of students in the experimental group compared with 61% of the control group experienced dysmenorrheal symptoms. The researchers did not differentiate between primary and secondary dysmenorrhea in their study protocol; it was not blind for students and could possibly increase bias probability. However, the prescribed exercises were effective in reducing menstrual symptoms and were important to perform on daily base.

Other studies have shown that dysmenorrhea was decreased in athletes who started sport activities prior to menarche. Furthermore, after initiating sport activity there has been observed improvements in the symptoms of dysmenorrhea, and that sportswoman who had participated in heavy physical activities had less symptomatic menstrual cycles [18]. Moreover, performing exercise reduced the intensity of pain, pain frequency, and the amount of analgesics medication. This had a positive association with the results of current study [1]. Perceived stress is considered to be a critical element in the relationship between exercise and treatment of dysmenorrhea. There was significant dose-response and temporal associations between perceived stress in one menstrual cycle and the incidence of dysmenorrhea in the following cycle. There are several studies that have shown considerable correlation between tensional stress in life and premenstrual symptoms [23]. The role of exercise therapy as a tool for reducing stress and biochemical changes in the immune system was considered extensively as well [13]. Physiologic mechanisms through which exercise might improve symptoms resulting from the menstrual cycle are not clear. However, some hypotheses are being proposed for its explanation. Izzo and Labriola [18] proposed that the increase in the blood flow and metabolism of the uterus during exercise may be effective in the reduction of dysmenorrheal symptoms. In another words, improved metabolism is a factor in the reduction of symptoms. It is also suggested that increased menstrual pain by uterine muscle contraction is derived from a nervous system that is innervated by the sympathetic nerve Hence, stress through hyperactivity of sympathetic nerve system via the increase contractibility of uterine muscles may lead to menstruation symptoms. Consequently, it might be possible to reduce dysmenorrheal symptoms by decreased sympathetic over-activity through exercise. Another hypothesis suggests that therapeutic exercise can increase the secretion of endorphins from the brain, and these materials in turn raise the pain threshold of the body [8].

It has been suggested that therapeutic exercise is helpful for the treatment of primary dysmenorrhea through various modes such as decrease stress, attenuate menstrual symptoms through increase of local metabolism, and increase local blood flow at the pelvic level and increase of endorphin production. It is a multidimensional problem and has various aspects that are a combination of organic, psychological, and sociocultural factors that result in its symptoms. However, findings of current research illustrate that exercise may have a key role in alleviating these problems. Age was an important element in the intensity of perceiving menstrual changes. With increasing age, decreases in pain level, negative states, impaired concentration, and behavior swings have been reported [2]. The findings of this study illustrate that girls with primary dysmenorrhea report less pain than the non-exercising group, which is in accord with Aganoff *et al.* [2]. However, the results contradict the findings of Metheny and Smith [23] who reported higher levels pain and negative moods with performing regular exercise in dysmenorrheal girls.

Exercise in various forms including stretching, aerobic exercise, free exercise, or competitive athletic performance has been believed to improve or even completely resolve primary dysmenorrhea for half a century. Studies were performed to prove the presence of such a relationship; however, each one had methodological handicaps and researchers were led to contradictory results, so there is a need to do more research. In particular, blind studies are needed to eliminate the psychological effects of exercise from its physical effects. The type and level of physical activity and frequency of movement was under control for every subject in the present study. However, as the nature of this research suggests, it is not possible to control this factor entirely. It is also suggested that further research be conducted in different age groups and in different treatment regimens. Furthermore, future research should be done in such a way that take into account the measurement of psychosocial and stress variables, until findings derived from a study purely demonstrate the role and effects of stretching on primary dysmenorrhea. A certain limitation of this study is the cross-sectional nature of the research, as it does not reflect any temporal changes. Furthermore, the study was performed on a relatively small sample; therefore, generalizations of results in terms of the entire female population ought to be made with caution.

Summing up, the findings of this study suggest that there is a beneficial impact of physical exercise on menstrual cycle symptoms. Whether or not the effects of exercise could be long-term should be the subjects of further research. According to the results of this study, performing 8 weeks of selected stretching exercises reduces pain intensity, diminishes pain duration, and decreases the consumption of analgesics drugs in students with moderate-to-severe primary dysmenorrhea during the menstruation cycle.

References

1. Abbaspour Z., M.Rostami, S.H.Najjar (2006) The effect of exercise on primary dysmenorrheal. *J.Res.Health Sci.*, 6:26-31.
2. Aganoff J.A., G.J.Boyle (1994) Aerobic exercise, mood states and menstrual cycle symptoms. *J.Psychosom.Res.*, 38:183-192.
3. Banikarim C., M.R.Chacko, S.H.Kelder (2000) Prevalence and impact of dysmenorrhea on Hispanic female adolescents. *Arch.Pediatr.Adolesc.Med.*, 154:1226-1229.
4. Berek J.S., E.Novak (2007) Berek & Novak's Gynecology. Lippincott Williams & Wilkins Philadelphia, USA
5. Chiou M.H., H.H.Wang (2004) The relationship between dysmenorrhea and menstrual attitudes among female students in vocational nursing schools. *Hu.Li.Za.Zhi.*, 51:45-52.
6. Daley A.J. (2008) Exercise and primary dysmenorrhea: A comprehensive and critical review of the literature. *Sports Med.*, 38:659-670.
7. Daley A.J. (2009) The role of exercise in the treatment of menstrual disorders: The evidence. *Br.J.Gen.Pract.*, 59:241-242.
8. Dawood M.Y. (2006) Primary dysmenorrhea: advances in pathogenesis and management. *Obstet.Gynecol.*, 108:428-441.
9. DeCherney A., M.L.Pernoll (1994) Current obstetric & Gynecologic diagnosis & Treatment.. Lange Medical Book Series, Tufts University, Boston, Massachusetts, USA.
10. Esfandiary F.K. (1988) Adolescent dysmenorrhea. *J.Pediatr. Health Care.*, 2:29-37.
11. Fox E.L., D.K.Mathews (1981) The Physiological Basis of Physical Education and Athletics. Saunders College Pub., Philadelphia, USA.
12. Golomb L.M., A.A.Solidum, M.P.Warren (1998) Primary dysmenorrheal and physical activity. *Med.Sci.Sports Exerc.*, 30:906-909.
13. Golub L.J., H.Menduke, W.R.Lang (1968) Exercise and dysmenorrhea in young teenagers: a 3-year study. *Obstet.Gynecol.*, 32:508-511.
14. Gordley L.B., G.Lemasters, S.R.Simpson, J.H.Yiin (2000) Menstrual disorders and occupational, stress, and racial factors among military personnel. *J.Occup.Environ.Med.*, 42:871-881.

15. Harel Z., F.M.Biro, R.K.Kottenhahn, S.L.Rosenthal (1996) Supplementation with omega-3 polyunsaturated fatty acids in the management of dysmenorrheal in adolescents. *Am.J.Obstet. Gynecol.*, 174:1335-1338.

16. Harlow S.D., M.Park (1996) A longitudinal study of risk factors for the occurrence, duration and severity of menstrual cramps in a cohort of college women. *Br.J.Obstet.Gynaecol.*, 103:1134-1142.

17. Israel R.G., M.Sutton, K.F.O'Brien (1985) Effects of aerobic training on primary dysmenorrheal symptomatology in college females. *J.Am.Coll.Health.*, 33:241-244.

18. Izzo A., D.Labriola (1991) Dysmenorrhoea and sports activities in adolescents. *Clin.Exp.Obstet Gynecol.*, 18:109-116.

19. Jarrett M., M.M.Heitkemper, J.F.Shaver (1995) Symptoms and self-care strategies in women with and without dysmenorrheal. *Health Care Women Int.*, 16(2):167-178.

20. Johnson J. (1988) Level of knowledge among adolescent girls regarding effective treatment for dysmenorrhea. *J.Adolesc. Health Care,* 9:398-402

21. Locke R.J., M.P.Warren (1999) Exercise and primary dysmenorrhea. *Br.J.Sports Med.,* 33:227.

22. Mastrangelo M.A., M.L.Galantino, L.House (2007) Effects of yoga on quality of life and flexibility in menopausal women: a case series. *Explore (NY).* 3:42-45.

23. Metheny W.P., R.P.Smith (1989) The relationship among exercise, stress, and primary dysmenorrhea. *J.Behav.Med.*, 12: 569-586.

24. Norton P.A., M.Peterson (1997) Menstrual disorders and other common gynecology. *Hum.Reproduct.Clin.Pathol.Pharmacol.* 4:255-259.

25. Roostayi M.M. (2000) Physiotherapy and exercise therapy in women and obstetric. *Tehran: Sana Nashr Pub.* pp: 25-27.

26. Rumball J.S., C.M.Lebrun (2004) Preparticipation physical examination: selected issues for the female athlete. *Clin.J.Sport Med.*, 14:153-160.

27. St George I.M., S.Williams, P.A.Silva (1994) Body size and the menarche: the Dunedin study. *J.Adolesc.Health.,* 15:573-576.

Changes in strength abilities of adolescent girls: the effect of a 3-year physical education curriculum

Renata Czarniecka [1], Katarzyna Milde [2], Paweł Tomaszewski [2]

[1] Department of Physical Education Methodology, [2] Department of Statistics and Computer Sciences, The Jozef Pilsudski University of Physical Education, Warsaw, Poland

Summary

Study aim: To evaluate changes in strength abilities of adolescent girls that underwent a 3-year physical education curriculum.

Material and methods: The research participants comprised 141 girls aged 13.3 ± 0.35 years who participated in a 3-year physical education curriculum (PEC). Evaluation was based on the following EUROFIT Testing Battery tests: standing broad jump, handgrip strength, sit-ups, and bent arm hang. After the completion of the curriculum, changes in strength abilities of the participants were evaluated. Test results were compared to reference values for the population of Polish girls.

Results: After the 3-year PEC, research participants obtained significantly better results in all analyzed tests. At the beginning of the PEC, participants performed significantly worse in comparison to the reference values for the standing broad jump and bent arm hang tests, and better in the handgrip strength test. After the completion of the PEC, the participants performed significantly better in the sit-up and handgrip strength tests compared to reference values; for the standing broad jump and bent arm hang tests, they performed closer to the reference values.

Conclusions: While the development of student physical fitness is achievable through physical education lessons at school, innovative teaching methods and professional and creative approaches on the part of teachers are necessary.

Key words: Strength abilities – Physical education curriculum – Girls

Introduction

Proper physical fitness, which determines healthy development of adolescent girls, can be achieved through regular physical activity of adequate intensity and duration. According to the 2008 guidelines of the European Comission [16], school-aged youth should participate in moderate to vigorous daily physical activity for 60 minutes or more. However, many researchers [5,7,8,13] have found that moderate and vigorous physical activity constitutes about 47% of physical education lesson time in primary schools and 40% in secondary schools. Studies also indicate that the effective time of physical activity for girls has significantly decreased in high school. Research done by Nader [10] has shown that actual effective time of student physical activity during a 45-minute physical education lesson is about 25 minutes. Moreover, Dudley *et al.* [5] have found that girls spend about 31% of the lesson sitting. This means that during a physical education lesson, the average intensity of student physical activity corresponds to the "sustaining effort," which does not develop motor skills [10]. National tests of children and youth conducted every 10 years also indicate a low effectiveness of physical education at schools. The test from 1999 showed a significant drop in physical activity performance compared to the results from 20 years ago [11]. These data are disturbing, since the physical fitness of an adult largely depends on his or her upbringing and development during childhood and youth. Therefore, values acquired during childhood will determine lifestyle well into old age [1].

With the aforementioned deficiencies of scholastic physical education in mind, a special physical education curriculum (PEC) for high schools was created. The curriculum was implemented between 2007 and 2010 in 4 state high schools in Łowicz, Łódzkie Province. The curriculum only included girls, because studies have shown that adolescent girls have a much lower need for physical activity than adolescent boys [10,13]. The aim of the PEC was to develop independence in girls and encourage them to take on additional physical activity apart from school lessons. This paper focuses on evaluating changes in strength abilities of adolescent girls undergoing the PEC. The development of strength abilities is especially intense during adolescence. At the same time, changes in the maturing body (a rapid gain of body weight and changes in

Author's address Dr Renata Czarniecka, Department of Physical Education Methodology, University of Physical Education, Marymoncka 34, 00-968 Warsaw, Poland

body proportions) make it difficult for girls to engage in physical activities that require overcoming own body, i.e., the activities that are used to develop strength abilities [17]. Thus, the aim of the study was to assess changes in strength abilities of adolescent girls that underwent a 3-year physical education curriculum.

Material and Methods

Research participants comprised 141 girls aged 13.3 ± 0.35 years undergoing a 3-year physical education curriculum (PEC). It was assumed that in each successive year, girls undergoing the PEC would personally engage in an increasingly wider scope of duties related to conducting a physical education lesson. Initially, the participants conducted only selected exercises or short sections of a lesson, whereas in the final stage of the PEC, participants designed and conducted a whole lesson under a teacher's supervision. Proper implementation of the PEC and the achievement of expected results required appropriate supervision on the part of teachers. Therefore, all teachers (members of the project development team) conducted a sample lesson that was observed and later discussed by the author of the project and other teachers involved in the PEC.

Participants' strength abilities were evaluated based on 4 strength tests of the EUROFIT Testing Battery [4]: SBJ (standing broad jump), HGR (handgrip strength), SUP (sit-ups), and BAH (bent arm hang). The tests were conducted at the beginning of the PEC (October 2007) and following its completion (May 2010). In addition, the participants underwent basic anthropometric measurements, i.e., the measurement of body height, body mass, from these the BMI values were calculated.

Due to considerable discrepancies between empirical distribution and normal distribution, body mass and BAH values underwent logarithmic and square root transformation, respectively. HGR results were analyzed using relative values, i.e., in relation to participants' body mass. To compare the obtained results against reference values for the Polish population, the participants' anthropometric parameters and the results of the participants' strength tests were normalized against the functions of mean and standard deviation for age computed for the sample of Polish girls [14]. The body height and body mass proportions of research participants were compared to percentile ranks for standard body mass, body height, and to BMI for girls with a normal amounts of fat tissue [15]. The significance of changes for the mean values of the analyzed parameters after the completion of the PEC was assessed using Student's t-test for paired samples. The differences between mean values for the participants and for the reference sample were evaluated using Student's t-test for independent samples. The level of $\alpha = 0.05$ was considered significant.

Results

Table 1 presents the mean values (±SD) of participants' somatic parameters and strength test results recorded before and after the PEC. Research participants were considerably taller and heavier than girls in the reference sample ($p<0.001$), both before and after the PEC. Furthermore, participants' BMI values exceeded the reference values by 0.89 SD ($p<0.001$) at the beginning of the PEC and by 0.66 SD ($p<0.05$) following its completion.

Table 1. Mean (±SD) values of somatic and strength variables recorded in girls (n=141) before and after 3-year physical education curriculum

Variable	Before	After
Body height (cm)	160.3 ± 6.4	165.7 ± 5.6***
Body mass (kg)	51.6 ± 11.6	58.0 ± 11.9***
Body mass index	20.0 ± 3.8	21.1 ± 3.8***
SBJ (cm)	154.5 ± 21.6	165.6 ± 23.5***
HGR (kg)	27.4 ± 5.4	28.9 ± 5.2***
SUP(n)	22.0 ± 4.3	25.0 ± 4.2***
BAH (s)	6.9 ± 8.7	8.3 ± 11.1*

Legend: SBJ - Standing broad jump; HGR - Handgrip strength; SUP - Sit-ups; BAH - Bent arm hang; Significantly different from the *Before* value: *$p<0.05$; ***$p<0.001$

A comparison of the participants' performance during strength abilities tests before and after the PEC showed that participants performed considerably better in all the conducted tests after participating in the PEC for 3 years The greatest and most significant ($p<0.001$) increase (approximately 20%) in the results was observed for the bent arm hang test, although the average time of hanging remained relatively short (8.3 s), and the results varied greatly between participants. In the sit-up test, participants improved performance by an average of 3 sit-ups (from 22 to 25 sit-ups). The improvement in the standing broad jump and handgrip tests was relatively lower, though statistically significant ($p<0.001$), corresponding to around 7% and 5% of the initial values, respectively.

Figure 1 shows the average results of fitness tests compared to reference values for the population of Polish girls. At the beginning of the PEC, the girls performed considerably worse in the standing broad jump and bent arm hang tests (by approximately 0.25 and 0.45 SD, respectively), but performed significantly better (by approximately 0.95 SD, $p<0.001$) in the handgrip strength test, compared to the reference sample. After 3 years of the PEC, the girls performed significantly better ($p<0.001$) in the sit-up and handgrip strength tests compared to the reference sample, and performed closer to the reference sample in the standing broad jump and bent arm hang tests (by approximately 0.09 and 0.35 SD, respectively).

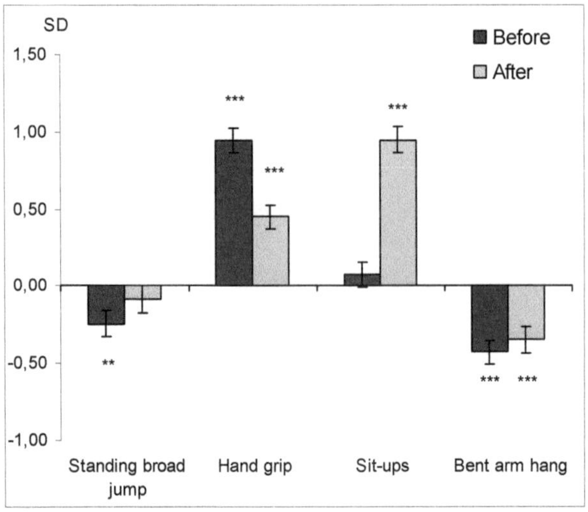

Fig. 1. Mean (±SE) values of fitness variables recorded in studied girls (n=141) before and after 3-year physical education curriculum standardized against functions of mean and standard deviations for age calculated for girls from Polish population [14] (horizontal line – 0)

Significantly different from the girls from Polish population: ** $p<0.01$; *** $p<0.001$

Discussion

This paper focused on evaluating changes in strength abilities of adolescent girls who underwent a 3-year physical education curriculum (PEC). Analysis of the obtained results showed that girls who underwent the PEC improved their strength abilities. The observed changes took place in all the analyzed fitness tests, with the greatest improvement taking place in the bent arm hang test. However, it must be taken into account that the observed changes, in addition to the effects of the PEC, may have been enhanced by the subject's ongoing physical development and strength-ability development, since both of these developments are especially intense during adolescence. Nevertheless, the PEC's effectiveness was supported by the decrease in the difference between the performance of the participants and the performance of the reference sample. It should be assumed, therefore, that the observed changes in participants' strength abilities can primarily be attributed to the implementation of the PEC. The observed reduction of the difference in BMI values between the subjects and the reference samples may also constitute a positive effect of the PEC. Similar results have been obtained by Chiodera *et al.* [3], who, after implementing their PEC in primary schools, observed positive changes in participants' physical fitness, but did not observe changes in BMI values despite a general-population tendency for body mass gain. In addition, Gutin *et al.* [6], after a year-long FitKid fitness curriculum for younger school-age children, observed improvement in both physical fitness parameters and body composition parameters. However, after the holiday period, the values of these parameters dropped to the levels observed for non-participating children. The above findings suggest that even innovative physical education curricula are not enough to guarantee the proper development of physical fitness, meaning that children and adolescents should be physically active not just at school, but during their spare time as well. That is why such curricula should include the promotion of a healthy lifestyle.

Positive results coming from the PEC may have been realized because participating teachers were able to systematically improve their teaching methodology during the 3 years the curriculum was implemented. To this end, monthly meetings were organized during which the participating teachers not only familiarized themselves with the aims of the PEC and its methods of implementation, but also presented their achievements and discussed the results their students. The meetings allowed for an ongoing assessment of the PEC and provided means for homogenizing the methods used by participating teachers. The relationship between a teacher's level of vocational competence and the effects of their work with children and adolescents is further confirmed by the findings of other researchers who implemented innovative solutions and physical education curricula, both in Poland and in other countries. For instance, Sallis *et al.* [12], observed a relationship between the physical fitness of 9-year-old students and the competence of teachers implementing the SPARK curriculum, i.e., specialized teachers, teachers trained to conduct physical education lessons, and untrained teachers working with students in kindergarten through third grade. Positive effects were observed for physical fitness tests (abdominal muscle strength and endurance) in groups of children under the supervision of teachers with the highest qualifications. Additionally, these groups made much more efficient use of lesson time through an increased amount of time spent on moderate and vigorous physical activity. Similar observations have been made by McKenzie *et al.* [9], who concluded that the effectiveness of the standard physical education curriculum in schools depends largely on teacher qualifications and on the location where the lesson takes place. Therefore, professional physical development curricula should be adjusted to local needs and conditions.

The improvement of participants' strength abilities could also have been affected by the teachers' use of the "improve your last score" method for assessing participant fitness. According to Przewęda and Dobosz [11], the level of motivation is 1 of 3 factors (next to constitution and motor abilities) that affect physical fitness, as assessed by outdoor fitness tests. The implementation of the above method motivated the girls to work on their physical fitness and to perform better and better during tests.

The effects of the 3-year PEC show that the development of motor abilities in adolescent girls can be effectively shaped by physical education lessons at school. This requires a specially designed curriculum and evaluation method. The evaluation method should motivate students to undertake physical activity beyond physical education lessons at school. Also important is to support teachers by systematically analyzing their work and directing it. This is substantiated by the experience of other researchers implementing innovative solutions and physical education curricula [2,3,6,8,12]. Their experience shows that taking part in physical education lessons that are appropriately designed and conducted unconventionally stimulates a child's physical development, facilitates the acquisition of new motor abilities, and creates a habit of regular physical activity that will last into adulthood. To summarize the research results: the 3-year PEC seems more efficient at improving strength abilities and physical development of girls. It can also be concluded that despite a low effectiveness of physical education lessons, the development of student physical fitness is achievable within the confines of physical education at schools; however, this requires using innovative teaching methods and a professional and creative approach to the subject on the teacher's part.

References

1. Barnett L.M., P.J.Morgan, E.van Beurden, J.R.Beard (2008) Perceived sports competence mediates the relationship between childhood motor skill proficiency and adolescent physical activity and fitness: a longitudinal assessment. *Int.J.Behav.Nutr. Phys.,* 5:40.

2. Boyle-Holmes T., L.Grost, L.Russell, B.A.Laris, L.Robin, E.Haller, S.Potter, S.Lee (2010) Promoting elementary physical education: results of a school-based evaluation study. *Health Educ.Behav.,* 37:377-389.

3. Chiodera P., E.Volta, G.Gobbi, M.A.Milioli, P.Mirandola, A.Bonetti, R.Delsignore, S.Bernasconi, A.Anedda, M.Vitale (2008) Specifically designed physical exercise programs improve children's motor abilities. *Scand.J.Med.Sci.Sports,* 18:179-187.

4. Council of Europe (1993) EUROFIT – European Test of Physical Fitness (2nd ed.). Strassbourg.

5. Dudley D.A., A.D.Okely, W.G.Cotton, P.Pearson, P.Caputi (2012) Physical activity levels and movement skill instruction in secondary school physical education. *J.Sci.Med.Sport,* 15(3): 231-237.

6. Gutin B., Z.Yin, M.Johnson, P.Barbeau (2008) Preliminary findings of the effect of a 3-year after-school physical activity intervention on fitness and body fat: The Medical College of Georgia Fitkid Project. *Int.J.Pediatr.Obes.* 3:3-9.

7. McKenzie T.L., S.J.Marshall, J.F.Sallis, T.L.Conway (2000) Student activity levels, lesson context, and teacher behavior during middle school physical education. *Res.Q.Exerc.Sport,* 71(3): 249–259.

8. McKenzie T.L., J.F.Sallis, J.J.Prochaska, T.L.Conway, S.J.Marshall, P.Rosengard (2004) Evaluation of a two-year middle-school physical education intervention: M-SPAN. *Med. Sci.Sports Exerc.,* 36(8):1382-1388.

9. McKenzie T.L., E.J.Stone, H.A.Feldman, J.N.Epping, M.Yang, P.K.Strikmiller, L.A.Lytle, G.S.Parcel (2001) Effects of the CATCH physical education intervention: teacher type and lesson location. *Am.J.Prev.Med.* 21(2):101–109.

10. Nader P.R., National Institute of Child Health and Human Development Study of Early Child Care and Youth Development Network (2003) Frequency and intensity of activity of third-grade children in physical education. *Arch.Pediatr.Adolesc.*Med., 157(2):185-190.

11. Przewęda R., J.Dobosz (2003) Growth and physical fitness of Polish youths in two successive decades. *J.Sports Med.Phys. Fitness* 43(4):465-474.

12. Sallis J.F., T.L.McKenzie, J.E.Alcaraz, B.Kolody, N.Faucette, M.F.Hovell (1997) The effects of a 2-year physical education program (SPARK) on physical activity and fitness in elementary school students. *Am.J.Public Health,* 87:1328-1334.

13. Singerland M., J.Oomen, L.Borghouts (2011) Physical activity levels during Dutch primary and secondary school physical education. *Eur.J.Sport Sci.,* 11(4): 249-257.

14. Stupnicki R., J.Dobosz, P.Tomaszewski, K.Milde (2005) Standardisation of somatic and physical fitness variables. *Phys. Educ.Sport,* 49:72-79.

15. Stupnicki R., P.Tomaszewski, K.Milde, J.Czeczelewski, M.Lichota, J.Głogowska (2009) Body fat-based weight norms for children and youths. *Pediatr.Endocrinol Diabetes.Metab.* 15:139-143.

16. EU Physical Activity Guidelines (2008) Recommended Policy Actions in Support of Health-Enhancing Physical Activity http://ec.europa.eu/sport/library/doc/c1/pa_guidelines_4th_consolidated_draft_pl.pdf

17. Żak S. (1994) Developmental conditionings of selected motor abilities of children and youth from Cracow population. *Antropomotoryka* nr 11:3-40.

Body image of adolescent boys

Jakub Turski [1], Joanna Głogowska [1], Marcin Wilczkiewicz [2], Romuald Stupnicki [3]

[1] The Jozef Pilsudski University of Physical Education in Warsaw; [2] Department of Physical Education, University of Rzeszów; [3] University College of Physical Culture and Tourism, Pruszków, Poland

Summary

Study aim: To compare the perception of own body by adolescent boys with an external assessment.
Material and methods: Two groups of boys (45 from Warsaw, aged 15 – 16 years, and 49 from a small town in South-Eastern Poland, aged 16 years) were studied by using standard body image templates containing 9 shapes. Every boy indicated the perceived shape and that he wished to have. The external assessment was done by the same investigator and that assessment served to classify boys as underweight (n = 4), normal (n = 51) or overweight (n = 39; Shapes 1 – 2, 3 – 4 and 5 – 9, respectively) and to correlate the scores with BMI.
Results: The external and self-assessments were concordant in overweight boys, the desired shapes being significantly lower only in Group 1. The percentage of overweight boys was significantly ($p<0.05$) higher in Group 1 than in Group 2. "Normal" boys from Group 1 significantly ($p<0.001$) overrated their body shape compared with external rating. External ratings of body shape significantly correlated with BMI values in both groups alike ($r = 0.82$, $p<0.001$).
Conclusions: The presented approach to body shape studies may contribute to preventing biosocial disorders in adolescent boys brought about by thoughtless striving for an ideal shape promoted by mass media.

Key words: Body image – Body shape – Adolescents – Boys

Introduction

Body image has been defined as the perceived body size and shape, and the attitude towards them [6,27]. Three factors are believed to contribute to shaping body image: physical (weight-height proportions and age-related changes), interpersonal (relations with parents and mates) and emotional [10]. Thompson [24] turns attention to physiological changes associated with growth, development and adolescence, as well as the perception of the community to those changes and to socio-cultural factors (attributing the beauty features to slim, fit bodies). Also, other factors – family, friends, mass media, etc., contribute to shaping body image. An important role is played by parents, who shape dietary habits and perceptions of body attractiveness. In case of even slight disorders in appetite or in negative perception of child's body, the parents are expected to provide adequate support [2].

The growth-related changes in body height and mass may often induce a distorted perception of own body. The model male and female bodies promoted in mass media induce in adolescents a lack of self-confidence with respect to own body [8]. Teenagers keep confronting their bodies with the ideal ones and strive, often in vain, to attain the ideal and this leads them to detesting their bodies to the minute details [11]. In effect, adolescents experience serious difficulties with an adequate self-assessment of own bodies [16,21].

Inasmuch the size and shape of a body are genetically determined, which limits possible control, stunt bodies are usually perceived as undesirable [19]. This may additionally lower self-perception in subjects with overweight or obesity, especially in the adolescence period.

Both male and female youths are impressionable by mass media but they differ in goals – boys prefer to have a stronger shape and girls a slimmer one. In addition, male preferences are more diversified than those of women, e.g. wrestlers are robust and well muscled, basketball players are extremely tall, marathon runners are slim and supple – all those shapes are socially acceptable.

Adolescents are particularly sensitive to their outlook. When they consider their bodies as not fitting the ideal notion, they may regard themselves as ugly and unattractive and this may lead to obsessions that everybody appraises them critically. They often disregard their positives and misjudge the external appraisal. This decreases their self-confidence and may, in turn, result in civilisation diseases, e.g. bigorexia or obesity. The aim of this study was thus to assess the perception of own body by adolescent boys and to confront that perception with an external, objective rating.

Author's address Prof. Romuald Stupnicki, Stryjenskich 10/199, 02-791 Warsaw, Poland

Material and Methods

Two groups of schoolboys were studied: 45 from Warsaw, aged 15 – 16 years (Group 1), and 49 from a small town in South-Eastern Poland, aged 16 years (Group 2). Their body height was measured with a stadiometer (accuracy of 0.1 cm) and body mass using medical scales (accuracy 0.1 kg). The values of BMI were computed and related to Polish reference data [23].

Every boy was shown the template of male body shapes (Fig. 1) and was requested to indicate the shape he thought he had, the shape he wished to have; an external rating was made by us. Boys rated as having shapes 1 or 2 were classified as underweight (U), those having shapes 3 or 4 as normal (N), and shape 5 or higher as overweight (O).

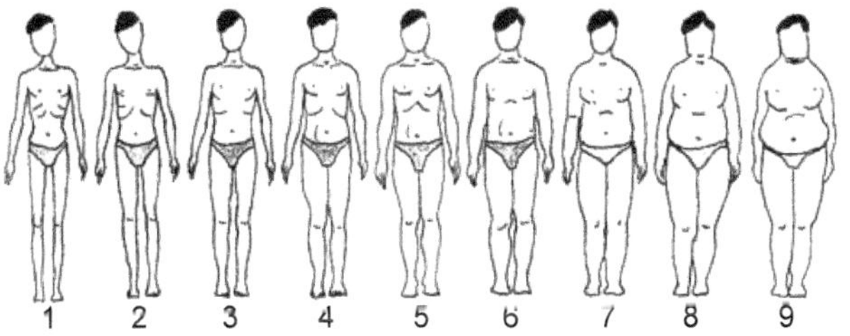

Fig. 1. Template of male body shapes [12]

Student's *t*-test for dependent data was used to assess the significance of differences between ratings. Chi-square function in the logarithmic form [22] was used to assess the significance of differences between frequencies. The level of p≤0.05 was considered significant.

Results

Mean values (±SE) of ratings of body image of boys are presented in Figs. 2 and 3. Boys classified as having normal body shape wanted to be heavier (p<0.01) and the same tendency was noted in underweight boys (n = 4 only). Overweight boys from Group 1 wanted to be lighter than they thought they were (p<0.001), unlike those from Group 2 whose desired shape did not differ from the perceived one.

The two groups of boys significantly differed from one another in some features of body image. The frequency of overweight Warsaw boys was significantly (p<0.05) greater than that of boys from Group 2 (53 and 30%, respectively) and mean BMI of those overweight boys tended to be also higher (24.4 ± 3.5 and 22.6 ± 2.2, respectively; p = 0.10). Warsaw boys of "normal" body size significantly (p<0.001) overestimated their body shape compared with the external rating; no such difference was noted in Group 2.

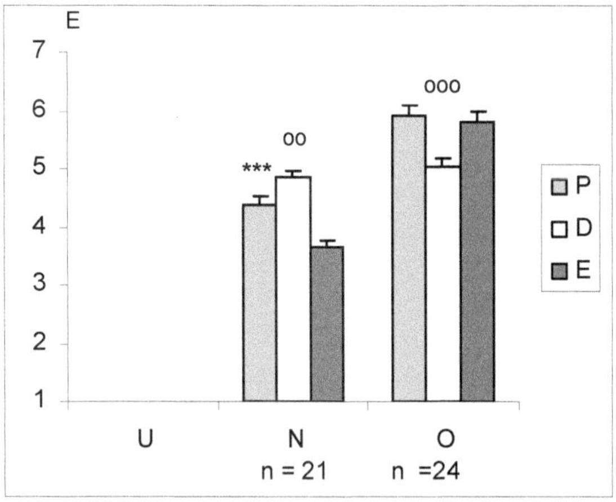

Fig. 2. Mean values (±SE) of body image ratings of boys from Group 1 (n = 45)

Legend: U – Underweight; N – Normal; O – Overweight; P – Perceived body image; D – Desired body image; E – External rating of body image; *** Significantly (p<0.001) different from E-rating; Significantly different from P-rating: °° p<0.01; °°° p<0.001

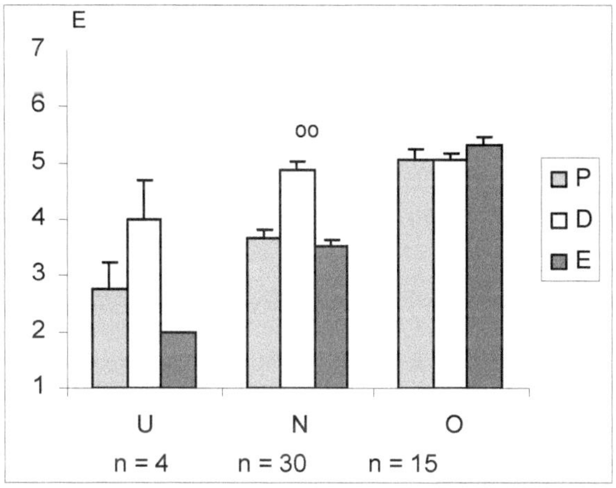

Fig. 3. Mean values (±SE) of body image ratings of boys from Group 2 (n = 49)

°° Significantly (p<0.01) different from P-rating; For explanations of other symbols see Fig. 2

The numbers of boys classified by their BMI values as underweight, normal or overweight + obese are shown in Table 1. The prevalence of overweight subjects was markedly (p<0.01) higher in Group 1 than in Group 2 (20 and 4%, respectively).

Table 1. Numbers of boys aged 15 – 16 years in various weight categories as classified by BMI

Category	Group 1 (n = 45)	Group 2 (n = 49)
Underweight	2	5
Normal	34	42
Overweight + Obese	9	2*

* Significantly (p<0.01) different from Group 1

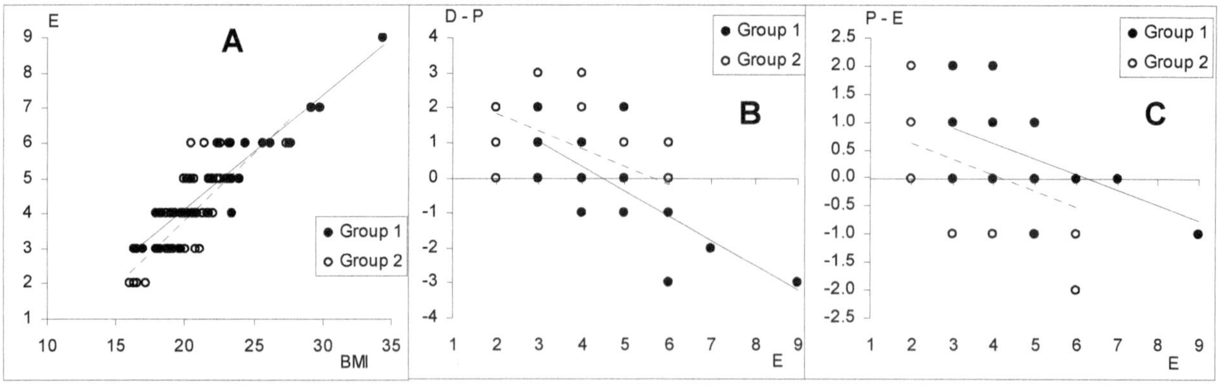

Fig. 4-A. Relationship between the external rating of body image (E) and BMI in two groups of boys aged 15 – 16 years (Group 1: n = 45; Group 2: n = 49)
Fig. 4-B. Differences between the desired and perceived body image vs. external rating of body image in two groups of boys aged 15 – 16 years
Fig. 4-C. Differences between the perceived and external ratings of body image in two groups of boys aged 15 – 16 years

External ratings of body shape significantly correlated with BMI values in both groups alike ($r = 0.82$, $p<0.001$; Fig. 4-A). The differences between the desired and perceived body shapes, as well as those between the perceived ones and external ratings, negatively correlated with the external ratings. Regarding the former relationship (Fig. 4-B), the average zero difference (D - P) corresponded to the external body shape rating equal to 4.5 in Group 1; Group 2 did not differ significantly in that respect. In contrast, both groups differed significantly ($p<0.001$) in the other relationship (P - E vs. E); the regression lines were parallel to one another and intersection points, or average zero differences, were shifted by two body shape ranks (4 and 6.2 for Groups 2 and 1, respectively; Fig. 4-C).

Discussion

The presented results suggest that non-overweight urban boys, unlike those from a small town, overrate their body shapes by nearly one degree in the 9-point scale. That inadequate perception of own body is probably characteristic of the adolescence period, when the system of values and body perception are being shaped, and supports the reports of other authors [16,21]. The between-group differences in body size distribution could have been due to between-region differences in social inequalities, the economic standards in Warsaw being higher than those in the province. Similar results were reported by Zaborskis *et al.* [28] who found differences between e.g. United States and Lithuania in body perception.

Adolescents are particularly susceptible to "ideal body" models, their peers and mass media having the most effective influence [5,14]. In effect, adolescent boys may not objectively assess their bodies which, in turn, may result in not accepting them [7,13,26]. The fact that boys of "normal" build (Shapes 3 and 4), especially the urban ones, tended to be heavier is disquieting as it might increase the risk of uncontrolled diets, exhausting training or even of pharmacological supplements. Such boys believe that a slim but muscular and strong body is a prerequisite to overcoming all obstacles, to make new contacts, to achieve recognition and prestige [1,15,25]. Despite all those sacrifices, only few of them achieve the perfect body, the other ones remain disillusioned and the efforts they made induce sadness and embarrassment and may result in eating disorders [12,20].

Studies on schoolboys, whose body shapes deviate from the "normal" ones, indicate their low self-esteem, low social adaptivity and signs of environmental isolation [17]. Similar results were noted in obese subjects whose social rejection was associated with lower self-esteem and self-perception compared with their mates [3]. Negative perception of own body may induce permanent anxiety and an urge to apply specific diets [4,18].

Summing up, adolescent boys strive for gaining weight in order to shape a pretty, muscular body, like the ideal one promoted by mass media; such attempts may, however, bring about diverse disorders. Therefore, a good insight into the body shape perceptions, especially in the adolescence period, is essential in preventing possible disorders. The presented data may be of assistance in attaining that effect.

References

1. Andersen A.E., L.Didomenico (1992) Diet vs. shape content of popular male and female magazines: A dose-response relationship to the incidence of eating disorders? *Int.J.Eat.Disorders,* 11:283-287.

2. Ata R., A.Ludden, M.Lally (2007) The effects of gender and family, friend, and media influences on eating behaviors and body image during adolescence. *J.Youth Adolesc.*, 36:1024-1037.

3. Ball G.D., J.D.Marshall, L.J.McCargar (2005) Physical activity, aerobic fitness, self-perception, and dietary intake in at risk of overweight and normal weight children. *Can.J.Diet.Pract. Res.,* 66:162-169.

4. Beneditto M.C., C.Tordera, C.Botella Arbona (2003) Body image and restrictive eating behavior in adolescents. *Ann.Pediatr.,* 58:268-272.

5. Cash T.F. (1994). Body Image and weight changes in multisite comprehensive very-low-calorie diet program. *Behav.Therapy,* 25:239-254.

6. Cash T.F., T.Pruzinski (1990) Body Images: Development, Deviance, and Change. Guilford, New York.

7. Collins M.E. (1991) Body figure perceptions and preferences among preadolescent children. *Int.J.Eat.Disorders,* 10:199-208.

8. Dion K., E.Berscheid, E.Walter (1972) What is beautiful is good. *J.Personal.Soc.Psychol.,* 24/3:285-290.

9. Fallon A.E., P.Rozin (1985) Sex differences in perception of desirable body shape. *A.Abnorm.Psychol.,* 94:102-105.

10. Garner D.M. (1997) The 1997 body image survey results. *Psychol.Today*, January:30-84.

11. Garner D.M., P.E.Garfinkel (1981) Body image in anorexia nervosa: Measurement, theory, and clinical implications. *Int.J.Psychiatry Med.,* 11:263-284.

12. Higgins T. (1987) Self-discrepancy: A theory relating self and affect. *Psychol.Rev.,* 94:319-396.

13. Laessle R.G., S.Kitel, M.M.Fichter, K.M.Pirke (1988) Cognitive correlates of depression in patients with eating disorders. *Int.J.Eat.Disorders,* 7:681-686.

14. Maes L., C.Vereecken, M.Johnston (2001) Eating and dieting. In: Health Behaviour in School-Aged Children: a World Health Organization Cross-National Study. Research Protocol for the 2001/02 survey. C.Currie, O.Samdal, W.Boyce, B.Smith (eds.) University of Edinburgh, Edinburgh pp.39-58.

15. Marzano-Parisoli M.M. (2001) The contemporary construction of perfect body image: Body building, exercise addiction, and eating disorders. *Quest,* 53:216-230.

16. Mulvihill C., A.Nemeth, C.Vereecken (2004) Body image, weight control and body weight. In: C.Currie, C.Roberts, A.Morgan, R.Smith, W.Settertobulte, O.Samdal, V.B.Rassmussen (eds.) Young People's Health in Context: International Report from the HBSC 2001/02 Survey. WHO Policy Series: Health Policy for Children and Adolescents No. 4, WHO Regional Office for Europe, Copenhagen:120-129 www.hbsc.org/publications.

17. Salmon G. (1998) Bullying in schools: self reported anxiety, depression, and self esteem in secondary school pupils. *BMJ,* 317:924-925.

18. Slade P. (1985) A review of body image studies in anorexia nervosa and bulimia nervosa. *J.Psychiatry Res.,* 19:255-265.

19. Smolak L., M.P.Levine (2001) Body image in children. In: J. K.Thompson, L.Smolak (eds.) Body Image Eating Disorders and Obesity in Youth. Assessment, Prevention, and Treatment. American Psychological Association, Washington DC, pp. 41-66.

20. Stice E., E.Schupak-Neuberg, H.E.Shaw, R.I.Stein (1994) Relation of media exposure to eating disorders symptomatology: An examination of mediating mechanizm. *J.Abnorm.Psychol.,* 4:836-840.

21. Stunkard A.J., J.Albaum (1981) The accuracy of self- reported weights. *Am.J.Clin.Nutr.,* 34:1593-1599.

22. Stupnicki R. (2008) Analysis and Presentation of Questionnaire Data. University of Physical Education Editions, Warsaw, Poland.

23. Stupnicki R., P.Tomaszewski, K.Milde, J.Czeczelewski, M.Lichota, J.Głogowska (2009) Body fat-based weight norms for children and youths. *Pediatr.Endocrinol.Diabetol.Metab.,* 15:141-145.

24. Thompson J.K. (2001) Assessing body image disturbance: measure, methodology, and implementation. In: J.K.Thompson (ed.) Body Image, Eating Disorders, and Obesity. An Integrative Guide for Assessment and Treatment. American Psychological Association, Washington DC., pp. 49-81

25. Thompson J.K. (1990) Body Image Disturbance: Assessment and Treatment. Pergamon Press, Elmsford NY.

26. Truby H., S.J.Paxton (2002) Development of the children's body image scale. *Br.J.Clin.Psychol.,* 41:185-203.

27. Williams, J.M., C.E.Currie (2000) Self-esteem and physical development during early adolescence. *J.Early Adolesc.,* 20:129-149

28. Zaborskis A., G.Petronyte, L.Sumskas, M.Kuzman, R.J. Iannotti (2008) Body image and weight control among adolescents in Lithuania, Croatia, and the United States in the context of global obesity. *Croat.Med.J.* 49:233-242.

Physical activity of soldiers in the Polish Armed Force's military administration units and special units

Andrzej Tomczak

Department of Physical Education, General Staff of the Polish Armed Forces, Warsaw; The Jozef Pilsudski University of Physical Education in Warsaw, Faculty of Physical Education and Sport in Biala Podlaska, Poland

Summary

Study aim: To determine physical activity levels of soldiers in military administration units and special units.
Material and methods: The research included 58 military administration soldiers (male) and 45 special unit soldiers. The average age of the military administration soldiers was 45.2 ± 5.54 years, whereas in the case of special unit soldiers it was 31.4 ± 4.40 years. The research tool employed was the International Physical Activity Questionnaire (IPAQ), long version, last 7 days.
Results: According to the adopted criteria, all special unit soldiers and 41.4% of the military administration soldiers were assigned a high level of physical activity ($p<0.001$). Of the researched soldiers in the military administrative units, 29.3% were assigned to the adequate level and 29.3% were assigned to the inadequate level. One in two soldiers from military administration units does not participate in mandatory physical education classes nor do they compensate for the shortage of physical activity in their leisure time.
Conclusions: Definite steps should be taken regarding broadly based promotion of health and physical activity among Polish Armed Forces soldiers.

Key words: Regular soldiers – Physical activity – IPAQ

Introduction

Numerous academic studies bear out the notion that in terms of one's health, physical activity functions as a preventive measure [5,6,13,17]. Undertaking physical activity plays an important role in the battle against the ever-increasing problems – seen both within a society and its armed forces – of being overweight, obesity, circulatory system diseases, and diabetes [1,4,8,16]. A lack of exercise and an unhealthy diet lead to being overweight or obesity. This disease of civilization affects about one-half to two-thirds of societies in highly developed countries [20]. As far as the Polish population is concerned, it has been estimated that being overweight and obesity affect about 50-60% of people [19]. It is the result of poor diet and low levels of physical activity, the effects of which Polish society has been suffering for years. Research conducted in 2003-2005 within the framework of the National Health Survey in Poland – Project WOBASZ – showed that about 30% of the Polish population does not do any physical exercise that lasts for more than 30 minutes. Furthermore, based on the analysis of the results of Eurobarometer surveys conducted in 2010, it was determined that only 3% to 6% of Polish males aged 25-45 years regularly undertake physical activity, and only 19% with some regularity [18]. In comparison to the male population of the European Union, these results are significantly lower (in the EU from 7% to 9% and 31%, respectively). The ever-increasing lack of exercise among the Polish children and teenagers constitutes an alarming phenomenon [3]. In the future, it could lead to an increased percentage of overweight or obese people.

Being a regular soldier requires special psychophysical predispositions, which are first evaluated as part of a qualification procedure for candidates wanting to join the armed forces of the Republic of Poland, and then periodically during their subsequent military service. According to legal requirements, a regular soldier is to have his or her physical fitness evaluated annually. If the soldier obtains an unsatisfactory mark in 2 consecutive years, he or she will suffer formal consequences. Until 2012, it was considered a mandatory discharge from military service; beginning in 2012, it results in lowering an overall score to satisfactory on the periodical evaluation. The soldier evaluated as such is required to participate in physical education classes in order to maintain physical fitness, thus allowing the soldier to effectively perform official duties. The main objective of these classes is to develop and enhance motor abilities, physical skills, and psychophysical dispositions. The secondary objective is to develop a habit of regular participation in physical recreation.

Author's address Dr Andrzej Tomczak, General Staff of the Polish Armed Forces, Rakowiecka 4a, 00-904 Warsaw, Poland

Thus far, the results of research upon which the levels of physical activity among soldiers were determined differ. In 2008, research employing the International Physical Activity Questionnaire was conducted among soldiers of land forces that took part in training at the Training Center for Land Forces. Based on the research results, those soldiers were given a high grade and an adequate level of physical activity [9]. Additional research, conducted by Migasiewicz *et al.* [10], showed that almost 46% of soldiers from elite units such as the 25th Air Cavalry Brigade were not interested in any physical activity whatsoever [10]. Furthermore, Sokołowski *et al.* [15], after having conducted research among the candidates for non-commissioned officers of the land forces, assigned to more than half of them an inadequate physical activity level [15]. The results of this research should not come as a surprise, since soldiers come from a certain society and they are a reflection of it. They go through the same education system. Therefore, their attitudes towards physical activity are, therefore, more or less the same as the greater society. Possibly, attitudes vary based on the upbringing received at home. However, as far as commitment to matters related to physical activity is concerned, there are higher expectations in the case of soldiers than society at large, as soldiers are in a profession that requires better physical fitness and mental endurance to begin with. The aim of the conducted research was thus to determine physical activity levels of soldiers from military administration units and special units.

Material and Methods

The research included 58 soldiers (male) from organizational units that together make up the Ministry of National Defense (in this paper conventionally referred to as military administration) and 45 soldiers (male) from special units. The average age of the military administration soldiers was 45.2 ± 5.5 years (aged 33 – 58 years), whereas in the case of special unit soldiers it was 31.4 ± 4.40 years (27 – 44 years).

The research tool employed was the International Physical Activity Questionnaire (IPAQ), long version, covering last 7 days [21]. The research was conducted in November. It had been decided that it was a typical military period during which there was no active preparation for a physical fitness assessment. The research did not include those soldiers who had gone on an official trip or doctor's leave within at least 10 days prior to the questionnaire. Research participants were provided with guidelines on how to complete the questionnaire.

A detailed analysis encompassed the answers provided by the participants to questions from the 2 parts of the questionnaire: part 1 – "Job related physical activity" and part 4 – "Recreation, sport, and leisure-time physical activity." The mean time of a given physical activity was calculated as well as the intensity rates corresponding to the multiples of basal metabolic rate (Metabolic Equivalent of Task, MET). The overall level of physical activity was determined based on the adopted criteria [21].

In order to compare the mean values of the duration of individual activities, a Student's *t*-test for independent samples was employed; fraction differences were assessed with the use of a chi-square test. For the assessment of significance of difference, $\alpha = 0.05$ was adopted.

Results

The conducted research showed considerable differences in the levels of physical activity undertaken by soldiers from special units and military administration units. The difference can be observed both in the intensity of the undertaken physical activity as well as its duration (Tables 1 and 2). In practicing their profession, the military administration soldiers devote about three-quarters less time for physical activity, either intensive or moderate ($p<0.001$), as compared to special unit soldiers. Similarly, in their leisure time, the military administration soldiers devote less time to physical activity than the special unit soldiers (about 45% less of time for intensive physical activity and 75% less for moderate physical activity; $p<0.05$).

Table 1. Physical activities undertaken by the special units (n = 45) and military administration (n=58) soldiers during their professional duties (mean ±SD)

Physical activities	Special units	Military administration
Intensive		
Days/week	4,8 ± 0,7	1,2 ± 1,6*
Minutes/day	99,7 ± 45,7	30,0 ± 38,5*
Moderate		
Days/week	3,7 ± 2,0	1,1 ± 1,6*
Minutes/day	65,3 ± 39,6	20,2 ± 37,1*
Walking		
Days/week	4,9 ± 1,3	2,2 ± 2,3
Total time of walking	42,0 ± 19,6	36,7 ± 36,0

* Significantly ($p<0.001$) different from Special units

All special unit soldiers who participated in the research stated that while practicing their profession they undertook intensive and moderate activity as well as walking (which lasted more than 10 minutes per individual event). However, in the case of the military administration soldiers, 61% of participants undertook intensive activity, 66% moderate activity, and 50% walking, all types of activities being significantly different ($p<0.001$) than those of the special unit soldiers. Significantly more soldiers from the special units, as compared to the military administration soldiers, declared undertaking leisure time physical activity, both intensive (88% and 60% respectively, $p<0.001$) and moderate (55% and 34% respectively, $p<0.05$). About 80% of participating soldiers, regardless of the nature of their service, declared undertaking activity related to walking.

Table 2. Physical activities undertaken by the special units (n = 45) and military administration (n=58) soldiers in their leisure time (mean ±SD)

Physical activities	Special units	Military administration
Intensive		
Days/week	3,75 ± 2,0	1,74 ± 1,81**
Minutes/day	74,2 ± 42,2	41,5 ± 41,4*
Moderate		
Days/week	1,73 ± 1,60	0,42 ± 0,7**
Minutes/day	48,4 ± 43,5	31,0 ± 43,1
Walking		
Days/week	3,7 ± 2,6	3,6 ± 2,7
Total time of walking	41,2 ± 31,8	38,7 ± 25,3

Significantly different from Special units: * $p<0.05$; ** $p<0.001$

The mean value of MET for the special unit soldiers, calculated together for job-related and leisure-time activities, amounted to 8624 ± 2275 MET (5083 MET – job, 3540 MET – leisure). It was significantly ($p<0.001$) higher than the one observed among the military administration soldiers, i.e. 2630 ± 1286 MET (1385 MET – job, 1245 MET – leisure). According to the adopted criteria, all soldiers from the special units and 41.4% of soldiers from the military administration were assigned a high level of physical activity. Of the researched soldiers in the military administrative units, 29.3% were assigned to the adequate and the same fraction to the inadequate level.

Discussion

The Physical Culture Regulations for the Armed Forces of the Republic of Poland state that the special unit soldiers should have 6 hours of physical education classes per week, whereas other soldiers should have at least 4 hours. Analysis of the research results showed that active duty military administration soldiers devoted approximately 50 minutes per week to intensive and moderate activities. It proves that they do not participate in the mandatory physical education classes. Furthermore, intensive and/or moderate activities are only undertaken by approximately 60% of those soldiers. The data is not optimistic in light of general health recommendations, which state that only physical training that results in energy expenditure of over 2000 kcal/week constitutes the minimum recommended value for the prophylaxis of the diseases of civilization. The obtained results indicate that only 1 in 3 soldiers from military administration units fulfills the minimum recommended energy expenditure for the prophylaxis of the diseases of civilization, whereas the average weekly energy expenditure of the military administration soldiers comes close to the above-specified minimum.

According to the research conducted by Piątkowska [14], in "the last seven days" 53.4% of Polish society did not undertake any intensive physical activity; 39.8% did not undertake moderate physical activity. The values are similar to those determined in European Union countries (57.4% and 40%, respectively). The population percentage of the European Union countries that declared a high level of physical activity is quite varied. It ranges from 44.2% (the Netherlands) to 22.9% (Sweden), and in the case of Poland it amounts to 33.5%. At the same time, a low level of physical activity was attributed to 27.9% of Poles [14]. Generally speaking, it can be stated that the representative levels of physical activity in Polish society correspond to the levels seen in military administration soldiers. Their physical activity level is also similar to the level determined for the personnel in executive management, out of which only 27% fulfills the recommended physical activity minimum needed to lead a healthy lifestyle [11]. If we are talking about regular soldiers, it seems that all soldiers should demonstrate a high physical activity level. Such a level guarantees proper physical preparation needed to perform official duties both at home and abroad (military missions). In light of the results presented in this paper pertaining to own research as well as other studies conducted by different authors, greater emphasis should be placed on the promotion of a healthy lifestyle within the Armed Forces of the Republic of Poland through the introduction of special programs promoting physical activity and a healthy lifestyle. Soldiers should be obliged to undertake regular physical activity not only by the "awareness of the necessity to stay fit," but also by an obligatory annual physical fitness assessment. However, considering current physical fitness assessments, which vary based on age, gender, military unit and official post, achieving the minimum physical fitness level (a satisfactory mark) does not require soldiers to undertake regular physical activity. Additionally, a certain paradox can be observed: despite being assigned to the identical official post (e.g., platoon or a company commander), soldiers of different ages or different sexes undergo different physical fitness assessments, the difference being in exercises and norms. In light of the statement above, a question must be posed as to the purpose of physical fitness assessment among soldiers. The criticism regarding the lack of logic here has been voiced for many years in the circles of the military physical culture during conferences organized by the Polish Association of Physical Culture, Physical Culture Section of the Armed Forces. The most common justification for the physical fitness assessments being different based on gender included the anatomical and physiological differences between male and female soldiers. However, there are numerous examples, both within sports and the uniformed services, which show that properly selected and trained women achieve better results than the average male. The introduction of a uniform physical fitness assessment for all soldiers and correlating the physical fitness norms to the requirements of a post that a soldier is supposed to hold (regardless of gender) is fully substantiated. Another issue that needs to be resolved is related to a rational necessity for the universal introduction of task-oriented physical fitness assessments. Resolving these matters should contribute indirectly to the increase in the level of physical activity and also indicate which forms of physical activity should be undertaken by soldiers (task-oriented psychophysical preparation).

Considerable differences can also be seen in relation to marks obtained on annual physical fitness assessments by soldiers from special units and military administration units. Generally, the former group, despite more stringent criteria, obtains very good marks, whereas in the military administration group, good marks prevail as well as a higher rate of doctor's leaves.

In the Polish Armed Forces, only military pilots currently receive special attention concerning physical fitness, health training, and the prophylaxis of the diseases of civilization. They participate annually in fitness camps that last for 3 weeks. During that time, participants' physical stamina and fitness are evaluated, and classes are offered on different forms of physical recreation, physical education, and health promotion. According to the results of research conducted in 2008, military pilots confirmed that classes in health promotion considerably enhanced their knowledge about a healthy lifestyle [16].

Soldiers from military administration units, whose job is sedentary, belong to a risk group as far as the diseases of civilization are concerned. Therefore, a minimizing factor should encompass regular participation in physical education and recreation classes. An associated, albeit separate, matter is to determine whether those soldiers who do not participate in mandatory physical education classes should be allowed to undergo physical fitness assessment. They constitute a risk group that can suffer injuries while undertaking sporadic physical activity with greater intensity dictated by the circumstances.

Analysis of the results of the research conducted for the purposes of this paper indicates that a commonplace opinion that the armed forces are physically active is not true. In general, only soldiers from special units devote a lot of time to physical activity. The reality is more disturbing in the case of soldiers from military administration units. This professional group, as well as others, should receive care from the physical culture specialists within the Armed Forces of the Republic of Poland and the military health services.

While we move towards a small and professional army, each soldier's health and physical fitness are valuable. Thus, all soldiers should be regularly acquainted with the tenets of health training, and these should be integrated into practice and everyday life. That is why it is worth considering including all personnel of the Polish Armed Forces in a few days of fitness training that which would encompass practical recreational activities as well as information about diet, individual physical training, and threats related to an overweight and sedentary lifestyle. Analysis of results pertaining to the research conducted on numerous participants shows that physical activity plays an important role in decreasing the occurrences of the diseases of civilization as well as mortality [7,12]. Carlsson *et al.* [7]. with their research on the lifestyles of twins, also proved that it is not genetic factors that are the main factors in maintaining good health, but rather physical activity. It refutes a commonplace opinion that says that genes are mostly responsible for our health and we ourselves do not have a real impact on it. Instead, as it turns out, our health is to a great extent in our hands.

Summing up, the obtained research results constitute an alarming warning, which should motivate physical education specialists and military health services to take definite steps regarding broadly based health promotion among regular soldiers, since 1 in 2 soldiers assigned to military administration units does not participate in the mandatory physical education classes nor compensates for the shortage of physical activity in leisure time.

References

1. Adams R.A., T.Higgins, S.Potter, S.A.Evans (2012) The effect of physical activity on haematological predictors of cardiovascular risk - evidence of a dose response. *Clin.Hemorheol. Microcirc.*, 52(1):57-65.

2. Bergier J., L.Kapka-Skrzypczak, P.Biliński, P.Paprzycki, A.Wojtyła (2012) Physical activity of Polish adolescents and young adults according to IPAQ: A population based study. *Ann.Agric.Environ.Med.*, 23;19(1):109-115.

3. Biernat E., R.Stupnicki, B.Lebiedziński, L.Janczewska (2008) Assessment of physical activity by applying IPAQ questionnaire. *Phys.Educ.Sport*, 52, 46-52.

4. Blair S., Y.Cheng, J.Holder (2001) Is physical activity or physical fitness more important in defining health benefits? *Med.Sci.Sport Exerc.*, 33(6 Suppl):S379-399.

5. Blair S. N., H.W.Kohl, R.S.Paffenbarger, D.G.Jr Clark, K.H.Cooper, L.W.Gibbons (1989) Physical fitness and all-cause mortality: a prospective study on healthy men and women. *JAMA*, 3;262(17):2395-2401.

6. Bouchard C., J.P.Depres (1995) Physical activity and health: atherosclerotic, metabolic, and hypertensive diseases. *Res.Q. Exerc.Sport.*, 66(4):268-275.

7. Carlsson S., T.Andersson, P.Lichtenstein, K.Michaelsson, A.Ahlborn (2007) Physical activity and mortality: Is the association explained by genetic selection? *Am.J.Epidemiol*, 166(3): 255-259.

8. Henrykowska G., A.Tomczak (2008) Prevention of overweight and obesity among military aircraft staff. In: M. Kozioł-Montewka, S. Spisacka (eds.) Współczesne zagrożenia zdrowia. PWSZ, Biała Podlaska, pp. 165-176.

9. Mierzejewski R. (2008) Evaluation of the level of the land-forces solders' physical activity on the base of the International Physical Activity Questionnaire (IPAQ) (English abstract). In: E. Szczepanowska, M. Sokołowski (eds.) Psychical activity and nutrition as the conditions for health promotion. Wyd. Wielkopolska Wyższa Szkoła Turystyki i Zarządzania w Poznaniu, Poznań, pp. 225-232.

10. Migasiewicz J., P.Kukulski, K.Kurzawski (2007) Interest in sports of the cadre from selected units of the Polish Army. In: M. Sokołowski (ed.) Biosocial effects of military service as basic for further improvement of future physical education and sports programmes. AWF Poznań, pp. 397-404.

11. Nawrocka A., A.Pronczuk, W.Mynarski, W.Garbaciak (2012) Physical activity of top level managers in the context of the public health recommendations. *Med.Pr.*, 63(3):271-279.

12. Nocon M., T.Hiemann, F.Müller-Riemenschneider, F.Thalau, Roll S., Willich S.N. (2008) Association of physical activity with all-cause and cardiovascular mortality: a systematic review and meta-analysis. *Eur.J.Cardiovasc.Prev.Rehabil.*, 15(3):239-246.

13. Paffenbarger R.S.Jr, R.T.Hyde, A.L.Wing, I.M.Lee, D.L.Jung, J.B.Kampart (1993) The association of changes in physical activity level and other lifestyle characteristics with mortality among men. *N.Engl.J.Med.*, 328(8):538-45.

14. Piątkowska M.E. (2012) Self-rated physical activity across Europe - Poland and other European countries. *Biol.Sport*, 29(1): 23-31.

15. Sokołowski M., M.Mrozkowiak, A.Kaiser. (2009) International physical activity questionnaire (IPAQ) as a tool to assess the potential regular soldiers. In: M.Sokołowski (ed.) Contemporary tasks, problems and perspectives of physical education in the army. Polish Scientific Physical Education Association Section of Physical Education in the Army, Warsaw, pp. 349-355.

16. Tomczak A., A.Sigłowa (2008) Health promotion of Polish military pilots during fitness trainings in Military Training and Fitness Centres. In: E.Zderkiewicz (ed.) Cultral behaviours conditioning wellness. Lublin, pp. 203-212.

17. Warburton D., C.W.Nicol, S.Bredin (2006) Health benefits of physical activity: the evidence. *CMAJ*, 174(6): 801-809.

18. www.dms.msport.gov.pl/app/document/file/1558/Eurobarometr_pl.pdf?field=file1

19. www.estymator.com.pl/WYNIKI/WAGA_I_NADWAGA_POLAKOW__raport.pdf

20. www.eufic.org/article/pl/page/RARCHIVE/expid/25/

21. www.ipaq.ki.se/downloads.htm.

Immediate cardiovascular effects of pranava relaxation in patients with hypertension and diabetes

Ananda Balayogi Bhavanani, Madanmohan, Zeena S, L Vithiyalakshmi

Advanced Centre for Yoga Therapy Education and Research (ACYTER), JIPMER, Puducherry, India

Summary

Study aim: To assess immediate cardiovascular effect of pranava pranayama in the supine position in patients with concomitant hypertension and diabetes.
Material and methods: Twenty-nine established patients having both hypertension and type 2 diabetes and attending regular therapy sessions were recruited and randomly allotted to pranava or control groups. Heart rate (HR) and blood pressure (BP) were recorded before and after 10 minutes of "sham relaxation" in the control group and 10 minutes of pranava pranayama in the study group.
Results: Significant ($p<0.05$) decreases of blood pressure and heart rate were observed. However, responses in the pranava and control groups were different: systolic pressure, pulse pressure, as well as mean pressure significantly decreased in the pranava group and this was not observed in the control group.
Conclusions: Pranava pranayam in the supine posture produces an integrated relaxation response, clinically valuable in patients with hypertension and diabetes.

Key words: Yoga relaxation – Pranava pranayama – Hypertension – Diabetes

Introduction

Comprehensive reviews have reported that Yoga is potentially beneficial for patients with hypertension (HT) and diabetes mellitus (DM), and that it reduces the risk profile in such populations [7,8]. Another review of relaxation therapy concluded that relaxation therapy is useful in the clinical management of HT, especially for those individuals with high BP despite pharmacological treatment [9]. Earlier studies from our laboratories have demonstrated that shavasan, a yogic relaxation technique, reduces load on the heart in normal subjects by blunting sympathetic responses with enhanced parasympathetic activity [11], while yogic relaxation training for a month reduces blood pressure (BP) and restores autonomic regulatory reflex mechanisms in hypertensive patients [20]. We have recently reported immediate beneficial effects of sukha pranayama on cardiovascular parameters in patients with HT after just 5 minutes of the technique [4].

Pranava pranayama is an important technique of the Gitananda tradition, involving slow and deep inhalation with conscious use of complete yogic breathing (mahat yoga pranayama), followed by an audible vibratory resonance of a prolonged AUM chant. This technique is usually done in the sitting position and is one of the practices taught in the comprehensive yoga therapy schedules imparted for HT and DM patients at ACYTER, JIPMER, in Puducherry, India. As the supine position is normally used for relaxation, the present study was designed to determine the immediate cardiovascular effects of pranava pranayama while resting in the supine position.

Material and Methods

The present study was conducted at the Advanced Centre for Yoga Therapy Education and Research (ACYTER), established in JIPMER, Puducherry, India. Ethical approval has been obtained by ACYTER from the Institutional Ethics Committee for studies on the effect of yoga therapy on HT and DM. The present pilot study was conducted as part of this larger study on the effects of yoga therapy in patients with HT and DM.

Twenty-nine patients receiving standard medical care for both essential HT and type 2 DM, and who were attending regular yoga therapy sessions for more than a month at ACYTER, were selected for this study by random sampling. Patients with secondary HT and those with history / signs and symptoms / laboratory reports suggestive of nephrological, neurologic, and ophthalmologic complications due to HT or DM were excluded from the study.

Author's address Dr Ananda Balayogi Bhavanani, Advanced Centre for Yoga Therapy, Education and Research (ACYTER), JIPMER, Pondicherry - 605006, India

For this study, 15 of the patients were male and 14 of the patients were female; the average age was 56.66 ± 10.9 years, the average BMI was 25.99 ± 3.5. All subjects were receiving standard medical management for more than 3 years with antihypertensive and oral antidiabetic medications under the supervision of consultants in the department of medicine at JIPMER. Patients on medication were selected, as it has been previously suggested that the combination of relaxation and medication has the maximum effect [6].

Subclassification of the subjects according to JNC VII [17] revealed that based on either systolic pressure (SP) or diastolic pressure (DP) values, 16 were in the prehypertensive range, 7 in Stage I HT, and one in Stage II HT, even with regular medication. This is pertinent, as a previous review had concluded that relaxation therapy is useful in the clinical management of HT, especially for individuals with high BP despite pharmacological treatment [9].

Informed consent was obtained by one of the investigators and the subjects were then randomly allotted to either the pranava or control groups. There were 8 males and 7 females in the pranava group with an average age of 53.47 ± 12.5 years. The control group consisted of 7 males and 7 females with an average age of 60.07 ± 7.9 years. The difference in age between groups was statistically insignificant (p = 0.103)

Subjects were familiarized with the study protocol and then given 5 minutes of supine rest. Heart rate (HR) and BP were then recorded from their left upper arm in the supine position using a non-invasive semi-automatic BP monitor (CH-432, Citizen Systems, Tokyo, Japan) with an instrumental accuracy of ± 5% for HR and ± 3 mm Hg for BP.

It has previously been suggested that one needs a sham treatment group rather than a mere nonspecific relaxation or "no treatment" control group when studying and comparing effects of psycho-physiologic therapies [5]. Hence, in the present study we have used a "sham relaxation" control group that performed 10 minutes of simple supine resting for the first and last 2 minutes; they were given verbal commands suggesting relaxation of different body parts from feet to head for the intervening 6 minutes. HR and BP were recorded again at the end of the 10 minutes of "sham relaxation." The pranava group, on the other hand, performed 10 minutes of supine rest that included simple conscious resting in shavasana for the first and last 2 minutes with a performance of pranava pranayama for the intervening 6 minutes. The technique of pranava pranayama involves the performance of 3 rounds of slow and deep yogic breathing into low chest, mid chest and upper chest, followed by the prolonged audible rendition of the akara, ukara, and makara nada (Aaa, Uuu, and Mmm sounds), respectively, during exhalation phase. Following this, subject performs 3 rounds of the complete yogic breathing (mahat yoga pranayama) technique with an audible rendition of omkara nada (AUM sound) during exhalation phase. The time taken for the exhalation with nada is approximately 3 times the time taken for each inhalation, thus maintaining a ratio of 1:3. After completing pranava pranayama, which took approximately 6 minutes, the subject continued to rest in the supine position for another 2 minutes, before post-intervention HR and BP were recorded. Pulse pressure (PP) was calculated as the difference between systolic pressure (SP) and diastolic pressure (DP), mean pressure (MP) as DP + 1/3 PP, rate-pressure product (RPP) as HR × SP / 100, and double product (Do P) as HR × MP / 100.

All data passed normality testing by Kolmogorov-Smirnov Test and was therefore analyzed using ANOVA for repeated measures followed by Tukey's test (*post hoc*). Effects of *Group* (pranava, control) and *Measurement* (pre, post) as well as their interaction were assessed. Statistical analysis was done using STATISTICA 9.1 (StatSoft, USA). The level of α=0.05 was considered significant.

Results

The mean ± SE values of cardiovascular variables before and after performance of pranava pranayama and "sham relaxation" control are presented in Table 1. Significant changes of means (*Measurement* effect) were observed for all variables tested except DP, while the effects of *Group* were not found. Significant interactions of *Group*×*Measurement* occurred for SP ($F_{1,27}$ = 17.69, $p<0.001$), PP ($F_{1,27}$ = 26.06, $p<0.001$) and MP ($F_{1,27}$ = 6.63, $p<0.05$). Interactions revealed differential responses in the pranava and control groups. Post-hoc tests showed that SP, PP, as well as MP decreased significantly in the pranava group; this was not observed in the control group.

Discussion

Enhanced cardiac parasympathetic tone is postulated to be an important mechanism underlying the beneficial effects of the relaxation response [15]. It has also been suggested that a holistic and complete sympathovagal homeostatic development is possible only by the practice of yoga in its true form and spirit [13]. A previous study conducted by our laboratories reported significant blunting of cold pressor-induced increase in HR, BP, and RPP following the practice of shavasan, thus giving evidence that shavasan reduces the load on the heart by blunting the sympathetic response along with an enhanced parasympathetic activity [11].

Table 1. Immediate effect of pranava pranayama in supine position on cardiovascular variables in patients having concomitant hypertension and diabetes (mean ± SE)

Variable	Pranava Group (n=15)		Control Group (n=14)		Pre-post changes	Int.
	Pre	Post	Pre	Post		
HR (beats/min)	77.5 ± 3.3	75.3 ± 3.1	84.8 ± 3.5	80.0 ± 3.5	***	–
SP (mm Hg)	134.3 ± 3.8	124.7 ± 3.2 ººº	136.3 ± 4.1	138.3 ± 4.2	*	***
DP (mm Hg)	77.2 ± 1.3	74.9 ± 1.2	77.4 ± 2.2	76.9 ± 1.6	–	–
PP (mm Hg)	57.1 ± 3.7	49.9 ± 3.0 ººº	58.9 ± 3.2	61.4 ± 3.5	*	***
MP (mm Hg)	96.2 ± 1.7	91.5 ± 1.5 ºº	97.0 ± 2.6	97.4 ± 2.2	*	*
RPP	104.5 ± 5.9	94.2 ± 4.9	116.3 ± 6.9	111.3 ± 6.7	***	–
Do P	74.8 ± 3.7	69.1 ± 3.2	82.7 ± 4.7	78.3 ± 4.5	**	–

Legend: HR - Heart rate; SP - Systolic pressure; DP - Diastolic pressure; MP - Mean pressure; PP - Pulse pressure; RPP - Rate-pressure-product; Do P - Double product; Int. - *Group×Measurement* interaction; Significantly different from pre-test: ºº $p<0.01$, ººº $p<0.001$; Significant effect: ** $p<0.05$, ** $p<0.01$; *** $p<0.001$. All baseline comparisons between groups were insignificant with $p>0.05$.

A review of relaxation therapy in the treatment of HT reported that task awareness adds to the treatment effect and suggested that relaxation therapy is useful in the clinical management of HT, especially for individuals whose BP remains high despite pharmacological treatment [9]. Most yogic relaxation practices have a task awareness element associated with them: as the performance of pranava pranayama while relaxing in the supine position is done with conscious awareness, it may be producing its beneficial effects in a similar manner to those of task awareness.

A study by Goldstein *et al.* [6] concluded that relaxation without drugs, although somewhat more effective than self monitoring alone, did not reduce BP as much as the combination of relaxation and medication. Interestingly, just as with our present study, they also found no significant changes in HR between groups. The significant decrease of HR in our control group may have been due to a reduction in physiological arousal that had been previously reported to occur from both guided relaxation and supine rest in a previous study [19].

Analysis of variance revealed significant interaction between group and measurement for SP, PP, and MP. The decreases of mean values of these variables were significantly greater in the pranava group as compared to the control group. This may be due to a decrease in venous return and resultant decrease in cardiac output occurring as a result of the prolonged exhalation phase in pranava pranayama producing a mild Valsalva-like effect due to the increased intrathoracic pressure and decreased preload to the heart. A previous study from our laboratories also reported that pranayama training of 3-month duration modulated ventricular performance by increasing parasympathetic activity and simultaneously decreasing sympathetic activity [18].

We have previously suggested that conscious deep breathing with prolonged exhalation and audible chanting during pranava pranayama may contribute towards a normalization of autonomic cardiovascular rhythms [3]. The beneficial effect of audible chanting in restoring these autonomic cardiovascular rhythms has been reported earlier [2]. It is plausible that the prolonged, audible chanting of the pranava in the present study may be producing a similar improvement in baroreflex sensitivity resulting in the normalizing of such autonomic cardiovascular rhythms.

The effects of interaction between group and measurement were not observed for RPP and Do P. However, the actual difference in Do P was greater in the pranava group (7.2%) as opposed to the control group (4.7%). This shows a trend that suggests further statistical significance of interaction could be achieved with a larger sample size. RPP and Do P are especially important in patient care, as they are indirect indicators of myocardial oxygen consumption and load on the heart, thereby signifying a lowering of strain on the heart [12]. RPP also provides a simple measure of overall heart rate variability (HRV) in hypertensive patients and is a surrogate marker in situations where HRV analysis is not available [14]. Reduction in RPP is thus representative of enhanced HRV power, implying better cardiac autonomic regulation in our subjects having concomitant DM and HT that are both major risk factors implicated in the causation of cerebrovascular accidents as well as other cardiovascular and neurological complications. Hence, this technique can be considered a means of primary prevention in this high-risk population, as we may be preventing the occurrence of future untoward and adverse events of high mortality and morbidity.

Pranava pranayama involves the audible chanting of the aaa, uuu, and mmm sounds and when performed in the supine position is strikingly similar to the deep relaxation technique (DRT) popularized by SVYASA University, Bangalore [19]. A previous study from SVYASA reported that DRT improves sustained attention and reduces the state of anxiety [10], while another reported a decrease in sympathetic activity with significant reduction in O_2 consumption, HR, and skin conductance along with decreased low-frequency (LF) power and increased high-frequency HF power of the HRV spectrum [19]. Satyapriya *et al.* [16] reported an increased HF band of the HRV spectrum along with a decreased LF band and LF/HF ratio during and after a guided relaxation period in pregnant women indicating improved sympathovagal balance. This improvement in sympathovagal balance following similar yogic relaxation techniques such as DRT is possibly one of the mechanisms behind the positive changes seen in our subjects. Hence, the reduction in RPP in our subjects having concomitant HT and DM implies a better autonomic regulation of the heart that is clinically valuable from both a qualitative and quantitative perspective.

Performance of pranava pranayama in the supine position may induce an integrated relaxation response similar to the one suggested by Benson *et al.* [1]: a wakeful hypometabolic state induced by simple, non-cultic mental techniques or by traditional meditational practices. They attributed this to an integrated hypothalamic response ("relaxation response") consistent with a state of decreased sympathetic nervous system activity. They have also reported that regular elicitation of the relaxation response is useful in the management of hypertensive subjects who are already on drug therapy. Based on our findings we suggest that pranava pranayama in the supine position can achieve the same benefits in those having concomitant HT and DM.

References

1. Benson H, B.R.Marzetta, B.A.Rosner, H.M.Klemchuk (1974) Decreased blood-pressure in pharmacologically treated hypertensive patients who regularly elicited the relaxation response. *Lancet*, 303:289-291.

2. Bernardi L., P.Sleight, G.Bandinelli, S.Cencetti, L.Fattorini, J.Wdowczyc-Szulc, A.Lagi (2001) Effect of rosary prayer and yoga mantras on autonomic cardiovascular rhythms: comparative study. *BMJ*, 323:1446-1449.

3. Bhavanani A.B., Madanmohan, S.Zeena, I.V.Basavaraddi (2012) Immediate cardiovascular effects of pranava pranayama in hypertensive patients. Indian *J.Physiol.Pharmacol.*, (in press)

4. Bhavanani A.B., Madanmohan, S.Zeena (2011) Immediate effect of sukha pranayama on cardiovascular variables in patients of hypertension. *Int.J.Yoga Ther.*, 21:73-76.

5. Frankel B.L., D.J.Patel, D.Horwitz, W.T.Friedewald, K.R.Gaarder (1978) Treatment of hypertension with biofeedback and relaxation techniques. *Psychosom.Med.*, 40(4):276-293.

6. Goldstein I.B., D.Shapiro, C.Thananopavaran (1984) Home relaxation techniques for essential hypertension. *Psychosom.Med.*, 46: 398-414.

7. Innes K.E., C.Bourguignon, A.G.Taylor (2005) Risk indices associated with the insulin resistance syndrome, cardiovascular disease, and possible protection with yoga: a systematic review. *J.Am.Board Fam.Pract.*, 18:491-519.

8. Innes K.E., H.K.Vincent (2007) The influence of yoga-based programs on risk profiles in adults with type 2 diabetes mellitus: a systematic review. *Evid.Based Complement.Alternat.Med.*, 4(4):469-486.

9. Jacob R.G., H.C.Kraemer, W.S.Agras (1977) Relaxation therapy in the treatment of hypertension. A review. *Arch.Gen. Psychiatry*, 34(12):1417-1427.

10. Khemka S.S., N.H.Rao, R.Nagarathna (2009) Immediate effects of two relaxation techniques on healthy volunteers. *Indian J.Physiol.Pharmacol.*, 53:67-72.

11. Madanmohan, K.Udupa, A.B.Bhavanani, N.Krishnamurthy, G.K.Pal (2002) Modulation of cold pressor-induced stress by shavasan in normal adult volunteers. *Indian J.Physiol.Pharmacol.*, 46: 307-312.

12. Madanmohan, K.Udupa, A.B.Bhavanani, C.C.Shatapathy, A.Sahai (2004) Modulation of cardiovascular response to exercise by yoga training. *Indian J.Physiol.Pharmacol.*, 48: 461-465.

13. Pal G.K. (2008) Role of sympathovagal balance in achieving an effective homeostasis. *Biomedicine*, 28:67-68.

14. Prakash E.S., Madanmohan, K.R.Sethuraman, S.K.Narayan (2005) Cardiovascular autonomic regulation in subjects with normal blood pressure, high-normal blood pressure and recent-onset hypertension. *Clin.Exp.Pharmacol.Physiol.*, 32:488-494.

15. Sakakibara M., S.Takeuchi, J.Hayano (1994) Effect of relaxation training on cardiac parasympathetic tone. *Psychophysiology*, 31(3): 223-228.

16. Satyapriya M., H.R.Nagendra, R.Nagarathna, V.Padmalatha (2009) Effect of integrated yoga on stress and heart rate variability in pregnant women. *Int.J.Gynaecol.Obstet.*, 104:218-222.

17. Seventh Report of the Joint National Committee on Prevention, Detection, Evaluation, and Treatment of High Blood Pressure (2004) US Department of Health and Human Services. NIH Publication No. 04-5230. http://www.nhlbi.nih.gov/guidelines/hypertension/jnc7full.pdf

18. Udupa K., Madanmohan, A.B.Bhavanani, P.Vijayalakshmi, N.Krishnamurthy (2003) Effect of pranayam training on cardiac function in normal young volunteers. *Indian J.Physiol.Pharmacol.*, 47:27-33.

19. Vempati R.P., S.Telles (2002) Yoga based guided relaxation reduces sympathetic activity in subjects based on baseline levels. *Psychol.Rep.*, 90(2):487-494.

20. Vijayalakshmi P., Madanmohan, A.B.Bhavanani, A.Patil, K.Babu (2004) Modulation of stress induced by isometric handgrip test in hypertensive patients following yogic relaxation training. *Indian J.Physiol.Pharmacol.*, 48:59-64.

Acknowledgements

The authors thank the Director, MDNIY and Director, JIPMER for their support. This study was possible because ACYTER has been established as a collaborative venture between Morarji Desai National Institute of Yoga (MDNIY), New Delhi and JIPMER, Puducherry with funding from Department of AYUSH, Ministry of Health and Family Welfare, Government of India.

Prevalence of faulty posture in children and youth from a rural region in Iran

Maghsoud Eivazi Gh [1,2], Amin Alilou [1], Solmaz Ghafurinia [1], Sara Fereydounnia [3]

[1] Physiotherapy Department, Faculty of Rehabilitation Sciences, Tabriz University of Medical Sciences, Iran; [2] Physiotherapy & Rehabilitation Department, Okan University, Tuzla Kampusu Istanbul, Turkey; [3] Physiotherapy Department, Faculty of Rehabilitation Sciences, Tehran University of Medical Sciences, Iran

Summary

Study aim: To assess the presence of musculoskeletal deformities in lower extremities and to detect faulty posture in schoolchildren living in a rural region of Iran.
Material and methods: 172 schoolchildren aged 5-20 years, including 66 boys and 106 girls were screened deviations in the musculoskeletal system. Furthermore, the postural muscles including the hamstring and gastroc-soleus were examined for finding any shortness.
Results: The prevalence of cervical lordosis (22.6% vs. 6.1%), forward head posture (24.1% vs. 9.1%) and thoracic kyphosis (27.8 % vs. 7.6%) was significantly higher in girls than in boys. The prevalence of cervical lordosis, FHP, thoracic kyphosis, and genu varum increased with age; in the case of genu valgum, the situation was reversed. Genu varum was almost twice as frequent in girls as in boys (44.4% vs. 25.8%; $p<0.01$), while the genu valgum was more frequent ($p<0.001$) in boys than in girls (13.6 and 2.8, respectively). No significant age or gender-dependent differences were found for hamstring shortness (29%), gastroc-soleus shortness (21%), genu recurvatum (22%), and hallux valgus (31%).
Conclusions: Faulty posture and lower limb deformities were highly prevalent in school children in this rural region. More attention should be paid to implementing school-based screening programs aimed at early detection of any musculoskeletal-related abnormalities and taking preventive steps to reduce their negative consequences.

Key words: Faulty Posture – Children – Visual assessment

Introduction

Faulty posture is common in children and teens with a wide spectrum of symptoms and causes [7,8,15,24]. Multiple intrinsic and extrinsic factors may influence posture in children such as age, sex, height, weight, hereditary factors, the physical environment of a child, socioeconomic level, psychosocial and emotional factors, physiological changes during puberty, improper postural habits, the presence of the pain, and the testing environment [3,21,24]. Any deviation from the standard postural alignment causes excessive loads on the articular structures and weakening periarticular soft tissues like muscles, tendons, ligaments, and fascia by stretching and tethering them beyond their normal limits [20], resulting in possible heel pain, back pain and neck pain as well as structural deformities of the spine and intervertebral disk degenerations [10,30]. Therefore, early detection of musculoskeletal alterations has been a challenging task for different medical specialists [7,8,11].

Epidemiologic studies have shown that musculoskeletal problems due to any structural deviations in children are very common. The combination of hyper pronation with genu recurvatum has been considered a risk factor in recurrent knee injuries and anterior cruciate ligament ruptures in athletes due to structural malalignment and altered neuromuscular functions [4,13,19,29]. Foot problems, including hallux valgus and heel pain, are common in children with different rates of incidence (17.4%-80.0%) and gender specific tendency [17].

Although several studies have been undertaken in school children about the prevalence of faulty posture and lower limb deformity, the prevalence of postural abnormalities and lower limb deformities has never been thoroughly examined in the rural region of Turkmanchay, Iran. It is a suburb of Mianeh, one of the oldest cities in eastern Azerbaijan in northwestern Iran. This region was selected by authorities at Tabriz University of Medical Science for screening and detecting any health problems, including musculoskeletal disorders in children, and then presenting

Author's address Amin Alilou, Physiotherapy Department, Faculty of Rehabilitation Sciences, Tabriz University of Medical Sciences, Tavanir-Str, 51576-35411, Valiasr, Tabriz, Iran

a report as a small part of the larger project. This study was designed to detect any postural abnormalities in the spinal region and lower limb deformities in school-aged children by visual observation and to explore any associations with age and gender.

Material and Methods

Participants: A total of 172 children including 66 boys and 106 girls with no known impairment of the musculoskeletal system affecting the vertebral column or the limbs were screened in this study. Participants were students at primary, intermediate, and secondary schools (ages ranging from 5 to 20 years old) in the Turkmanchay region in Mianeh, Iran. The prevalence of faulty posture and lower limb deformities were assessed in boys and girls as well as in 3 different age groups: A) 5-10 years old (n = 23); B) 11-15 years old (n = 93); C) 16-20 years old (n = 49). The body mass of each child was measured by medical scale with an accuracy of 0.01 kg. Body height was measured by a hanged meter with an accuracy of 0.1 cm. Basic characteristics of studied subjects are presented in Table 1.

Table 1. Characteristics of studied subjects (mean±SD)

Variable	Boys (n = 66)	Girls (n = 106)
Age (years)	12.5 ± 2.1	13.1 ± 3.0
Body height (cm)	149.2 ± 11.0	149.6 ± 17.7
Body mass (kg)	41.3 ± 11.6	44.5 ± 12.4
BMI (kg/cm^2)	18.1 ± 3.8	19.9 ± 3.4

Inclusion criteria included: good general health; no report of pain, systemic disease, or neurological disease; no evident musculoskeletal injury or trauma; agreement to participate in this research. The criteria for exclusion were the presence of any joint stiffness and any obvious deformity. All participants had received detail information about the aims of study and had signed a consent form or received parents' permission to take part in this project. Ethical approval for performing research was obtained from the Ethical committee in research deputy of Tabriz University of Medical Sciences.

Procedure: Before performing the survey, the aims of the survey were described to school authorities. With due respect to local customs and national ethics, the screening program was designed to give the least amount of inconvenience and disturbance to students and the school schedule; therefore, each child was examined with suitable clothing. The child was instructed to stand in zero anatomic position and relax posture with face forward, arms at side, hands face forwards, and forearms in mid-position between supination and pronation.

Visual posture assessment: The participants in this study were qualitatively evaluated by physiotherapy students who had short-term training in the field of musculoskeletal problems. The examiners had a postural assessment sheet and were requested to mark any abnormality according to observation. The girl subjects were evaluated by female therapists and boys by male therapists. The subjects were asked to stand in the sagittal and frontal plane. Musculoskeletal total body screening was carried out without using a plumb line or any other postural graphic devices.

Anterior view: The position of feet, knees, and legs were observed in this view. Bowlegs or knocked knee (genu valgum and genu varum) were noted in this view as well. In addition, hallux varus or valgus and the presence of any callosities were recorded on the postural assessment sheet [20].

Lateral view: In this view, the presence of the forward head posture (FHP), any abnormalities in cervical lordosis, pathologic thoracic kyphosis, and the presences of genu recurvatum were recorded on the postural assessment sheet [20].

Muscle shortness evaluation: For detection of gastrocsoleus muscle shortness participants were asked to lie down on the bed; an examiner extended the participant's knee and while holding it in extended position, dorsi flexed the participant's ankle. If the examiner should be able to reach at least 10° to 15° of dorsi flexion by goniometer it was considered normal. Otherwise it was regarded as shortened gastrocnemius and abnormal [20].

For assessment of hamstring shortness in the 90-90 straight leg raise test, subjects were asked to lay down on a bed with both hips in 90° while the knees are bent. The subject grasped behind the knees with both hands to fix hips at 90°of flexion, then actively extended each knee respectively as much as possible. We considered 10° to 20° short of extension as normal flexibility of hamstrings by goniometer, otherwise it was considered abnormal [20].

Statistical analysis: Due to the relatively small sample size, the data was analyzed by age and gender independently. All analyses were performed by using SPSS v.15. Chi-square test was used to assess between-group differences. The level of α=0.05 was considered significant.

Results

The prevalence of soft tissue and postural abnormalities observed in the studied boys and girls is presented in Table 2. FHP posture was found to be more frequent ($p<0.01$) in the female group as compared with their male counterparts (24.1% vs. 9.1%). Moreover, cervical lordosis and thoracic kyphosis were more common in girls than in boys (respectively: 22.6% vs. 6.1%; $p<0.01$, and 27.8 % vs. 7.6%; $p<0.001$), which means the girls showed a greater tendency for spinal abnormalities.

Table 2. Frequency (%) of soft tissue and postural abnormalities observed in studied boys and girls

Variable	Boys (n = 66)	Girls (n = 106)
Cervical lordosis	6.1	22.6**
Forward head posture	9.1	24.1**
Thoracic kyphosis	7.6	27.8***
Hamstring shortness	28.8	31.5
Gastroc-soleus shortness	27.3	16.7
Genu recurvatum	28.8	19.8
Genu valgum	13.6	2.8**
Genu varum	25.8	44.4**
Hallux valgus	39.4	27.4
Dorsal calluses	33.3	23.5

Significantly different from respective value observed in boys: ** $p<0.01$; *** $p<0.001$

Total knee abnormality, including genu varum, genu valgum and genu recurvatum, was reported in a slightly more than half the students. Genu varum was the most common postural abnormality in the children with its preponderance in female students (44.4%), which was almost as twice as much in male students (25.8%; $p<0.01$), while the genu valgum was more frequent ($p<0.001$) in boys than in girls (13.6 and 2.8, respectively). Foot deformities including the presence of hallux valgus and dorsal callosities were reported in about 32% and 27% of the subjects, respectively, and were not gender-dependent.

As shown in Table 3, the prevalence of cervical lordosis, FHP, thoracic kyphosis, and genu varum increased with age; in the case of genu valgum, the situation was reversed. No significant age-dependent differences were found for hamstring shortness (29%), gastroc-soleus shortness (21%), genu recurvatum (22%), and hallux valgus (31%). Dorsal calluses were the most frequent among the subjects aged 11-15 years (34.4%).

Discussion

A child is not an adult in miniature and is not presumed to have an adult's standard alignment, as greater range of mobility and flexibility take place during growth and development. It is possible that this greater flexibility in a child may create transitional observation in the child's alignment that could be considered an abnormality in an adult [24]. In other words, it may be a physiologic entity rather than a pathologic one. Because this survey was a cross-sectional study and not longitudinal one, it was not possible to assess this connection. However, this study aimed at determining the prevalence of faulty posture and lower extremity deformities in school children in a rural district of Iran. The results show that more than 50% of the study subjects had some kind of foot or knee problems and poor posture. In the present study, we did find that the occurrence of the vertebral faulty posture was more common in girls than in boys. In the knee area, the prevalence did not follow any particular pattern but genu valgum was more frequent in boys and genu varum vice versa. This prevalence pattern may mirror the association of other musculoskeletal conditions, like shoulder and low back pain [31], which we unfortunately did not examine in our subjects. However, a shortage of health services in the studied region, parents' inability to pay for private

Table 3. Frequency (%) of soft tissue and postural abnormalities observed in 3 age groups

Variable	5-10 years (n = 23)	11-15 years (n = 93)	16-20 years (n = 49)
Cervical lordosis	4.3	14.0	26.5*
Forward Head Posture	8.7	9.7	32.7*###
Thoracic kyphosis	0.0	16.1*	34.7***#
Hamstring shortness	26.1	26.9	34.7
Gastroc-soleus shortness	13.0	24.7	18.4
Genu recurvatum	17.4	24.7	20.4
Genu valgum	21.7	7.5	0.0**
Genu varum	21.7	34.4	51.0*
Halux valgus	30.4	34.4	26.5
Dorsal calluses	7.0	34.4**	22.4

Significantly different from the group of 5-10-year-olds: * $p<0.05$; ** $p<0.01$; *** $p<0.001$ Significantly different from the group of 11-15-year-olds: # $p<0.05$; ### $p<0.001$

treatment, and a lack of access to general practitioner or physiotherapy services, plus a culture of a lack of healthy body awareness, may partly explain the high prevalence of deformities and poor posture in the examined children and youth.

In our study, cervical lordosis, FHP, and thoracic kyphosis were more common in girls than boys. With categorized age groups, we found that FHP and thoracic kyphosis more common in older age groups. According to Widhe [32], the relationship between thoracic kyphosis and lumbar lordosis was independent of gender and age at 5-6 years old, while at 15-16 years old kyphosis was significantly less pronounced in girls than boys. Nitzschke and Hildenbrand [23] reported an increased kyphosis in 12% of the girls and in 15% of the boys, while in the study Poussa *et al.* [27] the prevalence of thoracic hyper kyphosis (exceeding 45°) was the same in the 14-year-old girls and boys; at the age of 22 years it was more frequent in boys than in girls (9.6% vs. 0.9%). In the growth period from adolescence to adulthood, there was an increasing tendency of kyphosis in the male subjects but in females the opposite trend was found [27]. As a result, in their longitudinal study they found men to be more kyphotic than women. In a study by Mellin and Poussa [22] with 294 boys and girls aged 8-16 years old, it was found that the upper thoracic sagittal alignment was more vertical among girls. However, they could not find any significant age-related differences between boys and girls in this regard.

Ultrasonography research on children indicated that muscular balance in the knee joint is one of the factors affecting patellar position in the knee [16]. Disturbing muscular balance results in the faulty position of the patella. This may lead to patellofemoral joint pathologies in later years. Moreover, shortened hamstrings may cause walking with flexed knees and the hyper function of quadriceps, both of which might result in the stimulation of the patellar tendon to grow and cause a high standing of the patella. Erkula *et al.* [5] reported that in severe hamstring shortness, the knee's extensor mechanism is affected and patella is migrated cephalad, which may cause changes in posture, walking ability, and knee discomfort. They suggested performing a routine knee extension deficits exam in evaluating knee discomfort. In another study, limited hamstring flexibility has been suggested as a possible cause of lumbar pain in children [28]. However, Harreby *et al.* [12] in their study on Danish children found hamstring flexibility defect more than 40º in 12.2% of the subjects, and according to the authors the defect was very common in growing teenagers, but no correlation with low back pain was found. Brodersen [2] diagnosed back pain in 7% of children; knee and heel pain in 3%. However, in children with extension deficit of more than 40° degrees, the incidence of low back pain rose to 15%. Moreover, in their study 75% of boys and 35% of girls had short hamstrings and 13% had Achilles shortness. Another study indicated that the extensibility of the hamstring muscle affects thoracic and pelvic posture in young athletes, especially in maximal trunk flexion [18]. Fakhari *et al.* [6] in research on 3308 healthy girls reported that the prevalence of hamstring and calf muscle shortness altogether was more than 30% in secondary school children. They indicated that shortness of the calf muscle and the hamstring are present together and concluded that in the case of finding one defect we should look for the other one as well. Hamstring shortness was found in 79.4% of cases in a survey of 7781 children aged 6-12 years old [25]. In our survey, hamstring shortness was reported in nearly one-third of the subjects and gastroc-soleus shortness in 21%. Neither were age or gender dependent.

Babaei and Salehi revealed a significant association between foot disorders including hallux valgus, hallux rigidus, flat feet, and short gastroc-soleus [1]. Hoshina *et al.* [14] in their study reported 2 peak age periods in developmental hallux valgus: one in adolescence and the other one in the period between 40 and 50 years old. In both groups, hallux valgus was associated with the collapse of arch structure, but in the young group the causative factor was joint laxity, whereas in older group it was the degeneration of ligaments. They concluded that hallux valgus deformation continues to progress during adolescence, and its progression stops in the 50's, and therefore, it is instead an age-dependent deformity rather than a gender-specific one. However, in this study the prevalence of hallux valgus was not related to age or gender, and it amounted to about 31%. In contrast, in a musculoskeletal deviations survey performed in children in Utah, hallux valgus was found only in 9% of subjects, pronated foot in 38%, genu valgum in 34%, pes planus in 20%, and the incidence of genu recurvatum in 16% [11]. In turn, Penha *et al.* [24] reported the frequency of genu recurvatum among school children amounting to 54% while in this study it was about two times lower. Nevertheless, our data were to some extent in agreement with the findings of Penha *et al.* [24] and Pinho and Duarte [26], confirming that there was a progressive decrease of knee hyperextension during childhood development. In the present study, the rate of hallux valgus was neither age- nor gender-related.

Faulty posture and lower limb deformities appear to be considerable risk factors for musculoskeletal problems later in life and should receive more prophylactic and therapeutic attention. By detecting large numbers of children with musculoskeletal deviation we could demonstrate the absolute necessity for performing screening programs among Iranian schoolchildren. Many countries, like the United States, Australia, England, Sweden, Norway, Denmark and Japan, had started some musculoskeletal screening program about 4 decades ago. In countries like Japan and some states in the United States performing a screening program is mandatory [30]. Our findings suggest that there is a need for involving well- qualified health personnel in the school screening and preventive programs aiming at early detection and disease management/treatment, which prevents the progression of musculoskeletal problems in the adulthood period in a very effective and economical way. Furthermore, it is possible by performing an effective referral system to affect corrective intervention in time. Further, it can prevent unnecessary psychological trauma that in the growing period may cause irreversible results. These data appear to be innovative considering the fact that Iran's student population is about 14 million students in primary and secondary schools [33], and there is not a regular screening program for early detection of musculoskeletal abnormalities. Clinically it is important to know whether a subject or patient has any postural abnormality or asymmetry. Based on the results of this study, it is possible to trace the source of various abnormalities in adulthood to childhood. This method can be used for screening children in the early period and manage them with preventive measures. The findings of this study suggests that physiotherapists can play a very active role in detecting these postural abnormalities, especially in schoolchildren prior to their becoming a complex entity. The primary prevention process will also improve their professional skills and effectiveness.

While not diminishing the importance of the research, there are several limitations in the study that should be mentioned: first, it is a cross-sectional study and does not demonstrate any physiological variation during the development process of children, which is quite common in these periods. Second, this study was performed by senior physiotherapy students without much clinical experience. Additionally, involvement of more than one examiner due to religious principles adds the problem of inter-examiner reliability. Finally, because of the poor reliability of this type of assessment and the relatively small sample size, the obtained results should be interpreted and generalized with caution.

Summing up, using the observation method we detected that faulty posture and lower limb abnormalities are common in schoolchildren from rural region in Iran. Moreover, there was a predominance of faulty posture in girls and in older children. Therefore, local authorities, health professionals, and teachers should pay more attention to taking preventive steps to reduce negative, musculoskeletal-related consequences.

References

1. Babaei Gh.R., H.Salehi (2004) Study of the relationship between low back pain and foot disorders. *J.Sabzevar Univer. Med.Sci.*, 10:45-52.
2. Brodersen A., B.Pedersen, J.Reimers (1994) Incidence of complaints about heel-, knee- and back-related discomfort among Danish children, possible relation to short muscles. *Ugeskr.Laeger.*, 156:2243-2245.
3. Casarotto R.A., E.A.Liberti (1994) Dados antropométricos de pré-escolares da cidade de São Paulo. *Rev.Fisioter.Univer.São Paulo*, 1:27-33.
4. Charrette M. (2011) Excessive pronation and knee ligament injuries. *Dynamic Chiropractic.* 29:1-4.
5. Erkula G., F.Demirkan, B.A.Kilic, E.Kiter (2002) Hamstring shortening in healthy adults. *J.Back.Musculoskelet.Rehabil.*, 16:77-81.
6. Fakhari Z., M.Senobari, S.Jalaie (2008). Prevalence of hamstring and calf muscle shortness. *Modern Rehabil.*, 2(1):6-6.
7. Foster H.E., D.A.Cabral (2006) Is musculoskeletal history and examination so different in pediatrics? *Best.Pract.Res.Clin. Rheumatol.*, 20(2):241-261.
8. Foster H.E., L.Kay (2003) Examination skills in the assessment of the musculoskeletal system in children and adolescents. *Curr.Paediatr.*, 13:341-344.
9. Francis R.S. (1988) Scoliosis screening of 3,000 college-aged women: The Utah study phase 2. *Phys.Ther.*, 68:1513-1516.
10. Griegel-Morris P., K.Larson, K.Mueller-Klaus, C.A.Oatis (1992) Incidence of common postural abnormalities in the cervical, shoulder, and thoracic regions and their association with pain in two age groups of healthy subjects. *Phys.Ther.* 72:425-431.
11. Grivas T.B., M.H.Wade, S.Negrini, J.P.O'Brien, T.Maruyama, M.C.Hawes, M.Rigo, H.R.Weiss, T.Kotwicki, E.S.Vasiliadis, L.N.Sulam, T.Neuhous (2007) SOSORT consensus paper: school screening for scoliosis. Where are we today? *Scoliosis.* 2:17.
12. Harreby M., B.Nygaard, T.Jessen, E.Larsen, A.Storr-Paulsen, A.Lindahl, I.Fisker, E.Laegaard (1999) Risk factors for low back pain in a cohort of 1389 Danish school children: an epidemiologic study. *Eur.Spine J.*, 8:444–450.
13. Hertel J., J.H.Dorfman, R.A.Braham (2004) Lower extremity malalignment and anterior cruciate ligament injury history. *J.Sport.Sci.Med.*, 3:220-225.
14. Hoshino T., S.Inokuchi, N.Usami, E.Hiraishi, T.Hashimoto (1998) Juvenile hallux valgus in Japan: a radiographic comparison with older age groups. *The Foot.* 8:93-95.
15. Jandial Sh., H.E.Foster (2007) Examination of the musculoskeletal system in children – a simple approach. *Paediatr. Child Health.*, 18(2):47-55.
16. Jozwiak M., S.Pietrzak (1998) Patella position versus length of hamstring muscle in children. *J.Pediatr.Orthop.*, 18:268-270.
17. Krul M., J.C.Van der Wouden, F.G.Schellevis, L.W.van Suijlekom-Smit, B.W.Koes (2009) Foot problems in children presented to the family physician: a comparison between 1987 and 2001. *Fam.Pract.*, 26: 174-179.
18. Lopez-Minarro P.A., F.Alcid (2010) Influence of hamstring muscle extensibility on spinal curvatures in young athletes. *Sci.Sports*, 25:188-192.
19. Louden J.K. (1996) The relationship between static posture and ACL injury in female athletes. *J.Orthop.Sports Phys.Ther.*, 24:91-97.
20. Magee D.J. (1997) Orthopedic Physical Assessment, 3rd edition. WB Saunders, Philadelphia, USA.
21. McEvoy M.P., K. Grimmer (2005) Reliability of upright posture measurement in primary schoolchildren. *BMC Musculoskelet.Disord.*, 6:35.

22. Mellin G., M.Poussa (1992) Spinal mobility and posture in 8- to 16-year-old children. *J.Orthop.Res.* 10:211-216.

23. Nitzschke E., M.Hildenbrand (1990) Epidemiologic study of kyphosis in school children. *Z.Orthop.Ihre.Grenzgeb.,* 128:477-481.

24. Penha P.J., S.M.A.João, R.A.Casarotto, C.J.Amino, D.C.Penteado (2005) Postural assessment of girls between 7 and 10 years of age. *Clinics.* 60:9-16.

25. Permoda A., A.Permoda, B.Chudak (2010) The problem of occurrence of faulty postures in children and adolescents in the city of Zielona Góra and the region. *Zdr.Publ.,* 120(4):361-364.

26. Pinho R.A., M.F.S. Duarte (1995) Analise postural em escolares de Florianopolis-SC. *Rev.Bras.Ativi.Fis.Saude,.* 1:49-58.

27. Poussa M.S., M.M.Heliövaara, T.J.Seitsamo, M.H.Könönen, K.A.Hurmerinta, M.J.Nissinen (2005) Development of spinal posture in a cohort of children from the age of 11 to 22 years. *Eur.Spine J.,* 14:738-742.

28. Rodriguez P.L., F.M.Santonja, P.A.Lopez-Minarro, P.Sainz de Baranda, J.L.Yuste (2008) Effect of physical education stretching programme on sit-and-reach score in schoolchildren. *Sci.Sports,* 23:170-175.

29. Smith J., J.E.Szczerba, B.L.Arnold, D.E.Martin, D.H.Perrin (1997) Role of hyperpronation as a possible risk factor for anterior cruciate ligament injuries. *J.Athl.Train.* 32:25-28.

30. Troyanovich S.J., D.E.Harrison, D.D.Harrison (1998) Structural rehabilitation of the spine and posture: rationale for treatment beyond the resolution of symptoms. *J.Manipulative Physiol.Ther.,* 21:37-50.

31. Urwin M., D.Symmons, T.Allison, T.Brammah, H.Busby, M.Roxby, A.Simmons, G.Williams(1998) Estimating the burden of musculoskeletal disorders in the community: the comparative prevalence of symptoms at different anatomical sites, and the relation to social deprivation. *Ann.Rheum.Dis.,* 57:649-655.

32. Widhe T. (2001) Spine: posture, mobility and pain. A longitudinal study from childhood to adolescence. *Eur.Spine J.,* 10:118-123.

33. www.magiran.com/npview.asp?ID=1487254.

Acknowledgements

The authors thank the Green Umbrella Organization affiliated with the Cultural Deputy of Tabriz University of Medical Sciences for financial support in the screening process and sample collections. We would like to thank Amin Abdali and Fereshteh Jalalimanesh for their work in collecting data. Furthermore, we acknowledge the help of Dr. M. Ghojazadeh in reading the manuscript and helping with the statistical analyses.

PERMISSIONS

All chapters in this book were first published in BHK, by De Gruyter Open; hereby published with permission under the Creative Commons Attribution License or equivalent. Every chapter published in this book has been scrutinized by our experts. Their significance has been extensively debated. The topics covered herein carry significant findings which will fuel the growth of the discipline. They may even be implemented as practical applications or may be referred to as a beginning point for another development.

The contributors of this book come from diverse backgrounds, making this book a truly international effort. This book will bring forth new frontiers with its revolutionizing research information and detailed analysis of the nascent developments around the world.

We would like to thank all the contributing authors for lending their expertise to make the book truly unique. They have played a crucial role in the development of this book. Without their invaluable contributions this book wouldn't have been possible. They have made vital efforts to compile up to date information on the varied aspects of this subject to make this book a valuable addition to the collection of many professionals and students.

This book was conceptualized with the vision of imparting up-to-date information and advanced data in this field. To ensure the same, a matchless editorial board was set up. Every individual on the board went through rigorous rounds of assessment to prove their worth. After which they invested a large part of their time researching and compiling the most relevant data for our readers

The editorial board has been involved in producing this book since its inception. They have spent rigorous hours researching and exploring the diverse topics which have resulted in the successful publishing of this book. They have passed on their knowledge of decades through this book. To expedite this challenging task, the publisher supported the team at every step. A small team of assistant editors was also appointed to further simplify the editing procedure and attain best results for the readers.

Apart from the editorial board, the designing team has also invested a significant amount of their time in understanding the subject and creating the most relevant covers. They scrutinized every image to scout for the most suitable representation of the subject and create an appropriate cover for the book.

The publishing team has been an ardent support to the editorial, designing and production team. Their endless efforts to recruit the best for this project, has resulted in the accomplishment of this book. They are a veteran in the field of academics and their pool of knowledge is as vast as their experience in printing. Their expertise and guidance has proved useful at every step. Their uncompromising quality standards have made this book an exceptional effort. Their encouragement from time to time has been an inspiration for everyone.

The publisher and the editorial board hope that this book will prove to be a valuable piece of knowledge for researchers, students, practitioners and scholars across the globe.

LIST OF CONTRIBUTORS

Skip M. Williams, Kelly R. Laurson, David Q. Thomas and Dale D. Brown
Illinois State University

Dan Phelps
Hononegah High School, Illinois, USA

Anna Leś and Marta Gaworska
University of Physical Education, Warsaw, and European Association for Promoting Motor Activity 50+, Warsaw, Poland

Petra Jansen
Institute of Sport Science, University of Regensburg

Léonie F. Lange
Department of Anaesthesiology, Charité University of Medicine, Berlin

Martin Heil
Institute of Experimental Psychology, University of Düsseldorf, Germany

Estélio H.M. Dantas, Rejane Daoud and Mario C.S.C. Conceição
Human Motricity Biosciences Laboratory (LABIMH), Federal University of the State of Rio de Janeiro (UNIRIO), RJ

Alexis Trott
Laboratory of Molecular Aspects Associated to Genetic Diseases, University of Western Santa Catarina (UNOESC), SC

Rudy J. Nodari Jr.
Laboratory of Prognostic Aspects of Intervention and Care in Health and Human Performance, UNOESC, SC, Brazil

Joanna Piotrowska
Warsaw Academy of Tourism, Food and Hospitality, Warsaw, Poland

Faruk Yamaner , Hayrettin Gümüşdağ and Alparslan Kartal
Hitit University, School of Physical Education and Sports, Çorum

M. Gümüş
Zonguldak Karaelmas University, School of Physical Education and Sports, Zonguldak

A. Güllü
İnönü University, School of Physical Education and Sports, Malatya

O. Imamoğlu
19 Mayıs University, School of Physical Education and Sport, Samsun, Turkey

Brad Schoenfeld and Gül Tiryaki-Sönmez
Lehman College, Department of Health Sciences, The City University of New York, Bronx, NY, USA

Christopher R. Edginton
School of Health, Physical Education and Leisure Services, University of Northern Iowa, Cedar Falls IA, USA

Ming-kai Chin
HOPSports, Inc., Valencia CA, USA

Michał Bronikowski
Methodology of Teaching Physical Education Department, Physical Education University, Poznań, Poland

Hayrettin Gümüşdağ, Faruk Yamaner and Alparslan Kartal
Hitit University, School of Physical Education and Sports, Çorum

İbrahim Yıldıran
Gazi University, School of Physical Education and Sports, Ankara, Turkey

Marzena Malara and Grażyna Lutosławska
Department of Biochemistry, University of Physical Education, Warsaw, Poland

Joanna Okęcka-Szymańska, Elżbieta Hübner-Woźniak, Iwona Piątkowska and Marzena Malara
Department of Biochemistry, University of Physical Education, Warsaw, Poland

Agata Wężyk
Noffer Institute of Occupational Medicine, Łódź, Poland

Gül Tiryaki-Sönmez1, Brad Schoenfeld
Lehman College, Department of Health Sciences, The City University of New York, Bronx, NY, USA

Serife Vatansever-Ozen
Abant Izzet Baysal University, School of Physical Education and Sport, Department of Training Science, Bolu,Turkey

Elżbieta Biernat
Warsaw School of Economics, Warsaw, Poland

Ryszard Zarzeczny, Mariusz Kuberski, Agnieszka Deska, Dorota Zarzeczna and Katarzyna Rydz
Institute of Physical Culture and Tourism, Jan Długosz University, Częstochowa

Anna Lewandowska
Primary School No. 36, Częstochowa

Tomasz Bałchanowski and Janusz Bosiacki
Primary School No. 48, Częstochowa, Poland

Anna Czajkowska
Department of Physiology

Grażyna Lutosławska
Department of Biochemistry

Krzysztof Mazurek
Department of Sports Medicine, University of Physical Education, Warsaw, Poland

Jadwiga Ambroszkiewicz
Department of Newborn Screening, Institute of Mother and Child, Warsaw, Poland

Piotr Żmijewski
Department of Physiology, Institute of Sport, Warsaw, Poland

Mariusz Hrycyna
The Halina Konopacka University of Physical Education and Tourism, Pruszków

Jacek Zieliński
University of Physical Education, Warsaw, Poland

Joanna Burdzicka-Wołowik
Department of Psychology, The Jozef Pilsudski University of Physical Education in Warsaw, Faculty of Physical Education and Sport in Biala Podlaska, Poland

Sándor Bollók and Zsuzsanna Kalmár
Semmelweis University, Faculty of Physical Education and Sport Sciences, Budapest

Johanna Takács
Semmelweis University, Institute of Behavioural Sciences, Budapest, Hungary

Beáta Dobay
Selye University, Department of Physical Education, Komarno, Slovakia

Hamid Arazi
Faculty of Physical Education and Sport Science, University of Guilan, Rasht

Mohammad Azizi
Faculty of Physical Education and Sport Science, University of Razi- Kermanshah, Iran

Csaba Konczos, Zsolt Szakály and István Barthalos
University of West-Hungary, Faculty of the Apáczai Csere János, Győr

József Bognár and Zsolt Oláh
Semmelweis University - Faculty of Physical Education and Sport, Budapest

István Simon
University of West Hungary, Faculty of the Benedek Elek, Sopron, Hungary

Małgorzata Stachowicz and Katarzyna Milde
University of Physical Education, Warsaw

Marcin Janik
Department of Physical Education, University of Rzeszów, Poland

Joanna Sobiecka
Faculty of Motor Rehabilitation, University School of Physical Education, Krakow

Ryszard Plinta
Department of Physical Education and Sport, Medical University of Silesia, Katowice
Faculty of Physiotherapy, The Jerzy Kukuczka Academy of Physical Education, Katowice

Katarzyna Drobniewicz
Non-Public Health Care Centre „Alma Spei", Cracow

Jadwiga Kłodecka-Różalska
Department of Psychology, Institute of Sport, Warsaw

Katarzyna Cichoń
Non Public Health Care Centre for Autistic Persons „EFFATHA", Cracow, Poland

Pamela Hodges Kulinna
Mary Lou Fulton Teachers College, Faculty Affiliate Program of Kinesiology, Arizona State University

István Kun and Laszlo Toth
Faculty of Physical Education and Sport Science, Semmelweis University, Budapest, Hungary

Pantelis Theodoros Nikolaïdis
Laboratory of Human Performance and Rehabilitation, Department of Physical and Cultural Education, Hellenic Army Academy, Greece

Ahmet Ş. Őkmen
School of Physical Education and Sports, Mugla University, Mugla

İbrahim Erdemir
School of Physical Education and Sports, Balikesir University, Balikesir, Turkey

Efstathios Christodoulides
Department of Social Sciences, Faculty of Physical Education and Sport Science, Semmelweis University, Budapest, Hungary

Vassilios Diafas, Eleni Dimakopoulou, Vassiliki Diamanti, Danae Zelioti and Socratis Kaloupsis
Department of Physical Education and Sport Science, National and Kapodistrian University of Athens, Greece

Shyamal Koley and Santhosh B. Kumaar
Department of Sports Medicine and Physiotherapy, Guru Nanak Dev University, Amritsar, Punjab, India

Władysław Mynarski, Agnieszka Nawrocka, Michał Rozpara and Wiesław Garbaciak
The Jerzy Kukuczka Academy of Physical Education in Katowice, Poland

Alicja Kaiser
Wielkopolska Higher School of Tourism and Management, Poznań

Marek Sokołowski
University School of Physical Education, Poznań, Poland

Anna Mróz
Department of Physiology

Krzysztof Buśko
Department of Anthropometry, The Jozef Pilsudski University of Physical Education in Warsaw
Institute of Sport, Warsaw, Poland

Jerzy Saczuk, Agnieszka Wasiluk and Mirosław Zalech
The Jozef Pilsudski University of Physical Education in Warsaw, Faculty of Physical Education and Sport in Biala Podlaska, Poland

Timothy A. Brusseau
University of Utah

Pamela H. Kulinna
Arizona State University

Tiffany Kloeppel
Montclair State University

Matthew Ferry
George Mason University

Edyta Suliga
Institute of Public Health, Jan Kochanowski University, Kielce

Iwona Wronka
Department of Anthropology, Institute of Zoology, Jagiellonian University, Krakow

Romana Pawlińska-Chmara
Department of Biotechnology and Molecular Biology, Opole University, Opole, Poland

Dalwinder Singh
Department of Physical Education, Panjab University, Chandigarh

Sukhwinder Singh
University College, Dhilwan, Barnala, India

Małgorzata Grabara
Department of Recreation, Jerzy Kukuczka Academy of Physical
Education, Katowice, Poland

Shahnaz Shahr-jerdy
Department of Physical Education and Sport Sciences, University of Arak, Iran

Rahman Sheikh Hosseini
Tehran University, Tehran, Iran

Maghsoud Eivazi Gh
Physiotherapy Department, Faculty of Rehabilitation Sciences, Tabriz University of Medical Sciences, Iran
Physiotherapy & Rehabilitation Department, Okan University, Tuzla Kampusu Istanbul, Turkey

Renata Czarniecka
Department of Physical Education Methodology

Katarzyna Milde and Paweł Tomaszewski
Department of Statistics and Computer Sciences, The Jozef Pilsudski University of Physical Education, Warsaw, Poland

Jakub Turski and Joanna Głogowska
The Jozef Pilsudski University of Physical Education in Warsaw

Marcin Wilczkiewicz
Department of Physical Education, University of Rzeszów

Romuald Stupnicki
University College of Physical Culture and Tourism, Pruszków, Poland

Andrzej Tomczak
Department of Physical Education, General Staff of the Polish Armed Forces, Warsaw; The Jozef Pilsudski University of Physical Education in Warsaw, Faculty of Physical Education and Sport in Biala Podlaska, Poland

Ananda Balayogi Bhavanani, Madanmohan, Zeena S and L Vithiyalakshmi
Advanced Centre for Yoga Therapy Education and Research (ACYTER), JIPMER, Puducherry, India

Maghsoud Eivazi Gh
Physiotherapy Department, Faculty of Rehabilitation Sciences, Tabriz University of Medical Sciences, Iran
Physiotherapy & Rehabilitation Department, Okan University, Tuzla Kampusu Istanbul, Turkey

Amin Alilou and Solmaz Ghafurinia
Physiotherapy Department, Faculty of Rehabilitation Sciences, Tabriz University of Medical Sciences, Iran

Sara Fereydounnia
Physiotherapy Department, Faculty of Rehabilitation Sciences, Tehran University of Medical Sciences, Iran

Index